Another Twinkle in the Eye

Contemplating another pregnancy after perinatal mental illness

ELAINE A HANZAK

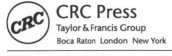

CRC Press
Taylor & Francis Group
Boca Raton London New York

CRC Press is an imprint of the
Taylor & Francis Group, an **informa** business

CRC Press
Taylor & Francis Group
6000 Broken Sound Parkway NW, Suite 300
Boca Raton, FL 33487-2742

CRC Press is an imprint of Taylor & Francis Group, an Informa business

Printed on acid-free paper
Version Date: 20150715

International Standard Book Number-13: 978-1-84619-888-5

Visit the Taylor & Francis Web site at
http://www.taylorandfrancis.com

and the CRC Press Web site at
http://www.crcpress.com

Contents

About the author

Since the publication of her autobiographical book *Eyes without Sparkle: a journey through postnatal illness* (Radcliffe Publishing, 2005), Elaine has become a leading expert by experience on the subject. She regularly appears in the media to increase awareness that mental illness can and does affect anyone. Her messages of hope through her interviews and writing have inspired others; her book has been described as a 'life saver', offering people hope for recovery. Elaine is in demand as a professional speaker to health professionals, students and other audiences looking for ways to cope with changes and resilience.

www.hanzak.com

Contributors

Dr Dawn Edge
Senior Lecturer/Associate Professor/Winston Churchill Fellow
Centre for New Treatments & Understanding in Mental Health
(CeNTrUM)
School of Psychological Sciences, The University of Manchester

Dr Carol Henshaw MB ChB MD FRCPsych
Consultant in Perinatal Mental Health
Liverpool Women's NHS Foundation Trust

Dr Fatimah Jackson-Best PhD
Global Health Research Post-Doctoral Fellow
University of Ottawa

Dr Jo Spoors
Senior Registrar, Perinatal Psychiatry
Tees, Esk and Wear Valleys NHS Foundation Trust

Dr Angelika Wieck FRCPsych
Consultant in Perinatal Psychiatry
Manchester Mental Health and Social Care Trust

Dr Elizabeth Boath Phd Adv UniDipCH BA(Hons) Adv EFT
Associate Professor in Health
Staffordshire University

Evelyn Burdon RN HV BSc
Cheshire Baby Whisperer

Michael Coote B Th BA (Psych) BA (Psych) Hons BA (Psych) Masters
Director and co-founder of S+ The Real Leadership Company

Debby Gould MSc Nursing BSc Midwifery (Hons)
Registered midwife and registered nurse
Director, Inside First Ltd

Dr Jane Hanley PhD RGN RMN Dip HV Dip Couns FRSPH
Hon Senior Lecturer
Swansea University

Pauline McPartland
Qualified Person-centred counsellor, Specialist practitioner and trainer
PMH
Manager PND Service
PSS, Liverpool

Katy Moss RMHN (7) Higher National Diploma in Nursing (Mental Health)
BA (Hons) in Mental Health
Team Leader and Specialist Perinatal Mental Health Nurse
Hull and East Yorkshire Perinatal Mental Health Liaison Team

Sue Peckham IAEBP (Acc) DHyp (Adv)
Clinical Hypnotherapist and co-creator of the Easyloss Weight Loss
Programme
Hampshire Hypnotherapy Centre

Julie Smith NNEB PGCE
Operational Development Manager/National Perinatal Lead
Family Action

Sharon Trotter BSc (Adv Studies in Midwifery)
Parenting Consultant and Founder of TIPS Ltd
Scotland, UK

Mark Williams
Founder of Dads Matter UK and Fathers Reaching Out
Social Enterprise Owner, Reaching Out Perinatal Mental Health

Acknowledgements

I am very grateful for the way that healthcare professionals have embraced me over the years since my first book, *Eyes without Sparkle: a journey through postnatal illness*, was published in 2005. My story was put into the public eye almost as soon as it was published. Within the first few months of it being printed, I was invited to speak on national television programmes and featured in national press. As a result I was in demand to speak at conferences. This was a lifestyle that did not fit with being a full-time teacher. I took a term off as sabbatical leave in the autumn of 2005 and have never returned to the classroom! Since then I have continued to learn, speak and write about this topic in order to spread awareness and improve the resources available for it. Initially I doubted my value especially when I would look at a list of delegates made up of doctors and professors! Who was I to address such an audience? Over time I began to appreciate that they did value my contribution. The more I learned, the more I had to share. This book enables me to include and pass on that knowledge. I appreciate being accepted by the health professionals as an 'Expert by Lived Experience'.

I also am indebted to the many people who have openly shared their experiences of perinatal (antenatal and postnatal) illness with me. This has given me the facts and motivation to represent them too when I speak and write. One lady called me 'every woman's advocate for postnatal depression (PND)'. I feel privileged to have been given such intimate details and insights into the lives of others. Several people have also commented that they are glad that I suffered as I did! They have explained that this is because I have been blessed with good communication skills to share the messages of suffering and the need for it to be alleviated. I admit that every now and then I have my 'supermarket moment' – when I question if I should still be talking about my experience of postnatal illness when my son is now 19. I go through some soul-searching questions around whether it is time for me to stop and do something else – for example, go and work in a supermarket. It is incredible how that same day I receive a message from someone sharing their story with me and how I either have or could positively influence their life or someone close to them. Thank you if you have ever sent me such a message – you have probably saved me from the supermarket application!

To the people who contributed to the survey for this book, I applaud and thank you for the time you took to answer the questions and for the candid and selfless way you did so. You have inspired me to write this book and I hope that I do you justice.

Without the love and support of my parents, Maureen and Lawrence Walsh, I may not have wanted a family of my own. They taught me what unconditional love is, along with the joys and pleasure that having a child can bring. They also have faced their own challenges over the years and yet have always been there for my siblings, Kevin and Claire, and me in our choices. Even if they have not agreed with our decisions in life they have always been our best supporters. They brought me up in a loving family and this is why I wanted children of my own. They continue to be a huge support to me in many ways and have encouraged me with this book. My appreciation is beyond words for all they continue to do.

My son Marius (formerly known as Dominic – he has chosen to use his middle name) also inspires and motivates me. I love having my siblings and I wanted him also to have that opportunity. The human heart has an unspecified amount of love to give. I would have liked him to have the joy of siblings too. During his teenage years, when his father and I divorced, he faced an unsettling time. Marius has emerged as a fine young man who fills me with pride. I appreciate his support over the years too for my passion around perinatal mental health. I admire the way in which he has allowed me to continue to be so public about my illness. I remember last year being invited to appear on *BBC Breakfast*, where the topic concerned mothers who are ill harming their babies. I told several million viewers about how I had almost thrown my son down the stairs when I was so distressed. I was extremely concerned that as a teenager he would not like this – I called Marius and his comment was 'Oh, was it the stairs thing? I'm fine about that!' Thank you for letting me help others.

I appreciate the support of the rest of my family and close friends who have continued to inspire me. It is such a joy and comfort to know that I have some people around me who, regardless of my choices in life, continue to give me their unconditional love and encouragement. My experiences over the last 10 years make me appreciate the saying that people come into your life for a reason, a season or a lifetime.

I am grateful to the media who have invited me to speak on television plus local and national radio along with the press. I acknowledge that I love the whole 'lights, camera, action' aspect and I do get a buzz from any article I have done. Having a photo shoot around Milan in Italy for a magazine was incredible – a coach load of tourists stopped and began taking pictures of me! One remarked, 'I don't know who she is, but she must be famous!' The main aspect that fills me with awe, hope and pride is because I want to reach out to those who have, or will have, a perinatal mental health issue. I want to be able to give them hope that they have an identifiable illness that can be treated and they will get better. Due to the marketing of my book *Eyes without Sparkle: a journey through postnatal illness*, I am aware that there are at least five ladies who are still alive because my book gave them the hope that they needed at such a crucial time in their own lives. I know because they have told me. When I see their postings on social media of happy family times and events, I have to fight the lump in my throat.

Since 2005 the impact of social media has grown beyond belief. Through Facebook, Twitter and LinkedIn I know that I, and many others, have been able to reach out to families in distress. Over the years I have been able to keep a blog going with references to any new information I have come across (www.hanzak.com/blog). Social media has led to a much bigger 'sisterhood' of sufferers who are all keen to help others. As I write this, a national campaign for a month of awareness around perinatal mental health is being planned by former sufferers and organisations in the UK. Most other illnesses do not have such a big majority of people who then wish to highlight the need for more services and offer help to others. Thank you to all those who continue to share their own experiences for the benefit of others.

Sadly there are some people who are no longer alive that have impacted on my life and purpose. Having been so ill that I lost almost all logical thought, I can empathise with the ladies who have taken their own life due to postnatal illness. I remember howling that I didn't want to die – I just wanted my brain to stop. I understand how your mind is whirring in such a state that all your usual rational thoughts are drowned and smothered by a tsunami of negative ones. For those left behind the pain will always remain about what they have missed and what has been lost. The families of Angela Harrison, Joanne Bingley and Emma Cadywould are amongst those who campaign for greater awareness and better facilities for new mothers. These three ladies had everything to live for yet their illness blinded them to it. Their loss motivates me incredibly because 'it could have been me'.

In recent years I am grateful for the flexible working arrangements I have with S+ The Real Leadership Company (formerly S+ Group). The work I do for them as Executive PA to Mike Coote (Co-founder and Director) and as a coach has given me the financial stability and time to complete this book.

I also wish to thank Radcliffe Publishing, as without their role in my first book, this second one may not have happened either. We can but wonder what the impact of this one will be.

Glossary

ADHD	Attention deficit hyperactivity disorder – a group of behavioural symptoms that include inattentiveness, hyperactivity and impulsiveness.
ASD	Autism spectrum disorder – a condition that affects social interaction, communication, interests and behaviour.
CPN	Community psychiatric nurse – a psychiatric nurse based in the community rather than a psychiatric hospital.
GP	General practitioner – medical doctor who treats acute and chronic illnesses and provides preventive care and health education to patients.
HCP	Healthcare professionals – persons who have special education in healthcare and who are directly related to provision of healthcare services.
HELLP syndrome	The medical term for one of the most serious complications of pre-eclampsia, in which there is a combined liver and blood clotting disorder. H stands for Haemolysis (rupture of the red blood cells); EL stands for Elevated Liver enzymes in the blood (reflecting liver damage); LP stands for Low blood levels of Platelets (specialised cells which are vital for normal clotting). HELLP is as dangerous as eclampsia (convulsions) and probably more common, although it is less easy to diagnose.
HV	Health visitors – professional individuals engaged in public health work within the domestic setting, predominantly found in countries with state-funded health systems.
Hypomania	(literally 'under mania' or 'less than mania') – a mood state characterised by persistent disinhibition and pervasive elevated (euphoric) or irritable mood but generally less severe than full mania. Characteristic behaviours are extremely energetic, talkative, and confident; commonly exhibited with a flight of creative ideas.
MBU	Mother and Baby Unit – an inpatient environment where mothers experiencing severe mental health difficulties can receive treatment and support while continuing to care for their baby.

NICU	Neonatal intensive care unit – also known as an intensive care nursery (ICN), is an intensive care unit specialising in the care of ill or premature newborn infants.
ObGyn	Obstetrician/gynaecologist – a physician specialist who provides medical and surgical care to women and has particular expertise in pregnancy, childbirth, and disorders of the reproductive system.
PE	Pre-eclampsia or preeclampsia – a disorder of pregnancy characterised by high blood pressure and a large amount of protein in the urine.
Perinatal	Pertaining to the period immediately before and after birth. The time period can vary. It is used in perinatal psychiatry terms as covering antenatal (pregnancy) and postnatal (up to 12 months post-delivery).
PICU	Paediatric intensive care unit (also paediatric) – an area within a hospital specialising in the care of critically ill infants, children and teenagers.
PND	Postnatal depression or postpartum depression (PPD) – a type of depression that affects some women after having a baby.
PP	Puerperal psychosis (Postpartum Psychosis, 'Postpartum onset Bipolar Disorder') – a severe mental illness, which has a sudden onset in the first few weeks following childbirth.
PTSD	Post-traumatic stress disorder – an anxiety disorder caused by very stressful, frightening or distressing events.
Somatic	Relating to the body, especially as distinct from the mind.
SPD	Symphysis pubis dysfunction or pregnancy-related pelvic girdle pain (PPGP) – pelvic pain that some women develop in pregnancy.
VE	Ventouse, also known as vacuum-assisted vaginal delivery or vacuum extraction (VE) – a method to assist delivery of a baby using a vacuum device.

Dedication

To my son Marius (formerly known as Dominic) who continues to be a huge sparkle in my life.

To my family and friends who have supported me in my passion for making early parenthood for others as happy and healthy as possible for all concerned.

To those who are no longer with us, yet their passing has motivated those left behind to build a better world.

To the current parents and those facing the decision to add to their families – I hope this book helps you to reach a decision that you are content with.

To the many dedicated healthcare professionals who strive to provide the best care and support to the people in their care.

I have been through hell – absolute hell – twice, but it has given me so much in return. I am not the person I was, but for the better. Despite suffering bereavement, divorce, moving house and other things in the last 3 years I have coped very, very well and never felt anything like I did after having my babies. I am now training to be a midwife and will qualify next year – it was my own experiences that led me down this path and for obvious reasons I have a particular interest in mental health around pregnancy. I wanted to take part in this survey as my fear over having another child was an immense issue for me for several years after having my first son. I was obsessed about it – I would dream about it, have nightmares, question it all the time. There were next to no resources out there for people in my position so I was very excited to hear about this project. It also makes me realise how far I have come! Best of luck to all those brave women and their families facing this reality.

Vicky, a mum

Reviews of *Another Twinkle in the Eye*

'This book is the best I have read about the topic of perinatal mental health. Elaine uses her own experiences and those of others to bring the theory to life. The very comprehensive list of symptoms of perinatal mental health problems will be hugely useful to sufferers, friends and family and healthcare professionals alike, and the chapter on things that people can do to support the mother who is unwell is both practical and realistic advice.

The advice given is balanced and facilitates the reader to make up their own mind rather than guide them in a particular direction, like so many self-help books ... I would highly recommend this book as a GP, a perinatal mental health sufferer and a mother. It is the book I have been wishing had been written to enable others to understand what is going on during a period of illness and how best to ask for help and support others who are suffering. Brilliant Elaine.'

DR STEPHANIE DEGIORGIO
GP with a special interest in perinatal mental health
Co-founder, Perinatal Mental Health Partnership

'This book is the perfect combination of personal experience, collected accounts from others, self-help advice, invaluable resource pack, and the latest research and evidence in the field, produced in an easy-to-read and accessible format. I will not only be recommending it to my team, but also to women who are making the difficult decision about future pregnancies in my clinic.

All healthcare professionals working with women of childbearing age will learn from this book and it will help to make their interactions more productive and more patient centred.'

DR GILES BERRISFORD FRCPsych
Consultant Perinatal Psychiatrist
Clinical Lead, Birmingham Perinatal Mental Health Service
Chair, Action on Postpartum Psychosis

'Covering just about every thought, emotion and practical suggestion necessary, this is a real must both for families and healthcare professionals. The book has been thoughtfully compiled into relevant and easy-to-access chapters making it possible to dip in and out whenever you feel the need for information and support on a specific aspect of the subject. Everything is addressed thoroughly without leaving the reader feeling overwhelmed. Medical conditions are explained well with the addition of a Glossary containing abbreviations of terminology used. Also included is an invaluable wealth of further reading, information and resources … A very important and much-needed resource which I am certain will be appreciated by so many people.'

LUCE
adventureswithmonster.wordpress.com

'In my opinion, every health professional and not just clinicians should read not only the first book [*Eyes without Sparkle*] but anything Elaine has to say on the subject.

[This is] another very informative book that, for me, brings an understanding of what being human is really like when faced with a very personal decision in a world of clinicians. It should be a standard reference book for GPs, hospital consultants and midwives.'

WILLIAM GREENWOOD
Chief Executive and Company Secretary
Cheshire Local Medical Committee Ltd

Introduction

It's not what happens to you, but how you react to it that matters.

Epictetus

The decision to bring a child into the world is rarely one that is taken lightly. So many factors are brought into consideration. When a previous pregnancy and early parenthood has resulted in poor maternal and/or paternal perinatal mental health, then making a conscious decision to have another baby is even more challenging.

I always wanted to have more than one child because as the middle child of three, I love the whole experience of having siblings and being part of a family unit. I wanted my son to have the same opportunity. My postnatal illness following his traumatic birth has been written in my previous book *Eyes without Sparkle: a journey through postnatal illness* (Radcliffe, 2005). Due to our experiences and his age, his father was not willing for us to have another baby even though I dearly wanted to. I can understand his reluctance as our experience first time was far from easy. I wanted to do it again, to hopefully enjoy it next time. He would not discuss it and eventually it became one of the main wedges that drove us apart and we divorced.

When our son was 13 years old I had to have a hysterectomy. I found that to be a very difficult reality as the operation took away my hope of being a mother again. The only aspect that made it easier was the gynaecologist explaining that I had too many fibroids and it was nature's way of letting me know that being pregnant again was something that would never happen to me.

On reflection I wish we had been given more information or guidance about what could have been possible had we both wanted another child. At my discharge appointment the psychiatrist simply said that if I ever was to become pregnant again the chances of me getting postnatal depression were higher. He also added that next time around 'everyone would be on my case'. My ex-husband focused on the first comment, and I on the second. The outcome was that it remained a taboo subject in his head and although I attempted to tell him on many occasions how important it was for me, it was something he refused to discuss and did not appreciate how much it meant to me.

I do not blame him, as he had witnessed the traumatic birth of our son, from which I was told I was lucky to be alive, and then I was so ill that I needed to be hospitalised for a psychotic illness. It is not surprising that he did not have the same 'rose-tinted specs' view I held of having a baby. It became an area in which there was no compromise. Along with my new career, as a result of my book being published, and other aspects, we drifted apart. I wonder if there had been a follow-up two years after discharge from the psychiatric team whether this matter could have been discussed. I wonder how many other relationships are affected years down the line, long after the crisis of the perinatal era has happened?

By sharing my story, many people have shared theirs with me. One question that has often landed in my email inbox has been the same dilemma faced by others. In some cases it is the father who wants another baby and the mother does not. Sometimes both do and are very scared about what may happen again. Others are in a panic when they unexpectedly fall pregnant. I discovered that, to date, there is only one book that covers this subject. It is by an American author, Karen Kleiman, *What Am I Thinking?*[1] I wanted to write a version for the UK that correlates to our healthcare system, although the emerged topics of conversations needed and aspects around this dilemma are applicable around the world.

My primary aim is to provide the facts, resources, discussion points and information to help people make an informed decision that they can comfortably live with. Each situation is as unique as the couple themselves and I want to provide them with the tools to make the best choice for them. I would never presume to tell anyone if they should or should not add to their family. I accept and acknowledge that what is right for one person, couple and family may not be right for others.

Through my speaking career that developed after the publication of my book, I have been privileged to address many healthcare professionals. They have often told me too that they would not know what to advise families faced with the decision to have another child. This book will also be a guide for them.

After my story was published in 2005, I was in demand as a speaker on the subject of postnatal depression. Readers of my book told me that they could relate to it at different levels. I was delighted to be interviewed and challenge the stereotypical view that someone who suffers from mental illness is usually weak, scruffy and maybe dribbles! One television producer even commented that she could not believe I was there to speak about postnatal depression because I looked glamorous. Another programme turned me down as they said I 'was too professional and not pathetic enough' to talk about mental illness! I admit that I love the media aspects and do get very excited to be asked.

The most important aspect is that awesome feeling of not knowing the impact of the interview or article. If just one person is helped by an interview where I show that mental illness does and can affect anyone and that you can make a full recovery, then it has been worth it.

Through my speaking career, I joined an association for fellow speakers and began a friendship with another man. He was an adventurer who then used his experiences to help others with their personal development. Clive Gott also had suffered a period of depression and when diagnosed, he declared to his GP: 'I can't be – I'm a motivational speaker!' We did some joint presentations to challenge the stigma of mental illness and to show that recovery is possible. My marriage failed and Clive and I became romantically involved, making plans for our future together. One Saturday evening he went up to bed early, saying he felt unwell. Twenty minutes later I heard a shout from him – I discovered he had suffered a fatal heart attack.

The shock and grief I felt in the months that followed taught me many lessons. The main one was that I now appreciated the physical pain and suffering that bereavement causes. Prior to Clive's death I had lost my grandparents, yet that is expected as part of the circle of life. I did not expect to lose a partner in my late forties. It made me appreciate how devastating the death of a new mother (or father) must be after the birth of a new baby. This motivated me even more to continue to do the work I do around raising awareness of poor parental mental health and hopefully to save lives.

It also made me appreciate that if bereavement occurs in pregnancy or around early delivery, how much more likely it is for the parent to suffer from depression. In grief I had many of the same symptoms I did with postnatal depression – an inability to sleep; a roller-coaster ride of emotions; loss of appetite; irrational thoughts and decisions. I also learned that many of the ways I had been advising people with maternal mental health issues to help themselves also applied to me in grief.

I learned too that one of my coping mechanisms is to write. As Clive had thousands of fans, they missed his regular blogging and I began to write about how I was getting through my days and nights. My blog has now had many tens of thousands of hits worldwide. At the time people told me that the ways I described to 'get through' were helping them through difficult places in their lives. It became cathartic for me and others. In retrospect I was too open and honest at times!

One very happy event that has inspired me too has been the arrival of my niece Sophie, on 14 February 2010. My younger sister Claire and her husband Martin had a wonderful wedding in a Cheshire castle. The fairy tale continued with their daughter. Sophie arrived three weeks early by an emergency section and Claire was poorly with HELLP syndrome, needing intensive nursing post-delivery. Our mum commented, 'Why can't my daughters do pregnancy and birth easily, like other people?' Sophie has brought joy to us all.

We were all very much on alert in the early days for Claire having postnatal depression. She was very healthy. As a mother she is so much more relaxed than I was. One aspect that she got right was the willingness to let the rest of the family share in the new arrival – unlike me. Sophie was bottle-fed due to Claire's illness, so that did make it easy for us to have her. The pleasure I have in spending time with my niece made me appreciate that I had unknowingly been selfish with my baby. I had wrongly believed that letting others look after him implied I was not managing. In fact, I deprived them of pleasure whilst I could have rested.

Through my work I became aware of the impact of suicide upon families. Joanne Bingley delivered her daughter Emily a few weeks after my niece Sophie was born. Tragically she took her own life as a result of postnatal illness. Her husband Chris set up a charity in her name as he wants the information and services around maternal mental health to be better. As a family they did not know how serious a condition it can be. At each milestone that we have celebrated with Sophie, it makes me aware of how sad it is that Joanne is not here to do the same with her delightful daughter. This inspires me more.

What I do want to do is explore the scenarios surrounding the (literally) life-changing and possible life creation that may or not happen in the decision to have a baby after a previously mentally unhealthy perinatal period.

Between 40% and 70% of women who experience postpartum psychosis decide not to have further children, often because of a belief that avoiding pregnancy can prevent them from experiencing further episodes of the illness.[2]

Having shared my experiences in *Eyes without Sparkle*, I can say that allowing other people to read and know about the personal experiences of others helps them to plan their own life and choices. I knew that this book then needed to be about more than just me!

My first approach was to ask for help and create a survey[3] for people who have faced or are facing the decision to add to their families. Using the replies consequently clarified exactly what parents felt they needed to know in making the decision, what help they wanted and their own outcomes. I was overwhelmed by the willingness of others to be so open. It clearly is a dilemma that many struggle with.

We often reflect in life on past decisions and allow our brains to wander down the 'if only' or 'what if' route. I turned 50 in August 2013. I often feel that 'if I knew at 25 what I know now' my life could have been very different. What are these pearls of wisdom and how can I help others?

- Life is constantly changing. Wherever we find ourselves 'now' is exactly that – now. If we are extremely happy, there will be something that pops up to change that. If where we are right now is challenging, at some point that too will change.
- Life is very precious. We cannot guarantee our time on this planet, so make

the most of every day. *Be* where you are at any given time, with the people you are with. The curse of technology – put that mobile phone down and be in the room with present company!

- Asking for help is a sign of strength. Other people genuinely like to help as it makes them feel good. Let them.
- Sharing your woes usually helps. Be careful who with and for how long though.
- If bad or sad things happen to you, accept that it is part of life. Have your 'wallow', find out what will help you through, and deal with it!
- As a little girl I used to sulk if I didn't get my own way or was unhappy about something. My dad used to say 'the only person you hurt when you sulk is yourself'. It took me many years to realise that! It is much better to communicate your feelings and thoughts, and look at the perspectives of others.
- The power of using positive thoughts and words can be incredible.

As I write this I am in a happy place in my life. My son has just completed the first year of his degree in photography. He continues to be a huge source of pleasure and love in my life. His teenage years were not easy for him and I am proud and thrilled at the closeness of our relationship now. I have my family close by and am able to be a regular part of my niece's life. My parents are very well and fill their retirement with their continued love and support for their children and grandchildren. Mum's retirement hobby is entering and winning competitions that keep us all entertained and them often on their travels!

I have a varied and interesting career. I have never returned to teaching. I am delighted that I am still asked to speak at conferences and training around maternal mental health, especially to students. Due to my attendance and involvement in many organisations over the last 10 years, my knowledge of the area and of the experts within it has grown.

Due to this I am honoured that when I asked for experts to add to this book, everyone I asked agreed willingly to do so if their schedule permitted. That way I hope it will give it the credibility that my role as 'expert by experience' may not. I have learned about many resources and examples of good practice over the years and I am delighted that this book gives me the opportunity to share them.

My part-time role as an Executive PA for a leadership company during the last three years is ideal for my high-detail and organisational skills!

My personal life is also very happy in that I am blessed with an amazing relationship with a wonderful man! We have much to plan and look forward to.

My life may not have followed my childhood storybook ideal of family life. I have reached a content place that my purpose in life is to help others to have a mentally healthy and happy early parenthood. If that means that as a result of this book you either do or do not add to your family, I wish you peace and contentment with your decision.

REFERENCES

1. Kleiman K. *What Am I Thinking?* Philadelphia, PA: Xlibris; 2005.
2. Bauer A, Parsonage M, Knapp M, *et al. The Costs of Perinatal Mental Health Problems.* London: Centre for Mental Health and London School of Economics; 2014. Robertson E, and Lyons A. Living with puerperal psychosis: a qualitative analysis. *Psychol and Psychother.* 2003; **76**: 411–31.
3. *See* Appendix 5 for survey questions.

PART 1

Reflection on the previous pregnancy, miscarriage or stillbirth

CHAPTER 1

Antenatal and postnatal mental health conditions

I felt completely detached from reality. Like I was in a bubble – behind a Perspex screen and the rest of the world was on the other side and I was totally trapped. I could see them but not reach them.

A mum

In this chapter I aim to outline some of the conditions that can happen in the perinatal period that affect mental health. As parents I hope you can identify with what happened to you and to others. For health professionals, I hope that this will help you to have a greater awareness and insight into the impact of these conditions and consequently why facing the decision to become pregnant again is likely to be difficult.

Before I became pregnant I had hardly heard of postnatal depression (PND). I may have read a small paragraph in the volumes of books and magazines I devoured whilst I was expecting, yet dismissed it as something that would not affect me. I had the misapprehension that I would be immune because my baby was desperately wanted; I was in a stable relationship; had a very comfortable home and lifestyle plus a supportive family. I had always been mentally well, was also incredibly organised and lived my life by lists! So it was a massive shock to be diagnosed with postnatal depression when my baby was four months old and to then develop puerperal psychosis three months later. I had never had any previous mental health challenges, so the whole process was a steep learning curve for me and those close to me. It is only since I suffered that I have increased my knowledge of mental illness and recognise how ignorant and wrong I had been in thinking 'I wasn't the type'. There seems to be a common belief that 'it won't happen to me'.

Of the people who responded to my survey, only around 50% of them knew anything about perinatal mental illness before or during their first pregnancy. Some were aware that 'baby blues' were common and that postnatal depression existed; they knew brief details of the symptoms and that it may affect your ability to bond with your baby. Like me, none had heard of puerperal or postpartum psychosis.

Sources of information came from:

- reading books, leaflets and magazines – this usually was very sparse in mainstream pregnancy resources
- media
- internet
- friends and family experience
- antenatal classes and appointments
- GP, midwives and maternity support workers
- professional experience – as a nurse, for example.

Only a small number felt that they knew enough before they became unwell, e.g. 'Had I heard of puerperal psychosis, it would have been less of a shock to receive a diagnosis of something totally unknown to me and my husband.'

I do wonder whether, if I had been given more details about possible mental health problems, I would have absorbed it when I was pregnant. I had a slight awareness yet dismissed it happening to me for the reasons I have outlined. Maybe it would be like considering divorce options when you are getting married! You do not want to know or think it will happen to you! We must also take into consideration the fine line between keeping parents informed and giving them too much information or details which could be distressing. The balance must be to give enough knowledge and resources to help parents realise that their mental health may be affected by pregnancy and birth then give them a pathway to follow if they do need help.

Here are some other comments from parents regarding knowledge of perinatal mental health when they were pregnant and what could have been better:

- I think that PND is glossed over. In lots of baby books it is given barely a small paragraph of information. I didn't know what it was at all. To my knowledge it was prolonged baby blues. Postnatal depression isn't glamorous or idealistic when planning for the arrival of your child really is it? That's not the reality and it should be addressed to each pregnant individual.
- Better prenatal classes with realistic information; less crowded and a more in-depth talk rather than very rushed.
- More information on signs and symptoms of PND and what to do if you experience them. Also to be told I may have been more likely to suffer with it because of my previous history of anxiety.
- To know that PND isn't as clear cut as I thought. I thought if you had it everyone felt the same.
- I needed the expertise of other women and mothers but I only knew that

retrospectively. I read too many 'expert opinions' but never knew I should have made time and space to consider the situation for myself.

- Nothing as I would have skimmed over the info thinking it wouldn't relate to me. I had no reason to think I would ever have mental health problems.
- More information about the signs of PND to look out for. On the other hand, if I had read up/known too much about PND beforehand it might have made me more anxious because I would have been worried I'd get it before I even did!
- Some knowledge of puerperal psychosis. I do not find the description that PP is severe postnatal depression to be that helpful – I felt many things, but never depressed! I would like to have had a debrief on what happened during my delivery and why labour was so protracted.
- I didn't know postpartum psychosis existed. I had clear insight into the fact that I was becoming increasingly manic – I have no doubt if this condition was more widely discussed I would have sought help. It is almost completely not mentioned in any of the popular baby bibles. I know it is rare, but it happens and can be severe. I think it deserves more of a mention.
- Some way of being able to mentally prepare for the stress of looking after a newborn and lack of sleep.

Here are some of the main mental health conditions that may be identified around pregnancy:
- previous or existing conditions before and during pregnancy
  - depression
  - anxiety
  - panic attacks
  - self-harm
  - eating disorders
  - personality disorders
  - mental illness, e.g. schizophrenia
  - body dysmorphic disorder
  - bipolar disorder
  - family history, e.g. 'My mother committed suicide when I was 14 years old and her father (my maternal grandfather) shot himself in the heart a year and a half later. I was never counselled.'
  - trauma, e.g. bereavement, witnessing or being abused
  - undiagnosed conditions that emerged after the birth, e.g. onset of bipolar disorder
  - loss of a baby, miscarriage or stillbirth
  - substance abuse related
  - mental challenges due to pain, e.g. pregnancy-related pelvic girdle pain (PPGP) or symphysis pubis dysfunction (SPD)
  - hormonal conditions, e.g. premenstrual syndrome
  - thyroid imbalance

- postnatal conditions:
  - ‣ baby pinks
  - ‣ baby blues
  - ‣ mild to moderate depression
  - ‣ severe depression
  - ‣ obsessive-compulsive disorder (OCD)
  - ‣ anxiety
  - ‣ puerperal psychosis
  - ‣ post-traumatic stress disorder
  - ‣ physical difficulties as a result of birth, e.g. bladder control, mastitis, that can lead to mental health issues, such as fear of leaving home.

There are many sources of information that describe these conditions in detail. I have listed some of them in the resource section at the back of the book. Two most recent collections of journal articles concerning these disorders, screening and treatments can be found in the *Best Practice and Research Clinical Obstetrics and Gynaecology* (January 2014)[1] and *The Lancet* (November 2014).[2]

I think that because the range of conditions are so different and the symptoms can vary so widely, this often makes it difficult for parents and healthcare professionals to approach this area. It is not as 'straightforward' as some physical conditions, e.g. getting appendicitis, when there are small number of indicative symptoms and only one or two alternatives for treatment. Sometimes people do not speak out because they consider what they are feeling is possibly normal. These are some of the emotions and thoughts that parents have described to me during or after pregnancy that have impacted their mental health. Not everyone is affected by all of these! As I compiled this list there were many that I could relate to and others that did not affect me. I hope that this table (*see* p. 13) does illustrate how wide the symptoms can be and also that they vary so much in level.

Here are some more detailed examples of how early motherhood can feel.

- During the first few weeks everything seemed okay but I started to dislike my son. Everything felt wrong and the only change was having him, so it must be his fault. During the summer – I can't remember (he was born in June) anything. My daughter started school in the September part time. I would take her then come home and hide under a blanket waiting for my son to wake and scream. I could never relax while he was asleep – I would be anxious knowing that he would wake soon. Every pregnant woman I saw, I wanted to scream at them, that they didn't know what they had done. I felt that everyone was looking at me and talking about me wherever I went.
- My feelings? Right now I am still fighting PND, I still feel like I'm failing my daughter, like I could be a better mum. I grieve for the first 10 months that I

A range of symptoms experienced and described by sufferers of perinatal mental illness			
Failure – self, baby, loved ones Disappointment Mix of disappointment and joy Mood swings	Exhausted Too tired to have feelings! Inability to sleep Unable to relax Inability to focus Loss of memory Struggle	Overwhelmed Stressed Anxious Tearful Panic attacks Nervous	Incompetent Worthless and unworthy of being a mother Helpless Ignorant Stupid Lack of confidence Unable to cope with everyday life Withdrawn Detached
Anger Aggressive Resentment Guilt Ashamed Bad mother Impatient	Isolated Lost Lonely – wanting someone to talk to Abandoned Vulnerability	Numb Don't remember Spaced out Dead inside Emptiness	Deep level of sadness Low Depressed Miserable Hopeless Blackness
Suicidal – hating life Everything felt wrong Moving strangely	Self-loathing at altered body image Ugly Loss of libido Self-hatred Over or under eating Weight loss or gain	Terror Scared Trapped Unable to socialise	'Going mad' 'Losing the plot' 'Going crazy' Never be 'normal' again Complete mess 'I did not feel like me' 'Zombie' 'Robot'
Shock Panic Confused Desperate Out of control – spiralling	Grief and loss – my freedom, my body, 'me', the experience I expected to have when the baby arrived	In pain – episiotomy, mastitis Self-harm	Manic Excessive energy Erratic Bizarre behaviour Compulsive talking Catatonic Irrational Paranoid Delusional Had hallucinations

(continued)

A range of symptoms experienced and described by sufferers of perinatal mental illness			
No instinct of how to soothe and care for baby	'Hitting a brick wall'	Concerns over loved ones	Content
Baby hates me	Being a fraud	Doubts and challenges with relationships	Happy
Lack of attachment/ bonding	Hostile		Excited
Overprotective of baby		Argumentative	Powerful
No feelings for baby			Special
Harsh feelings for baby, e.g. ugly			Elation
			Ecstasy

lived in a cloud and couldn't bond with her. I can't get that time back but I try to enjoy the days I have with her now.

- Crippling anxiety interspersed with feelings of absolute despair.
- I hated life and felt there was no point to it. I rationalised my death and worked out how everyone would be better off. The anxiety was the worst part as I felt it constantly and couldn't even be left in a room on my own. I was embarrassed of my daughter as I thought there was something seriously wrong with how she looked and I used to look through baby magazines and find babies that looked more like they could be mine (I was very ill at this point). I didn't understand what had gone wrong and why I had ended up with this freak baby and I constantly plotted on how I could get Social Services to take her away.
- I can remember seeing my husband carrying the baby around and feeling jealous and alone. Separated from them by an invisible glass wall.
- I could hardly leave the house because of anxiety and would just cry and cry. I wanted to die but knew that having no mum for my children would be worse than having the awful mum that I felt I was.
- I could not face the prospect of experiencing the anxiety and lack of control over my life that I had experienced with my baby. I don't think I could have coped with a second round, even with support and help. It would have pushed me too far and I would have taken drastic action if I had another child.
- I asked my partner to leave me and take the baby so they would be free of me. People were adamant that I was having a baby boy so two weeks after the birth I found myself crying that she wasn't my baby and someone must of gotten them mixed up. Everyone kept saying 'isn't it the best' but I couldn't say out loud 'no it's not'. I was unsure my partner wanted us there and felt unsure how the relationship would turn out.
- I was terrified of being on my own with three children and how I'd cope. I also realise looking back now that my horrible, racing, non-logical thoughts started back then as well. My husband and my dad were cutting the hedge and I was

paranoid that my baby would get hurt when he was nowhere near. Then it started – the horrible thoughts that I should cut my baby's head off. I find it very hard to talk about this as I would never have done anything to harm him at all.

- I wished that he (my baby) would die so that I could return to normal life. I felt like I was probably the only one feeling like this.

This certainly is not the outcome or pathway that we all anticipated of motherhood! This is not the image portrayed in the glossy magazines – although for many this is the reality. I believe that every parent at some point probably has at least one moment of 'what have we done?' yet we are led to believe that it is all plain sailing. This makes it difficult to admit your feelings if they are less than positive and is why many then suffer the guilt. I commend these ladies for being so open and honest – hopefully this will help others.

Let me add as encouragement that you can recover, which I and many others are proof of. For example:

- I am happy now! I never thought I would get out of that dark place but I did! I have to admit writing about all of this makes me feel very emotional.
- Now I feel well, mostly happy and thankful for small things.

The onset of deteriorating mental health can come at any time in the perinatal period. Studies[3] do indicate a peak immediately after delivery, especially for some of the more severe illnesses such as puerperal psychosis. The stories that were shared with me covered the whole period:

- From initial discovery of pregnancy as it was unplanned and family were very unsupportive.
- At 6 weeks pregnant, I felt very positive. After seeing the doctor who asked me where I was going to give birth, I went downhill from there.
- At the delivery – although looking back I think it started about 7 months into my pregnancy. I woke up one morning with a horrible feeling of absolute dread and the realisation that I didn't want this pregnancy anymore. I didn't tell anyone and just assumed it was hormones.
- After the birth I didn't feel the 'rush' of love that people talk about but presumed I was tired. Realistically though I knew when baby was about 4 weeks old, that I wasn't right and things should have altered.
- I knew almost immediately I felt strange, detached almost from the first night I found it impossible to rest or sleep. My mind was constantly racing and buzzing with unpleasant thoughts of the baby falling down stairs or being taken from me. I was constantly worrying and anxious the baby might die or be taken from me.
- Five or six days after birth I mentioned to my midwife that I felt really anxious and didn't like my son very much.

- Definitely after the first week. I started having severe panic attacks and thought I was dying!
- I didn't realise anything was wrong. I had lost my grip on reality, my husband and health visitor picked up on this around day 14.
- I didn't realise it until after my son was 3 months old. The health visitor had started making weekly visits and kept asking me to see my GP from 6 weeks. But I was determined not to be depressed or look like I was not coping. For the first 3 months I told everyone else, and myself that I just had a poorly baby.
- I think it was gradual, I remember wanting him to just not be there – no idea how this was going to happen. And then it would be better if I wasn't there, but then I would be leaving my daughter and I couldn't do that, so it was his fault.
- I didn't realise until I was diagnosed when he was seven or eight months old. I thought it would just go away but it didn't – it just got significantly worse.
- I was reading an article on postnatal depression, and kept thinking how most of the symptoms listed applied to me but I thought I was making a mountain out of a molehill and was looking for excuses for not coping.
- When I returned to work. I didn't want to leave my baby. I was anxious, very possessive of baby.
- I managed to conceal it at my 6 week GP check and so didn't ask for help until my baby was 11 months old and I was past breaking point.
- I tried to ask for help but didn't get a proper diagnosis until I had a breakdown after 24 months.
- I realised at about 3 or 4 months I think, though this is very blurry. A bit later, I confided in my partner but I did not go to the doctor until my son was around 2.

> The two key messages here are that we all need to be alert throughout the perinatal period for changes in mental health and also that the mother herself may be oblivious to changes.

I asked mothers who had recognised that they were not feeling or behaving as expected.

Who recognised PMHI	Example given by a mother
Self	• I had tried to hide it from everyone. I felt ashamed and unable to cope.
	• Me (I had talked to both my husband and my mum, who had both told me to 'stop being so soft, this is what it's like with a newborn – get used to it!')
	• I diagnosed myself on the internet. Googled PND and did a survey on the APNI site (Association for Postnatal Illness). After utter relief at feeling I wasn't mad, I went to the doctors (and lied – I was ashamed). I then called the midwife and told her everything and she immediately made an appointment with the GP who was great.
Husband/partner/ family and friends	• My husband, family and friends before any professional but they didn't know what it was.
Health visitor	• Had a check with the health visitor and filled in a questionnaire regarding postnatal depression.
	• I rang my health visitor unsure of how to react to my 2 year old crying and basically showing signs of what we see in depression. She instantly said could 'he could be reflecting you' and that's when I knew.
GP	• Although I did have to tell the GP what was wrong with me, and the GP asked me why I hadn't pointed this out before, but I stated that as I had never had a baby before, I thought everyone felt like I did.
Other healthcare professional	• Probably the crisis worker at the intensive care unit where I was initially taken before I was admitted to the psychiatric hospital.
Boss	• I came home and telephoned my boss to say that I could not get to work, and broke down sobbing. She asked me where my baby was and I told him he was safe with his grandma. Shortly after my husband and mum turned up and I was taken to the doctors.
Charity	• I called the APNI[4] helpline and spoke to a very helpful lady on the phone, who told me that I was suffering with PND and to go and see my GP. They sent me loads of information about my condition, and it made me realise that I did actually have a medical condition for the way I was feeling.
Social media	• I told a parenting forum where other mums urged me to see a doctor.

Some mental health issues were diagnosed quickly. Others took a while due to reluctance or denial of the mother to admit her feelings, e.g. 'I knew I wasn't right but I just assumed it was me being useless at motherhood and didn't want to admit it.' Other delays were due to the lack of appropriate action or resources from the healthcare professionals. I shall touch on this in a later chapter. The range of treatments that were offered varied depending on the severity and kind of illness and local resources.

Type of treatment	Example
None	• None as the doctor said that I had got through the worst bit and did not need medication. I suspect I did, for my anxiety, at that point.
Medication (e.g. antidepressant, antipsychotic, sedatives)	• I was offered antidepressants, which I took for 1 month only – I was worried I would become addicted to the medication, even on a mental level. Examples – Sertraline, Prozac, Lexapro, Seroxat
Support group	• I think at first I just felt like it was just me not being good enough especially as the one time I managed to get out of the house to a baby group and everyone had perfect babies, etc. What really helped me was going to a weekly group meeting run by the perinatal mental health service and feeling that I wasn't the only person with crazy thoughts who was going mad. I felt like I was normal and supported by others.
Community psychiatric nurse	• I had an amazing named nurse and team looking after me.
Relaxation classes	• I was an inpatient for a number of months having therapies like art, relaxation classes.

Other treatments that were mentioned included electroconvulsive therapy (ECT), counselling, cognitive behavioural therapy (CBT), health visitor listening visits, reading and attachment sessions.

See Appendix 3 for information on screening for perinatal mental health conditions.

Of the mothers who shared their stories with me, 69% received treatment at home and 31% in hospital.

Place of treatment	Type of treatment
Home	GP consultations, health visitor support Community Mental Health team – visits, groups Crisis team Family support
Hospital	Specialist Mother and Baby Unit General psychiatric unit/ward Private clinic

Most mothers preferred to be kept with their babies if they were hospitalised, in a specialist unit as close to home as possible. These are very limited around the country.[5] Some have commented that without the care here, they may have taken their own lives.

- Although the Mother and Baby Unit (MBU) was approximately 40 miles from home, it was the best solution for me and my baby as we could stay together. In the previous psychiatric units I was alone, with people experiencing a number of different mental health problems. I could only see my baby on arranged times and in inappropriate places such as the hospital café or a small hospital meeting room.
- I feel very bitter that I was separated from my child especially as there was a MBU at my hospital but no places at the time I needed help. I think this separation greatly added to my distress as did the surroundings in a general psychiatric unit – a new mother who has experienced physical distress during labour, plus a major operation (C-section) needs specialist care and handling at such a sensitive and precious time.

One mum commented that 'I needed time on my own – the private clinic helped me so much – being there saved my life.'

For others being at home with their baby and surrounded by supportive family and friends was the best solution, possibly with support in the community, e.g.:

- The support groups were held in a children's centre and being with others made me realise that I wasn't alone, and although my thoughts made no sense, they could understand. Also that PND appears in many forms – I had always believed it was if you had suicidal thoughts.

Some sufferers do go on to make a full recovery, as I did. Others may continue to have mental health issues. Either way, we are here to look at the aspects around considering having another baby after suffering from any of the above. After reading this chapter you may have thought it would be madness! Why would you even want to go back to that place again?

- I felt like someone had taken my old life away and replaced it with a life of anxiety, lack of sleep, unhappiness and an ongoing black mood.

Some people do decide that is enough of a reason for them, and they are content with that decision. As others have gone on to have another baby, we will now look at some of the risk factors involved and whether or not they can be minimised.

REFERENCES

1. O'Hara MW, Wisner KL and Joseph GF, editors. Perinatal mental health: guidance for the obstetrician-gynaecologist. *Best Pract Res Clin Obstet Gynaecol.* 2014; **28**(1): 1–188. Available at: www.bestpracticeobgyn.com/issue/S1521-6934(13)X0007-0
2. *Lancet.* 2014; **384**. Available at: www.thelancet.com/series/perinatal-mental-health
3. Doyle M, Carballedo A, O'Keane V. Perinatal depression and psychosis: an update. *Adv Psychiatr Treat.* 2015; **21**(1): 5–14. Available at: http://apt.rcpsych.org/content/21/1/5.full
4. APNI: http://apni.org
5. UK specialist community perinatal mental health teams (current provision) http://everyonesbusiness.org.uk/?page_id=349

FURTHER READING AND RESOURCES
Books

Church C. *I Blame the Hormones: a journey through female depression.* 2014. Available at: www.iblamethehormones.com/index.htm

Martini A. *Hillbilly Gothic: a memoir of madness and motherhood.* New York: Free Press; 2008.

Moyer M. *A Mother's Climb Out Of Darkness: a story about overcoming postpartum psychosis.* Amarillo, TX: Praeclarus Press; 2014.

Sharrock G. *Saving Grace: my journey and survival through postnatal depression.* Bloomington, IN: AuthorHouse; 2010.

Internet

- www.beatingbipolar.org/women_and_bipolar/
- www.postpartumprogress.org
- www.mypostpartumvoice.com/
- http://hope4ocd.com/foursteps.php

Film/DVDs

- Emily Atef. *The Stranger in Me/Das Fremde in mir* [film]. 2008.
- *Dark Side of the Full Moon: when new motherhood meets mental health complications in America, no one is listening* [DVD]. 2015. Available at: www.tugg.com
- PSS Parent and Baby Wellness Service, Liverpool. *Our Stories: Postnatal Depression* [DVD]. Available at: www.psspeople.com/whats-happening/news/stories-dvd-sale-now

Clinical research

- Robertson P. Experiences of postpartum mood disorders of women with more than one child. *The Family J.* 2013; **21**: 435–42.

   In this consensual qualitative research study, the postpartum mood disorder (PMD) experiences of 127 women who have more than one child were explored through an online survey. Implications for practice include an expansion in predictive factors and symptoms when screening for PMD and the identification of prevention and coping strategies useful in the education and treatment of women who experience PMD. We found evidence in the Maternal Health Study that depression in pregnancy and the first postnatal year significantly decreased the likelihood that women would have a second child at the 4.5 year postpartum follow-up.

● Woolhouse H, Gartland D, Mensah F, *et al*. Maternal depression from early pregnancy to 4 years postpartum in a prospective pregnancy. *BJOG*. 2015; **122**(3): 312–21.

Our findings indicate that maternal depression is more common 4 years after a first birth than at any time in the first 12 months postpartum. Women with one child at 4 years postpartum show higher levels of depressive symptoms than women with two or more children, a difference which is in part explained by greater levels of social adversity experienced by women with one child at this time. There is a need for the surveillance of maternal mental health to extend beyond the perinatal period, to encompass at least the first 4 years of parenting, and to incorporate a focus on social health. At a time when so much attention is given to the surveillance of child health, an increased focus on maternal health is warranted, particularly given the strong connections between maternal and child health outcomes.

Training

Visit http://marcesociety.com/resources/education/ for a wide range of training materials and resources for healthcare professionals.

CHAPTER 2

Risk factors and possible causes of perinatal mental illness

Accept that all of us can be hurt, that all of us can and surely will at times fail. Other vulnerabilities, like being embarrassed or risking love, can be terrifying, too. I think we should follow a simple rule: if we can take the worst, take the risk.

Joyce Brothers

It is common knowledge that by behaving in certain ways, e.g. smoking, we can adversely affect our health and increase our risk of vulnerability to certain diseases. My own grandfather suffered a horrible death by lung cancer, probably caused by his years of smoking. As a result I made the decision many years ago that I would never smoke and I do take every effort to look after myself (although I always know I should exercise more). So it followed that I would want to maximise every opportunity for my own health and my unborn child whilst I was pregnant. Yet when I approached this condition, my mental health was never even considered by me or anyone around me. I felt I prepared myself physically by taking folic acid, avoiding alcohol and eating a healthy, well-balanced diet. I do remember at my 'booking in' appointment with the midwife, at the start of pregnancy, being asked if either I or any member of my family had suffered from mental health problems. I said no; the box was ticked; end of topic. I was so ecstatic at finally being pregnant and skipped off to read, write lists and prepare for the baby.

Had I ever been pregnant again, my mental health would have been top of the agenda. How we learn by experience and knowledge! I now know too that because I suffered from a severe mental illness after pregnancy, I had around a 50% chance of it recurring in a subsequent one.[1] I originally did not think that anyone could have suspected that I might have become so ill after having my baby. I remain grateful to this day that I did receive treatment and recovered, albeit wiser. I never really thought it could have been prevented until I was interviewed on *Woman's Hour* for BBC Radio 4 in 2005. They had invited a leading perinatal psychiatrist, Margaret Oates, to the interview too. Afterwards Margaret told me she had read my story and concluded, 'It should never have happened to you – you should have been given individual, specialist care much sooner.' At other events, experienced healthcare professionals have commented that they were not surprised I had become ill either.

So what were their reasons? Physically I had a tough time. During the latter stages of pregnancy, I was ill with urinary tract infections and very exhausted. The birth was traumatic; I had a retained placenta, postpartum haemorrhage and needed surgery. At my six week check-up, I had to have more surgery for a D&C (dilation and curettage) as the neck of my womb had not closed. I developed mastitis several times, a condition that causes a woman's breast tissue to become painful and inflamed, as a result of breastfeeding. I was extremely sleep-deprived. Not only was the birth traumatic, there was considerable stress when my baby was four months old as he was hospitalised for suspected meningitis. It was finally diagnosed as a viral septicaemia (another name for blood poisoning that refers to invasion of bacteria into the bloodstream, and this occurs as part of sepsis). Along with all of that was my personality – I like to be busy, efficient and organised. I like to be tidy and to please and impress others. As a school teacher, I was used to planning, writing and completing tasks from lists then evaluating them. I attempted to maintain all this with a fractious baby and diminishing sleep. I had high expectations of myself and motherhood. I had the financial pressure to return to work when neither I nor my child were well enough. In hindsight, it wasn't surprising something had to give – that was my mental health.

So, if I had become pregnant again, I would have considered all of these points and looked at how, if possible, they could be minimised next time around. I strongly suggest that you and your healthcare professionals do this with regard to your situation. Although there will be the 'usual' decisions to be considered about having another baby (which we will look at later), let's look at those which have been proved to be risk factors for perinatal mental illness, which we know can have a huge effect on everyone concerned.[1] I have listed many references and sources of research in this chapter so that as a parent and as professionals you have the clinically, evidenced-based support to demonstrate that you may need additional care should you choose to have another baby.

PSYCHIATRIC AND PSYCHOLOGICAL FACTORS

Existing history of depression, psychiatric illness and/or premenstrual dysphoric disorder (PMDD)

There are examples of research, for example by Ryan and colleagues in 2005,[2] that found that having a personal history of depression or any other psychiatric disorder predisposes one to a greater risk of developing postnatal depression. Some women have suspected that if they have had problems with menstruation, they may also have perinatal mental health issues. I would agree that it makes sense that those women who are highly sensitive to hormonal changes would be more likely to experience mood problems all across the lifespan. Research in 2013[3] finds that there is an association between menstrual symptoms and a risk of postpartum depression.

Family history of depression

Studies have shown that having a first-degree relative affected by mental illness is also an added risk factor for perinatal mental illness.[4] One of the ladies in my survey commented that:

- My mother was an alcoholic and Grandma had electric shock therapy. Her mother also died in a mental health institution. I DID NOT DISCLOSE THIS due to the fear of being judged; my professional fear of it being recorded on my medical records and problems with travel, mortgage and life insurance.

The key point here is that although you cannot change your family history, if you are aware of anything, then disclose it. It may help add extra gravity to your requirements for additional support. You can use the reference[4] as a key indicator too.

Family history and/or personal diagnosis of bipolar disorder and/ or puerperal psychosis

Bipolar disorder, previously known as manic depression, is a condition that affects your moods, which can swing from one extreme to another (NHS Choices). The risk of developing puerperal psychosis is considerably higher than the general population if you have this condition.[5,6,7] There is a wonderful organisation that has a wealth of information and support on this specifically related to pregnancy and early motherhood. It is called Action on Postpartum Psychosis, APP (www.app-network.org). They have recently published a small booklet for women who have already had a diagnosis of bipolar disorder who are planning a baby for the first or subsequent time. As parents and professionals, I strongly urge you to contact them and discover their resources, if this area is relevant to you. They have some excellent forums, one-to-one email support and often are looking for people to be involved in research. This group is also invaluable for information and support if you have had puerperal psychosis with a previous pregnancy and want specialist advice. They will be able to tell you if there are specialist support services in your region. If not, then Professor Ian Jones, a perinatal psychiatrist and expert at APP, is happy to see any woman at high risk via the Cardiff University Psychiatry

Service if their GP or psychiatrist refers them (http://medicine.cf.ac.uk/psychological-medicine-neuroscience/cups/perinatal-psychiatry-service/).

The same team have produced an excellent online training film, *Identifying Women at risk – a learning programme for midwives* at www.beatingbipolar.org/perinataltraining/ I feel that this is worth looking at if you are a health professional working in this area.

Depression and anxiety during pregnancy

Some studies have shown that many women who have postnatal depression have symptoms of depression in pregnancy and therefore can be identified antenatally.[8] One study also looks at anxiety in pregnancy.[9] Many of the symptoms are similar to postnatal depression and often mums-to-be feel that they are 'wrong' to feel depressed because the expectation is to be happy during pregnancy. Remember that you would let the midwives know if you had physical, detrimental effects whilst pregnant so, again, be candid about your mental health. Look at www.babycentre.co.uk/a539921/depression-in-pregnancy for a good source of information and support.

Perinatal obsessive-compulsive disorder (OCD)

OCD causes women to experience severe anxiety, obsessions and compulsive behaviours. This can occur at any time, but the onset of OCD or worsening of symptoms has been associated with pregnancy and childbirth.[10] One specialist resource for this is Maternal OCD www.maternalocd.org/, where you can find useful information and support.

Post-traumatic stress disorder

> PSTD and mental health problems which result from childhood trauma, such as emotionally unstable personality disorder, can recur or worsen both during pregnancy and after childbirth. Research suggests that rates of PTSD are higher in pregnant women than in adult female population as a whole.[11] It is thought that the experience of being pregnant triggers the symptoms of these disorders, particularly for women who have experienced childhood abuse or sexual abuse and who may experience complex feelings as a result of becoming a parent, and the physical care experienced in pregnancy.[12] Post-traumatic stress disorder can also be triggered by childbirth, and is estimated to occur in approximately 3% of women after birth. Women are particularly at risk if they have an emergency caesarean, are admitted to high dependency or intensive care units, or if their baby dies.[13]

This paragraph is taken from *Prevention in Mind – All Babies Count: Spotlight on Perinatal Mental Health*,[14] a report by Sally Hogg for the NSPCC. I recommend this for healthcare professionals who want to improve services in their area.

Bereavement

I was very shocked that when I lost my partner, I realised how closely related the symptoms of my grief were to my symptoms of depression. This included lack of sleep; my over-zealousness at unnecessary physical activities; my feelings of loss and drowning. I recognised that I could easily have 'slipped' back into clinical depression as a result and the GP did offer me medication. I chose other ways to heal that I shall share later. It did occur to me that if you therefore suffer bereavement either whilst pregnant or during early motherhood, then the pain must be massive. You will need additional support, both practical and psychological. The turmoil of loss mixed with the joy of a new baby must be awful.

I strongly suggest bereavement counselling, e.g. www.cruse.org.uk/ It may be that you feel that you have never come to terms with the death of someone close to you from years earlier. It may help to deal with this before you consider another pregnancy. If a child is also grieving a helpful site is www.griefencounter.org.uk/

I have read that new mothers may also be more susceptible to perinatal mental health issues if they have lost their own mother, especially at an early age. I know how excited I was to share the news and every stage of my pregnancy with my mum. Her ongoing support and involvement with my son is a pleasure that I treasure. I know how painful I would have found this if she had not been alive.

I have never experienced the pain of losing a baby or having a miscarriage. I have listened to those who have and they have made me aware of the additional concern that this adds to another pregnancy. Many have gone on to give birth to healthy babies. Two organisations that have specific help are www.uk-sands.org/ and www.miscarriageassociation.org.uk/ and they especially offer guidance and support if you feel you want to try again. Often the fathers are missed out of this process, yet can also be deeply affected. They too may need additional support.[15]

If mourning of any prior miscarriage(s) or other loss(es) has not been addressed, there may be a resurgence of memories of the prior, lost pregnancies, along with feelings of increased anxiety during the current one.[16,17] At the moment there is a study starting at the University of Manchester, supported by the charity Tommy's, on 'Improving support in the next pregnancy after miscarriage'. It is aimed at being a useful guide to practice, once completed. A study published in 2013 explored 'Women's decision making and experience of subsequent pregnancy following stillbirth'.[18] They reported that 'these women employed a number of coping strategies not previously reported. These include 'taking an accepting stance in relations to pregnancy outcome, actively avoiding reminders of current pregnancy, living in the moment, resisting attachment through not acknowledging pregnancy, having ambivalence in relation to enjoying their subsequent pregnancy, preparing oneself for difficulties in subsequent pregnancy or further loss, thinking positively about the future, and recognising the positive impact of subsequent pregnancy'.

It is understandable that these ladies have increased anxiety if they have lost a previous baby, as their hopes, aspirations and dreams have been taken from them through miscarriage or stillbirth. Sometimes this can lead to a loss of confidence and self-esteem; isolation and feeling misunderstood. Remember that there is assistance with this process, so I encourage you to use it or direct those who need it.

SOCIAL FACTORS
Poverty and social exclusion
Studies show that rates of perinatal depression are higher amongst women experiencing social disadvantage. This may include isolation and poverty.[19] Findings suggest 'that postnatal depression may affect up to 42% of migrant women, compared to around 10–15% of native-born women. Common risk factors for PND amongst migrant women include history of stressful life events, lack of social support and cultural factors. With a growing number of babies born to immigrant mothers, greater awareness of PND amongst this group is needed in order to respond to their particular maternal mental health needs. Maternity providers should regard all recent immigrants as at high risk of PND and give closer observation and support as necessary'[20] (*see* Chapter 27).

Age
Age at time of pregnancy is a risk factor: the younger you are, the higher the risk. This can almost be twice as high for teenage mothers.[21] A useful document for healthcare professionals is by The Mental Health Foundation, www.mentalhealth.org.uk/content/assets/PDF/publications/young-mums-together-report.pdf

We also need to be mindful of the older mothers too. When I met Margaret Oates (see above), she said I was part of the classic 'conservatory set' who suffered from perinatal mental illness. She was involved in the Confidential Enquiry into Maternal and Child Health (CEMACH) 'Why Mothers Die'[22] who identified that professional women in their mid-30s with a stable career, lifestyle and relationship were the most likely to take their own life in early motherhood. Margaret suggested that these ladies were the most likely to have a big house with a conservatory. More recently at an event she described the same type of lady as having 'bi-folding doors from a large kitchen-diner onto the garden'. The message is that we must be aware of different social groups and ages and avoid expectations and judgements based on them.

Marital conflict/domestic violence
Studies have consistently demonstrated that dissatisfaction with the marital

relationship and the amount of social support from a spouse and other significant persons increases the risk of perinatal mental disorders.[23] Look at www.bestbeginnings.org.uk/domestic-abuse for more information and resources.

Stressful life events

As with non-puerperal depression, stressful life events have been shown to be associated with poor perinatal mental health. For example, a woman who is on maternity leave is likely to feel more vulnerable if her husband is made redundant than she would have if she herself were working full time.[24] Moving house and making any major decisions are best done at other times than during pregnancy and the early days of motherhood.

Ambivalence about the pregnancy: unwanted/unplanned

According to a recent study,[25] women with unintended pregnancies are four times more likely to suffer from postpartum depression at 12 months after the birth.

Assisted conception

I had no challenges in conceiving a baby, yet for some couples this is a major difficulty. The supposition would be that couples who have worked so hard to have a baby and gone through possibly years of fertility treatment, the highs and lows of becoming pregnant and then ultimately having a baby, would be completely joyful. For some this is the case, yet for those who do then suffer with their mental health, the additional guilt they feel may make this worse to admit to, for fear of appearing ungrateful. Research[26] has shown that assisted conception appears to be associated with a significantly increased rate of early parenting difficulties. Women who experience assisted conception may require additional support before and after their babies are born.

Substance misuse and history of poor or abusive parenting

In a review of research, it was found that there were high rates of postnatal depression among substance-using women and those with current or past experiences of abuse.[27] There is useful information at www.bestbeginnings.org.uk/drugs and www.drugscope.org.uk/resources/pregnancyguide

PHYSIOLOGICAL FACTORS
Traumatic birth and prematurity

Both parents can be affected by the birth experience particularly if there are added complications and/or prematurity due to the additional trauma and stress. I know that I felt out of control and never really understood until years later what had physically 'gone wrong'.[28,29] I will go into more detail later about this. Amongst the support resources are http://preemiehelp.com/ and www.

birthtraumaassociation.org.uk/. The Australian Foundation https://lifeslittle treasures.org.au/ is also very good.

Low self-esteem

The charity MIND www.mind.org.uk/ says that if your self-esteem is low, you may doubt your ability to cope as a new mother. When your baby cries, for example, you may think it is because of something you have done wrong – or because of something you haven't done. The way you think about yourself can put you at risk of developing PND.

Morning sickness

One young mother who developed puerperal psychosis felt that being constantly sick throughout her pregnancy robbed her of any feelings of joy. Grace Sharrock has written her complete story in *Saving Grace: my journey and survival through postnatal illness.*[30] She suffered with 'hyperemesis gravidarum', an extreme form of sickness that can leave a pregnant woman very weak and vulnerable. Recently the Duchess of Cambridge has increased awareness of this condition as she has been affected in both her pregnancies. There is a charity that offers support at www.pregnancysicknesssupport.org.uk/

Post-delivery complications

I attended a talk given by Amanda Williams who shared a study she and others had done.[31] I was shocked to discover the incidence of how many women, 12 months after giving birth, are still having problems with their bodies. This may include issues with bladder leakage, continence difficulties and pain with intercourse. The very alarming fact was that so many of these ladies suffer in silence as often they are too embarrassed to ask for help or consider it to be 'normal' after having a baby. Usually, with treatment all of the conditions can be solved. I was also surprised that ladies who had a Caesarean section also had problems. I had wrongly assumed that it would only be those who had a vaginal delivery.

What occurred to me was that if a new mum has issues 'down below' that make her unwilling or cautious to leave the house or affect her intimate relationship, this can greatly affect her social isolation and self-esteem. This could contribute to postnatal depression. It made me wonder how many ladies are still having concerns years later. Amazingly, I was having lunch with a friend recently and told her about this talk. She confessed that she has just had an operation recently to improve her situation – she has struggled since her first baby was born. He is 19!

If you are in practice, is this a question you ask new mums? If not, why not? If you are a mum of any age with issues in the perineal area, I encourage you to see your GP.

Lack of sleep

One of the studies that I particularly relate to is by Kathleen Kendall-Tackett,[32] because I had the first four out of the five aspects she lists as risk factors for perinatal mental health disorders. She concludes that stress, sleep disturbance, pain, psychological trauma and history of abuse are all key factors, with inflammation as the underlying risk factor. 'Postpartum women are particularly at risk because their inflammation levels are naturally elevated in the last trimester of pregnancy, and this elevation continues through the postpartum period.' It is a fascinating article and she outlines some strategies to reduce the risks. These will be referred to in later chapters.

There are further studies that say sleep has a big impact.[33]

Ongoing medical conditions

For women who have existing medical conditions, it follows that they may need extra care and attention due to this, for example diabetes. Ensure that all the relevant care procedures are in place so that any possible anxiety linked with it can be reduced. Thyroid conditions also need to be monitored, *see* www.btf-thyroid.org/index.php/campaigns/pregnancy/23-general-btf-articles/our-campaigns/169-thyroid-in-pregnancy-information

One condition that can be mistaken for a mental health problem is Dysphoric Milk Ejection Reflex (CD-MER). This is 'a condition affecting lactating women that is characterised by an abrupt dysphoria, or negative emotions, that occur just before milk release and continuing not more than a few minutes. D-MER is not postnatal depression or a postpartum mood disorder' (www.d-mer.org).

I trust that this chapter has given you some insight into some of the possible risk factors for developing perinatal mental health issues. If you would like to read further, one comprehensive source of much of the above is an article by Ruth Zager on 'Psychological aspects of high risk pregnancy'.[34]

We shall now move on to some ways to explore how these may be minimised and how to come to terms with what happened in the past.

REFERENCES

1. O'Hara MW, Swain AM. Rates and risk of postpartum depression – a meta-analysis. *Int Rev Psychiatry*. 1996; **8**: 37–54.
2. Ryan D, Milis L, Misri N. Depression during pregnancy. *Can Fam Physician*. 2005; **51**(8): 1087–93.
3. Buttner MM, Mott SL, Pearlstein T, *et al.* Examination of premenstrual symptoms as a

risk factor for depression in postpartum women. *Arch Womens Ment Health*. 2013; **16**(3), 219–25.

4. Rowan C, McCourt C, Bick D. Provision of perinatal mental health services in two English Strategic Health Authorities: views and perspectives of the multi-professional team. *Evidence Based Midwifery*. 2010; **8**(3): 98–106. Joint Commissioning Panel for Mental Health. Guidance for Commissioners of Perinatal Mental Health Services. London: Joint Commissioning Panel for Mental Health; 2012.

5. Oates M. *Perinatal Maternal Mental Health Services: recommendations for provision of services for childbearing women*. London: Royal College of Psychiatrists; 2001. Available at: www.rcpsych.ac.uk/usefulresources/publications/collegereports/cr/cr88.aspx

6. 4Children. *Suffering in Silence*. London: 4Children; 2011. Available at: www.4children. org.uk/Resources/Detail/Suffering-in-Silence

7. Heron J, O'Connor TG, Evans J, *et al*. The course of anxiety and depression through pregnancy and the postpartum in a community sample. *J Affect Disorder*. 2004; **80**: 65–73.

8. Sutter-Dallay AL, Giaconne-Marcesche V, Glatigny-Dallay E, *et al*. Women with anxiety disorders during pregnancy are at increased risk of intense postnatal depressive symptoms: a prospective survey of the MATQUID cohort. *Eur Psychiatry*. 2004; **19**(8): 459–63.

9. Mavrogiorgou P, Illes F, Juckel G. Perinatal obsessive-compulsive disorder. *Fortschr Neurol Psychiatr*. 2011; **79**(9), 507.

10. Seng JS, Low, LMK, Sperlich M, *et al*. Prevalence, trauma history, and risk for post-traumatic stress disorder among nulliparous women in maternity care. *Obstetrics and Gynaecology*. 2009; **114**(4), 839.

11. Wood J (2011). PTSD and Pregnancy. Available at: http://womensmentalhealth.org/posts/ptsd-and-pregnancy/

12. Joint Commissioning Panel for Mental Health. *Guidance for Commissioners of Perinatal Mental Health Services*. London: Joint Commissioning Panel for Mental Health; 2012.

13. Sutan R, Amin RM, Ariffin, *et al*. Psychosocial impact of mothers with perinatal loss and its contributing factors: an insight. *J Zhejiang Univ Sci B*. 2010; **11**(3): 209–17.

14. NSPCC. *Prevention in Mind: all babies count: spotlight on perinatal mental health*. London: NSPCC; 2013. Available at: http://everyonesbusiness.org.uk/wp-content/uploads/2014/06/NSPCC-Spotlight-report-on-Perinatal-Mental-Health.pdf

15. Theut SK, Pedersen FA, Zaslow MJ, *et al*. Pregnancy subsequent to perinatal loss: parental anxiety and depression. *J Am Acad Child Adolesc Psychiatry*. 1989; **27**(3): 289–92.

16. Theut SK, Pedersen FA, Zaslow MJ, *et al*. Perinatal loss and parental bereavement. *Am J Psychiatry*. 1989; **146**(5): 635–9.

17. Center on the Developing Child at Harvard University. *Maternal Depression Can Undermine the Development of Young Children: Working Paper No. 8*. Cambridge, MA, Center on the Developing Child. Available at: http://developingchild.harvard.edu/index. php/resources/reports_and_working_papers/working_papers/wp8/

18. Lee L, McKenzie-McHarg K, Horsch A. Women's decision making and experience of subsequent pregnancy following stillbirth. *J Midwifery Womens Health*. 2013; **58**(4): 431–9.

19. Deal LW, Holt VL. Young maternal age and depressive symptoms: Results from the 1988 National Maternal and Infant Health Survey. *Am J Public Health*. 1998; **88**: 266–70.

20. Collins CH, Zimmerman C, Howard LM. Refugee, asylum seeker, immigrant women

and postnatal depression: rates and risk factors. *Arch Womens Ment Health.* 2011; **14**(1): 3–11.

21. Reid V, Meadows-Oliver M. Postpartum depression in adolescent mothers: an integrative review of the literature. *J Paed Health Care.* 2007; **21**: 289–98.

22. Oates M, Cantwell R. Deaths from psychiatric causes in 2011 Centre for Maternal and Child Enquiries (CMACE). *BJOG.* 2011; **118**(Suppl 1): 132–203.

23. O'Hara MW. Social support, life events, and depression during pregnancy and the puerperium. *Arch Gen Psychiatry.* 1986; **43**: 569–73.

24. Paykel ES, Emms EM, Fletcher J, Rassaby ES. Life events and social support in puerperal depression. *Br J Psychiatry.* 1980; **136**: 339–46.

25. Mercier RJ, Garrett J, Thorp J, *et al.* Pregnancy intention and postpartum depression: secondary data analysis from a prospective cohort. *BJOG.* 2013; **120**(9): 1116–22.

26. Fisher JR, Hammarberg K, Baker HW. Assisted conception is a risk factor for postnatal mood disturbance and early parenting difficulties. *Fertil Steril.* 2005; **84**(2): 426–30.

27. Ross LE, Dennis CL. The prevalence of postpartum depression among women with substance use, an abuse history, or chronic illness: a systematic review. *J Women's Health (Larchmt).* 2009; **18**(4): 475–86.

28. Kendall-Tackett KA. Trauma associated with perinatal events: birth experience, prematurity, and childbearing loss. In: Kendall-Tackett KA, editor. *Handbook of Women, Stress and Trauma.* New York: Taylor & Francis; 2005. pp. 53–74.

29. CT Beck. (2003) Recognizing and screening for postpartum depression in mothers of NICU infants. *Advances in Neonatal Care.* 2003; **3**(1): 37–46. Available at: http://journals.lww.com/advancesinneonatalcare/Citation/2003/02000/RECOGNIZING_AND_SCREENING_FOR_POSTPARTUM.7.aspx

30. Sharrock G. *Saving Grace: my journey and survival through post natal depression.* Bloomington, IN: AuthorHouse; 2010.

31. Williams A, Herron-Marx S, Knibb R. The prevalence of enduring postnatal perineal morbidity and its relationship to type of birth and birth risk factors. *J Clin Nurs.* 2007; **16**(3): 549–61.

32. Kendall-Tackett K. A new paradigm for depression in new mothers: the central role of inflammation and how breastfeeding and anti-inflammatory treatments protect maternal mental health. *Int Breastfeed J.* 2007; **2**: 6. Available at: www.internationalbreastfeedingjournal.com/content/2/1/6

33. Ross LE, Murray BJ, Steiner M. Sleep and perinatal mood disorders: a critical review. *J Psychiatry Neurosci.* 2005; **30**: 247–56.

34. Zager R. Psychological aspects of high-risk pregnancy. *Global Library of Women's Medicine.* 2009. Available at: www.glowm.com/section_view/heading/Psychological%20Aspects%20of%20High-Risk%20Pregnancy/item/155

CHAPTER 3

Dealing with the past before we move into the future

> Oh yes, the past can hurt. But from the way I see it, you can either run from it, or ... learn from it.
>
> *Rafiki*

Have you seen the Disney film, *The Lion King*?[1] It is the story of the 'Circle of Life' based around a family of lions, particularly the main character called Simba. At one point he is debating about going back to the family he left behind with the 'wise' mandrill, Rafiki. Simba is scared to go back to his family because he will have to face the consequences of his past actions, which he has been running from for so long. Rafiki advises him with the statement above.

We all have that choice with the past – we can learn from it or run from it. There are other choices too – we can lock it away, bottle it up and pretend it never happened. We can distort our memories. The one thing we cannot do is undo the past or relive it. If a previous pregnancy was not the idyllic one that was hoped and planned for, perhaps there are some painful memories that need to be processed first? Then you or those you are helping will be able to reach the decision about having another baby or not, with greater contentment. Where there are specific areas that may need attention in order to make it better next time, e.g. at the birth, I shall cover them later in the book. Here, I would like to share with you some of the ways I have processed painful memories and some techniques that may help you to do so.

I had dreamed of a blissful motherhood for 32 years. In reality it was very hard due to all the pressures and events that unfolded. I always said I wanted another baby 'to do it properly next time'. After a while, when I had rationalised that I had not been a failure, I changed it to 'enjoy it next time'. For a few years I held onto the hope and desire that this would happen. As it did not, partially due to my now ex-husband's unwillingness, I struggled to come to terms with it. After the breakdown of our marriage, I faced a hysterectomy and I remember the turmoil I went through, as that meant my 'dream' of another baby would never happen. I interpreted my physical condition as a direct result of my broken marriage and that I was being punished! In the hours before my operation I remember writing a vitriolic email to my ex-husband blaming him for everything. I now am appalled I did that. I have apologised to him, yet that does not take away my regret at doing it. There were two of us in that once happy marriage and we both had our parts to play in it breaking up. No one picked up that I needed someone to listen to me about the emotional impact of having my womb removed. Yes, I had several years of awful periods and investigations showed I had fibroids. The gynaecologist explained that even if I did want more children, my body was telling me that this was not possible. At a surface level this did help because it meant that the choice was no longer mine. Maybe that was part of my struggle as the power had gone from me and I was being 'robbed' of something so precious to me?

Seeing my distress before the operation, a nurse sent for the hospital chaplain. She sat with me and listened whilst I poured my heart out about my postnatal illness and the impact. As a result, I did feel more peaceful going into the operation. In the recovery room, though, as I came round, I was aware I had blood loss and was in great pain. As the team were deciding what to do with me I remember getting so upset again that I was being punished! I was taken back into theatre. As the physical scars healed so did my deep disappointment at never having another child. It was no longer possible, so why torture myself about it? I had done enough of that. I have rationalised it because I cannot do anything about it, so it becomes a waste of thoughts and energy. I now know that the important thing is to focus on what I 'can do' in life.

I admit that writing this book is another way to let go of what did not happen for me. I cannot change the past. I have learned from it and it is that knowledge I want to share. If that helps others I feel it has been worthwhile. The fact that by sharing my story of postnatal illness and recovery has been influential in saving at least five lives and improving the lives of many others makes my experiences meaningful. I am not saying that every person who suffers from a mental health problem should share it – I am saying that it has helped me.

The second significant event I have had to deal with was the death of my partner. I have said before that I realised the connections between bereavement and depression during the months after he died. That era taught me that we only have 'now' and to make the best of every day. We can waste the present by dwelling too much on the past and spoiling what we have and where we are now. I read several books whilst I was grieving to help me through. I found the books by Elisabeth Kübler-Ross[2] particularly useful to recognise some of the emotional stages that I was going through. Here is a brief indication of how these stages[3] affected me during each traumatic period.

Stage of grief	Postnatal Illness	Bereavement
Denial	I felt I 'wasn't the type'; that it could not be happening to me. I had read all the books, I had planned meticulously. I became numb and drifted through days with little sense of purpose – either being hyperactive or morose. Life was overwhelming. I wore a 'mask' and acted in ways that I thought were expected of me.	Why him? He had so much still to give to others. It wasn't real – he would wake up and say it was just him having a laugh. I became hyperactive to avoid my real feelings. Life was overwhelming. I wore a 'mask' and acted in ways that I thought were expected of me.
Anger	It wasn't fair! Why me? Why had the birth gone so badly? Why didn't my baby sleep? Why was he so ill? What had I done to deserve this? Why did no one know that I was becoming so ill?	It wasn't fair! After all the heartache of the early days of our relationship, it seemed all to be going well. Why hadn't we sorted out the practical implications of this happening even though we had discussed them? Why did he lie to me that he would never leave me?
Bargaining	'If only' the birth had gone better; if only my baby had been well and slept well. 'What if' I hadn't needed to go back to work?	'If only' we had known how little time we had. 'What if' I had taken him to the hospital as I had suggested, on the day he died?
Depression	Feeling lost and questioning if there was any point in carrying on	Feeling lost and questioning if there was any point in carrying on
Acceptance	I have a healthy and happy son and a lifetime of being his mother to look forward to. The period of postnatal illness was a short one in comparison and 'worth it' for the outcome. Some people are unable to have any children – I have an amazing and happy son to cherish. I cannot go back and relive it again. I can enjoy the present and be excited about the future.	We had three years of fun, laughter and challenging experiences from which I have learned a great deal and which have led me to the contented place I am in now. He will not come back and neither will the lifestyle I had with him. I can look back and smile at the happy memories and am glad that the intense pain is no more. I can enjoy the present and be excited about the future.

I now recognise that I had tortured myself for years about the 'loss' of having another baby. I allowed myself to drown in pity and regret rather than focusing on all the positives in my life. When my partner died, it occurred to me how precious every day really is and that the person I hurt most with any negative thoughts was me! I am a person who likes to plan, so when my intended life's plan made changes, I had to let go of it in order to enjoy a new one. We cannot have certainty. I now 'go with the flow' much more and as a result I find I am more fulfilled and happy. If we allow ourselves to be free from all the negative thoughts, we create space for new, better ones. Think back to a time that you were having serious difficulties. Remember how every waking moment your thoughts would be directed to it? Then what happened when the crisis passed? Did you feel more able to function effectively? This is what I mean by 'letting go' and being able to deal with the past.

> Just let it happen. 'Letting go' can't be taught or explained, only experienced. It is not a numbered list or a step-by-step process like the stages of grief. Life is not neat and tidy. Things get emotional, dramatic, messy. 'Letting go' is an awesome intention and a beneficial practice. But it isn't easy. Take it moment to moment, day by day.[4]

So what would I suggest to help you let go of the hurt and pain of the past to help you create room for new thoughts and experiences?

> If you let go a little, you will have a little peace. If you let go a lot, you will have a lot of peace. If you let go completely, you will discover complete peace.
>
> Ajahn Chah[5]

Firstly, I would recommend that you need to recognise that you have choices to make. You can either accept the situation, change it or stay in the dilemma you are currently in. I believe that you either want to change or accept the issues, and this is why you are reading this book. So first make the conscious decision to 'let go' of the negative thoughts that are making you unhappy. Decide to stop the disillusion and illusion of your initial 'plan' and instead of procrastination, choose to take constructive actions. Trust that you, and the situation, will get better, even though you do not know what the actual outcome will be. Remember that I said that we cannot have certainty?

Next, I would say that you need to claim ownership and responsibility for where you are. Looking back, I did not do this. I clearly did not communicate well enough with my ex-husband about how important a second child was for me. I blamed him and I should have also acknowledged that I had a part to play. I considered myself as 'the victim'. I compared myself to others whom I envied, those having larger families, instead of being grateful for the many blessings I did have with my son.

This brings me onto my next point: forgiveness. It took me a long while before I forgave myself for what I thought had been a terrible start to motherhood – I had failed at what I most sought in life. I now know that I had been ill. If I had knowingly set out to behave and act as I did, then I would have deserved what happened. Perhaps people around me could have done things differently during my perinatal period – even if they could, holding onto anger or frustration would serve no purpose other than hurting myself even more. I do not believe that anyone maliciously set out to hurt me, so what would the point be of holding onto any grudges? I have also learned that there are always 'two sides to a coin', as the saying goes. It helps to consider others from their situation – perceptual positioning. For example, if you felt a healthcare professional was very rushed in how you were treated, consider what else they were maybe dealing with.

It is important to express your pain first, before you can leave it behind. Some people stifle their true negative feelings, e.g. sadness or anger. In time, this can have a pressure-cooker effect and they 'blow' at an unexpected time, leading to more problems. It is commonly believed that it is better to acknowledge your thoughts, really 'feel' them, process them and move on. Some ways to express these include:

1. Cry. Shout. Kick the cat – proverbially! Scream somewhere you cannot be heard. Let it out! Have the equivalent of a toddler tantrum. Just choose your time and place very carefully! I find I always feel better after a cry and there are scientific studies that prove this.[6]

2. Writing. This may be just an account to yourself that you write, tear up and ceremoniously burn or throw away. It could be a letter or email to a relevant person, to express how their actions have made you feel. You may decide not to send it. My advice is to give yourself a 'cooling off' period before you do post or press 'send', in case you then wish you had not done so. I wish I had done this with the letter I wrote to my ex-husband. Ask yourself if it will do any good by sending it. Some people like to write a journal or blog. I suggest an air of caution about making too much public as you can hurt others unnecessarily in the process, as I did with some of my blog posts after my partner passed away.

3. Talk to people. Sometimes simply sharing your thoughts with a trusted listener can help. A business contact of mine called me a few months after having her first child. She was going through all kinds of emotional distress because she thought her feelings were abnormal. All she needed was that one reassuring conversation to make her realise she was doing a great job of motherhood. For anxieties and concerns that go much deeper, I do recommend that you seek and have appropriate, professional counselling for the issue. If you feel you want to verbally 'rant' at someone, I recommend that you write your points down first. Give yourself some time (overnight?), then you will communicate to them better in a rational rather than a hysterical way.

4. When you are ready to, begin to give away practical items that maybe add to your pain. Start by putting them out of sight for a while, e.g. in a box in the loft. At a later date you may find it less painful to give them away or recycle them. Some people find it better to do it in one big 'clear out'. It is up to you. I hung on to my son's baby equipment for many years, 'just in case'. I used to sit with his baby clothes and sob my heart out for two reasons. One was for the 'loss' of the expected happy days and the other for

the maternal ache for them to be worn again. Eventually I had to let them go. It felt better to buy something good for us instead to create happy, new memories. I do still have a box of keepsakes that make me smile. Some I was able to pass onto my niece. Maybe one day I shall have grandchildren to love who will enjoy 'Daddy's toys'? Consider it as a way of spring cleaning your mind and environment. How does it feel to get rid of a tatty yet much-loved rug, to then have it replaced by a fresh, clean new one when you redecorate? Stuff is just that – stuff. Memories can never be lost in your heart and mind. Make space. One mum who decided not to have another baby said:

> One of the ways I dealt with this was to pass on many of the toys to our child minder. In doing so, I knew that our daughter would still get pleasure from them and play with them with younger children at the child minders. This made the wrench of giving the toys up much easier. Obviously I have my stash of special items, clothes etc. but you can't physically hang on to everything, unless a house with elastic walls is invented!!

5. Sing and use music to unleash your emotions! Allow yourself some time and tears to sob to sorrowful music. Think of the opening of the film *Bridget Jones's Diary*,[7] when she sings 'All by Myself' using a hairbrush as a microphone. When you are ready, flip to some more assertive ones, e.g. the classic has to be 'I Will Survive' by Gloria Gaynor. We now have the aptly named song 'Let it Go' from the Disney film *Frozen*. Now if ever there was a song to do a spin in the kitchen wearing your dressing gown – there it is! There is a fascinating article called '10 stress management lessons from *Frozen*'s Let it go'.[8] Have a read and it may help add even more power to your singing! Also have a look at www.barefootbeginnings. net/2014/02/23/songs-to-release-stress/

I find it useful to reflect on life's experiences and consider what I have learned from them. This can be especially useful if those experiences have been perceived as negative or caused you pain. Acknowledging what the situation has taught you is perhaps a way of getting closure on it. It may be that you have increased your self-knowledge and awareness. Postnatal illness taught me that I am capable of many things. It has given me a confidence that says: 'if I got through that, I can get through this'. It taught me the need to be candid. If I had only expressed my true feelings and fears earlier, and people had reacted accordingly, maybe I would not have become so ill. It has also helped me to come to terms with what happened to me after my son was born by learning more about the physical and emotional impact, e.g. what a retained placenta is. You may find it helpful to research what troubled you, although be aware of information overload. I have learned that worry is a waste of time and energy.

Worry pretends to be necessary but serves no useful purpose.

Eckhart Tolle[9]

I have learned that when something upsets me, I now realise I have two choices – do something or do nothing! If there is nothing to be done, why worry? It may be useful to reframe the situation instead. I will say more on this in the chapter on communication. If I can actively do something, I do it! I have found that focusing on the possible actions is much more fulfilling and beneficial than moping about things I am unable to impact on.

Incredible change happens in your life when you decide to take control of what you do have power over instead of craving control over what you don't.

Steve Maraboli[10]

Finally, and most importantly, I encourage you to focus on the present and have gratitude for the many blessings you do have in your life. This can be difficult when you are in a crisis; you feel overwhelmed or so deeply in a tunnel; you cannot see your way out. One inspirational man has a great way of looking at this. Nick Vujicic was born with no arms and legs, yet he has overcome so many obstacles to now be a husband and amazing father. Have a look at his website and YouTube films.[11]

Nick says in his book *Life without Limits*, 'the light at the end of the tunnel may just be around the next bend.'[12]

So what are some of the ways I have found helpful to achieve this?

1. List all of your achievements and positives in your life. You can begin with the fact you woke up this morning. Everything else is a bonus! The huge aspect to focus on is that even if you got off to a less than perfect start to parenthood, you have a lifetime ahead of you to make amazing new memories and happy times. Stop punishing yourself for what you feel you missed or 'should have' done. Start seeing what you have and could have in the future.

2. Look back on the time of your perinatal distress and recall all of the good things. Some people find this difficult as their memory of this time may have been lost. Focus on the things you can remember that you now can look back on … and smile. Even if the birth experience was not what you expected, or it took you a long time to bond with your baby, there will be some positives there. Accept them and be thankful.

3. If you have negative thoughts, perhaps you can consider writing them down (as above) and throwing them out. Another idea is to visualise a box or a shelf. As they come in your head, decide to put them there, and move on. Do this whenever you have the draining emotions of fear, anger and irritation.

4. Choose people who help you be the best you can be. Distance yourself

from those who appear to want you to join them in their pity or complaining party. It is so empowering and much more fun to be with people who are full of positive energy. Decide to be one too. Find things that make you laugh out loud and enjoy yourself thoroughly!

5. Find activities that help you be in the 'here and now'. Techniques include mindfulness (*see* Chapter 29), meditation, yoga, controlled breathing and exercise.

6. Remember that everything does not have to be done now! That is one of my weaknesses. When I decide to commit to something I can then get carried away into putting all my focus onto it. Writing this book is an example. I learned I have to pace myself (although I often need a reminder!) Little and often is the way to achieve bigger things. One small step at a time!

7. When you have completed small tasks, reward yourself. It may just be a cup of tea or booking an enjoyable event. The important thing is to recognise your strengths and celebrate them accordingly.

8. Some people find that saying or having reminders written around them of positive affirmations can help. These can be linked to thoughts and beliefs, e.g. 'It's wonderful that I am a good parent'.

9. Take action to help others. This may be deciding to help some of the charities involved in perinatal mental health. It may be taking your elderly neighbour a bunch of flowers.

10. Give yourself permission to be happy. Do you often sabotage contentment by being in a panic that because you are 'up' it won't last and you spoil it by predicting you will come 'down'? Perhaps you even self-doubt that you deserve to be happy? In the book *The Big Leap* by Gay Hendricks,[13] he says that we are our own worst enemy by putting the lid and limit on our happiness in this way. Go on – be brave! Allow yourself to smile.

You will find more suggestions under the NHS Five Ways to Wellbeing[14] and also in Chapters 29 and 30 in this book.

One mum told me how she processed the advice not to have another child:

- I'd like to share my GP's comments from when I was considering IVF to have another baby (because of the trauma of PP, we waited to have another baby. I was 38 when we had our daughter and had conceived immediately). When she was about 2.5 years, we tried for another baby but to no avail. After 6 months or so trying, we had some fertility investigations and it appeared I was perimenopausal. Then we looked into IVF. As part of this, the comments from the GP which seemed especially harsh at the time were basically 'What are you even considering IVF for? The IVF drugs are incredibly strong and you don't know what brought on your PP first time around. The IVF drugs could bring on another psychosis'. The point of this is not about IVF but about being thankful for what you have, and about celebrating the joy in the baby you do have. Most ladies with PP I assume felt like I did i.e. robbed of those precious early months with my baby. What the GP's words did for me was to shock me into seeing what I had got, not what I hadn't. I could then stop looking to the past and live in the present!!! I made damned sure I loved and experienced and cherished every minute that I had with our beautiful girl from that time on. PP had robbed me of those early months but I could do something to stop it from robbing me of any more time enjoying my baby. The control was with me. It so helped me to move forward. Harsh words but they worked.

I am often asked how I was able to 'let go and move on' by several people. I found this poem useful:

Letting Go Takes Love

To let go does not mean to stop caring, it means I can't do it for someone else.
To let go is not to cut myself off, it's the realisation I can't control another.
To let go is not to enable, but allow learning from natural consequences.
To let go is to admit powerlessness, which means the outcome is not in my hands.
To let go is not to try to change or blame another, it's to make the most of myself.
To let go is not to care for, but to care about.
To let go is not to fix, but to be supportive.
To let go is not to judge, but to allow another to be a human being.
To let go is not to be in the middle arranging all the outcomes, but to allow others to affect their destinies.
To let go is not to be protective, it's to permit another to face reality.
To let go is not to deny, but to accept.
To let go is not to nag, scold or argue, but instead to search out my own shortcomings and correct them.
To let go is not to adjust everything to my desires, but to take each day as it comes and cherish myself in it.
To let go is not to criticise or regulate anybody, but to try to become what I dream I can be.
To let go is not to regret the past, but to grow and live for the future.
To let go is to fear less and love more.

Author unknown

I can read this and in every suggestion that I find, I can relate it to myself. Can you?

Often people will say the cliché that 'time is a great healer'. There are also those who challenge that, by saying that over time you simply learn to live with the pain of the past better. I do believe that time *can* be a great healer, as long as we do something practical and realistic with it! Perhaps Mother Nature herself may have her role to play, as she did with me as I needed a hysterectomy. Another mum said:

> Trust Mother Nature. I am not religious at all but do feel that going into early menopause was possibly brought on by PP. I will never know this for sure, but by turning around how I look at this, it has really helped. Instead of getting frustrated with the apparent 'failure' of my body to allow us to have another baby, I see it as Mother Nature protecting me and telling me 'this is dangerous for you and so I am not going to let it happen again'.

My biggest tip to you for regaining a sense of contentment for your life is to visualise a time when you once were content. Remember how that made you feel. By taking some of the steps above, have faith that you will be there again. Which one will you begin with?

> Renew, release, let go. Yesterday's gone. There's nothing you can do to bring it back. You can't 'should've' done something. You can only DO something. Renew yourself. Release that attachment. Today is a new day!
>
> Steve Maraboli[15]

REFERENCES

1. www.imdb.com/title/tt0110357/quotes
2. Kubler-Ross E, Kessler D. *Life Lessons: how our mortality can teach us about life and living*. New York: Scribner; 2003.
3. http://grief.com/the-five-stages-of-grief/
4. Fajkus MM. *18 Fantastic Ways to Let Go*. Available at: www.elephantjournal.com/2014/06/18-fantastic-ways-to-let-go/
5. www.ajahnchah.org/
6. Bylsma LM, Vingerhoets AJJM, Rottenberg J. When is crying cathartic? An international study. *J Soc Clin Psychol*. 2008; **27**(10): 1080–1102.
7. www.imdb.com/title/tt0243155/
8. http://mumcentral.com.au/10-stress-management-lessons-from-frozens-let-it-go/
9. Tolle E. *A New Earth: awakening to your life's purpose*. New York: Penguin Group (USA); 2005.
10. Maraboli S. *Life, the Truth, and Being Free*. Port Washington, NY: A Better Today; 2009.
11. www.lifewithoutlimbs.org/
12. Vujicic N. *Life Without Limits*. Colorado Springs, CO: Waterbrook Press; 2010.
13. Hendricks G. *The Big Leap*. New York: HarperCollins; 2009.
14. www.nhs.uk/Conditions/stress-anxiety-depression/Pages/improve-mental-wellbeing.aspx

15. Maraboli S. *Unapologetically You: reflections on life and the human experience*. Port Washington, NY: A Better Today; 2013.

OTHER LINKS AND RESOURCES YOU MAY FIND USEFUL

- McGee P. *S.U.M.O. (Shut Up, Move On): the straight-talking guide to creating and enjoying a brilliant life*. Chichester: Capstone Publishing; 2006.
- http://psychcentral.com/blog/archives/2014/07/22/learning-to-let-go-of-past-hurts-5-ways-to-move-on/
- http://tinybuddha.com/blog/40-ways-to-let-go-and-feel-less-pain/
- www.masteryoflife.com/letgo.html
- http://bodyspiritandmind.co.uk/index.php/articles/80-general/849-27-life-changing-lessons-to-learn-from-eckhart-tolle
- Kleiman K. *Dropping the Baby and Other Scary Thoughts: breaking the cycle of unwanted thoughts in motherhood*. New York: Routledge; 2011.

PART 2

Decisions to be considered about another pregnancy

CHAPTER 4

Personal desire and situation

Making the decision to have a child – it is momentous. It is to decide forever to have your heart go walking around outside your body.

Elizabeth Stone

I love the expression (above) by American author, Elizabeth Stone. I know that even in the last couple of days, my parents have been concerned about my 54-year-old brother, currently in China, me at 51 being on the M6 motorway and my 42-year-old sister on her travels! Who says concern goes when the children are grown up? Equally there are the associated joys and knowledge that you have produced independent adults (who may need you from time to time). Pleasure and pain is all part of parenthood. If a previous perinatal period was more painful than it should have been, it follows that deciding whether to do it all again is likely to be an even bigger decision than before.

As you know by now, I always knew that I wanted more than one child. Even at my most ill, I doubt if this desire ever really disappeared for me – it was subdued for a while though. On reflection I would say that Marius was about four years old when I felt I would have been really ready again. I felt mentally and physically well and although I was aware of the financial aspects, I would have been happy to have made compromises. I felt I had learned so much more and would have been much more relaxed and open to help next time round. My ex-husband had other reasons for not wanting to go ahead. He felt he was too old; we had only just begun to have undisturbed nights of sleep; he didn't want to risk all the pregnancy/birth/postnatal issues again. I would never have tricked him into another child, so it never happened.

Any couple considering whether they should add to their family usually have a number of issues to consider and discuss – although I have been told that some simply say 'Should we?' as the proverbial twinkle in the eye is there and that's it! Yet in the circumstances we are looking at, it possibly takes a bit more thought than that, and that is why you are reading this or are wanting to help others with their decision. It is easy to find a list on the internet or in books of questions to consider before adding to your family. What I aim to do here is to take these aspects deeper.

PERSONAL DESIRE

I know that my maternal desire for children was a strong biological urge linked to experiences and pleasure of being one of three siblings. Many men also have similar feelings and want to create a secure and large family. There is no right or wrong. I would say that having another baby is better to be based on a 'want' rather than a need to 'fix' a situation, e.g. to 'save' a marriage. The arrival of a new baby represents huge changes for everyone. If you have not got that maternal or paternal urge, then that is okay too. There is no need to feel guilty about it. Having another child should be a mutual decision. If one partner 'tricks' the other by pretending to use contraception, it is very likely to build resentment into the relationship which is ultimately bad for the child.

RELATIONSHIPS

What is the relationship between the parents? Is it a strong, happy and loving one or one fraught with difficulties? In the ideal world it is obviously better for your mental health to contemplate another baby if you are secure and work together to maximise good mental and physical health for all the family. One of the mothers in my survey said:

- Husband hadn't wanted it, he only agreed because I said I just couldn't be happy with just one child. He was very anxious about it happening again, plus coping with a toddler at the same time.

I will explore this in more detail in the next chapter.

FERTILITY

We cannot always assume that just because you decide to try for another baby that it will happen to order. It may be that the previous time you conceived quickly or you needed treatment to do so. Either way, are you prepared for the emotional roller-coaster of trying and maybe being disappointed? If you do need to have fertility treatment, can you afford this financially and mentally?

YOUR MENTAL HEALTH

It may be that your healthcare professionals have advised you that it may cause you serious illness if you were to become pregnant again and they fear you would be unable to care for your children or yourself. I am in no position to criticise or question that. I know I reached a stage when I was no longer on medication and I felt well enough to try again. The length of time mothers in my survey felt it took them to recover depended on how ill they had been and how effective and/or immediate any treatment was. They stated periods between a couple of months to three years on average:

- From being put on antidepressants in December and starting the PND course in February I started to think more clearly around August. The doctor said it was good when I forgot to take my tablets as it meant that I wasn't so reliant on them.
- I felt a lot better after about 3 weeks of taking the antidepressants and stopping breastfeeding and felt able to cope to some degree on my own (my mother went home). However I continued to take antidepressants for about 2 years.
- Six months, once I stopped trying to overcome it with CBT and counselling, and took the Sertraline. It was like a light coming on.
- I took about 2 years for all the symptoms to disappear. I recall looking back over the first 6 months and thinking how much better I was, and that I was back to normal. After a year I did the same reflection and realised that I hadn't fully recovered at 6 months, as I knew that I had improved significantly up to 12 months.

I asked the mothers in my survey if they felt they had recovered from their perinatal mental illness. Like me, some felt that they had made a full recovery, although the experience had changed them. Some recognised a greater awareness of their mental vulnerability if they get tired or stressed; others have been left with the need for ongoing medication, e.g. due to being diagnosed with bipolar disorder. Several commented that they still are prone to anxiety, especially around menstruation. Sometimes mothers were aware of other stages:

- I recovered from the postnatal illness itself but I am still grieving for the lost times of joy I didn't have much of with my son as a baby.
- I thought I had recovered but started to have bad flashbacks and was very tearful two years after my son was born when my sister-in-law had a baby. I realised then that I hadn't really dealt with what had happened, and had just tried to block it away with the antidepressants.

Thirty-one per cent of the mothers I asked felt they had no long-term effects from their perinatal mental illness.

- I don't think you are ever the same – but in good ways as well. You have more compassion, empathy – you understand what depression really is and how it affects people.
- It has taken a long time to build my confidence again. I felt that I was incapable

of doing anything. I do feel panic in certain new situations and do have some times when I feel that I will cry but know how to recognise and manage my feelings.

- I believe I will never forgive myself, it has also left me a lot more resilient to leave my children, and my confidence and self-esteem are rock bottom.
- A feeling of vulnerability and lack of confidence in myself which I don't believe will ever go. I use to feel invincible – not any more.
- I will need to take lithium forever (can have a break for a second pregnancy if stable). I feel my brain never recovered to 100%. I describe it as 'it felt like my brain was completely wiped during the psychosis' and continues to rebuild itself now (3 years later). My ability to learn feels compromised and my ability to retain information is definitely not what it was before.
- Memory loss. Less-organised and efficient.
- Feelings of guilt. Although, this is reducing over time. I had to give up a job that I loved and will probably never return to it.
- I constantly feel I have a very distance relationship with my son. I don't feel as close to him as I feel I should be. I constantly blame myself for his tantrums.

The main question to ask yourself is where do you feel you are at? If you instinctively feel that you are not ready, then be honest to admit it. You may feel stronger in a few months. Revisit the decision then and accept that your feelings may change or not.

- I feel I am now out of the woods so to speak and I don't think I could risk it all again. Maybe I will feel different one day but for now we are happy just the three of us.

PHYSICAL HEALTH

There may be some conditions where medical advice is such that they strongly recommend that you do not become pregnant, e.g. certain heart conditions. If this is the case, seek specialist support and counselling from the team connected to that illness. Could your physical health be improved by increasing your fitness level? Consider the general pre-pregnancy guidelines for the need to limit alcohol intake and stop smoking.

AGE

You may feel that you or your partner are too old to want to begin all of the baby stages again. I know with every decade that passes that I do not have the energy I had previously. Equally, is age an attitude? My parents had my sister in their late thirties, just as their peers were drifting into middle-age. Now as grandparents to her lively 5-year-old, she keeps them mentally and physically 'young' like her mother did. It is well known that with age your fertility decreases, so there is always the pressure of time to consider. How long are you prepared to wait?

GAP BETWEEN CHILDREN

Some people like to have children close together so that they 'get over' all the baby stages sooner. Others like to leave gaps so they only cope with one set of baby needs at a time. After a perinatal mental illness healthcare professionals would probably suggest that it may be better to have an older sibling who has passed the 'baby' stage before you begin again.

SEX OF YOUR EXISTING CHILDREN

Some people may feel that they are willing to go on having children until at least one of each gender is born. For others, the sex of a child does not matter. How important is this for you? Is it an area of pressure or concern for you and/or your partner? Gone are the days when inheritance was only passed down the male side. One mother told me:

- I feel that the decision to not have another child is somewhat easier for me than others, as I have been blessed with a boy and a girl. I don't know if the decision would have been a lot harder if I only had one baby or 2 of the same sex.

DESIRE OF EXISTING CHILDREN AND THE EFFECT ON THEM

I always knew I wanted a baby brother or sister and pestered my parents for years! Other children are quite happy as they are. My son used to say he was lucky that he didn't have a younger sibling who may have broken his Lego creations! He says he can always find company and then go home to be quiet. The age of the existing children could also be a significant aspect. The older they are, possibly the more helpful they would be, yet also more sensitive and aware of difficulties if your mental health is affected. A useful book to help older siblings is *A Monster Ate My Mum* by Jen Faulkner.[1]

When I first did my presentations I asked my son to help me choose some family photographs. He was probably about 8 years old at the time. We found one of him looking very bewildered, taken on the Christmas Eve when I had been admitted to the psychiatric hospital. He looked at it and exclaimed: 'I've just thought. If I was the age I am now and all this had happened to you with another baby, I'd be a traumatised child!'

Perhaps that may have been enough to convince me that another baby may have been wrong for us. Yet I still say that I would have planned for plenty of support for us all to minimise any effects and would have risked it. I got better before and believed I would again. Other mums shared their thoughts on this:

- I think I could do it but I will never take the risk – my son is 'my everything'.
- I don't want another baby but I would be worried it would happen again. My son is nearly 7 and I couldn't risk what he might experience or go through if it did.

One couple did decide to have another child and concluded that

- As horrific as it is remember it is not your fault that it happened to you and just like other illness it rips through families and changes things. That is real life and real life involves children and family members learning to cope with these things. Life isn't all cotton wool and rose bushes. My children know they are loved and safe and they now have each other. They also have a good understanding of mental health and insight into how important it is to talk about problems and get help if you need it. PND has given me gifts I can pass on to them – awareness and tools to help them through life. I was so worried about the effects on my older child but it has given him far more than it ever took away.

CAREER

One of the mothers in my survey told me that:

- My career has taken a real hammering, I have still not achieved the salary I was on before I had postnatal depression. I feel like a failure.

I know that my teaching career was knocked because of my absences. Yet I also feel it made me a better teacher because I was now a parent and understood many of the issues faced by the families I was involved with. Many women feel that their career is affected by motherhood, even if it has gone without problems. You need to consider what means more to you. Is it okay for you to be more focused on children for a few years or not? Having seen my son off to university now makes me realise how fast the years go. Might it be worth considering that your partner considers a career break or change to support you all as a family? I explore this in detail, *see* Chapter 22.

REALITIES AND COMPROMISES

Are you ready to face the broken nights of sleep; the demands of feeding; changing about 10,000 nappies? Are you willing to make different arrangements than last time if it may improve your mental health? For example, getting help sooner with regards to sleeping challenges?

Financially are you prepared for the additional costs of bringing up another child? I know that next time round I would not have spent a fortune on brand new clothes and equipment that is needed for such a short time. Yes, there would have been some items already in our home, yet I would have been prepared far more to get good pre-loved items. What else could you look at to save costs? Perhaps negotiating a budget may help between you as a couple.

Are you prepared to have a different social life? I often think that families with young children have far more social activities than most of us adults! In taking children to swimming, dancing classes, etc. you certainly can make friends. It just is different from dinner parties and clubbing!

Are you prepared to expect the unexpected? What if you have a multiple birth? What if there are different complications next time? What if all goes smoothly?

Are you prepared to make compromises on your lifestyle? Is your home adequate?

> My mother had a great deal of trouble with me, but I think she enjoyed it.
>
> Mark Twain

FAMILY AND FRIENDS

What are their comments to you? How much is this influencing your decision? How much support will or won't they be able to offer? Have you asked them?

The responses in my survey of family and friends to the news that a mother was pregnant again, after having had a previous perinatal mental illness, were varied and extreme. At the negative side, one lady was asked: had she considered a termination? Others were shocked, surprised or critical. One lady told me that when she informed her mother that she was expecting again, she commented that 'it was not a very sensible thing to do'. She now dotes on her grandson and has always been a great support following the initial comment. Some had a neutral reaction and others were supportive, e.g.:

- Happy for me they were very supportive that I had the courage to get pregnant again.
- Positive – I was worried they would judge me but people wanted me to have another baby.

Some commented that others were concerned and anxious for them:

- Most were fine. Partner's parents were very anxious and felt it was the wrong decision.

I say much more on this topic in Chapter 20.

ARE YOU READY TO TIP THE BALANCE?

Is your life already okay as you are? Perhaps you feel that you have just come through a tough journey and that by repeating it you are possibly going to add strain to every aspect of your life? Ask yourself the opposite question – what if I/we do not have any more children? How do you see yourselves in 5, 10, 20 years?

In researching this chapter I came across an article online entitled '41 things to do before having a baby'.[2] It left me open-mouthed! If we all followed the advice to have all the exotic holidays; drive the best cars; live in top notch houses and get rid of clutter, for example, before we had any children we would be facing a population crisis! Of course all of these things, and more, do not make you necessarily any happier. Some of their suggestions, like going to Disneyland, are much more fun *with* children. I am now enjoying some of the items on this list now my son is away at university. I still say that the perinatal period is so short in comparison to a lifetime of 'family'.

Let's close this chapter with a positive comment from a mother who went on to have a second baby:

- Because I got the right help this time, my recovery was so much better than the first time and it's made me even stronger. I have my son – he is 6 now and the thought of not having him – well it's just awful to think of. The Consultant told me I was incredibly brave and I do feel brave now – 6 years on. I feel like if I hadn't have risked it then I would have got to the menopause with so many regrets – that I was too scared to follow my heart. I feel very lucky.

REFERENCES

1. Faulkner J. *A Monster Ate My Mum!* 2013. Available at: www.lulu.com/shop/jen-faulkner/a-monster-ate-my-mum/paperback/product-21305413.html
2. http://ideas.thenest.com/love-and-sex-advice/dealing-with-relationship-issues/slideshows/15-to-dos-before-baby.aspx

FURTHER READING AND RESOURCES

- www.telegraph.co.uk/women/mother-tongue/10245505/Infertility-My-unmet-desire-to-have-a-second-child-follows-me-like-a-shadow.html
- www.wikihow.com/Decide-Whether-or-Not-to-Have-a-Baby
- http://stayathomemoms.about.com/od/raisingyourchildren/a/Should-I-Have-A-Second-Baby.htm

CHAPTER 5

Additional concerns within the decision-making process due to past experience

Most of the important things in the world have been accomplished by people who have kept on trying when there seemed to be no hope at all.

Dale Carnegie

In the replies from my survey, 44% of couples did not want another baby after suffering from a perinatal mental health illness; 32% did. Nine per cent of mothers wanted another one and their partner did not. Twelve per cent of partners wanted another baby where the mother did not.

Their biggest concerns are based around mental health and its effects on all involved. Perhaps you share some of these? I list all of these comments with the aim to convince you that you are not alone in your concerns. I want to encourage you in acknowledging the areas of anxiety, as then we can find some possible ways to ease them. As healthcare professionals you may find these helpful in assessing and planning your services to address these needs.

One mum's response to being asked about her concerns highlights to me what mental turmoil this can create:

- Losing temper; hurting others' feelings; causing embarrassment; losing friends/family; losing respect; becoming more ill; having children taken; people thinking I'm a bad parent; losing partner; financial concerns due to not working; creating a stigma.

If you are reading this as a healthcare professional, please let this be an example to show how difficult it can be when faced with a maternal desire to have another baby when your head is battling with all these worries.

Area of concern	Comments from others
Repeat of same illness	• Getting ill again or worse. • If I get ill again my biggest worry is being apart from my first child if I had to go into hospital. • I was very scared that I could become sick again. I was also scared that I would spend the rest of my life in a Mental Health hospital. • Being so tired. The strain in my body. Postnatal illness risk. • Everything!! Baby being poorly again, me getting ill again physically and mentally! • Getting psychosis, becoming very depressed and not bouncing back as quickly as I do at the moment. • Is it too big a risk to have another baby and risk another serious depression – i.e. might I damage my son/lose my son into care/hurt my son or myself as a result? • A repeat of last time which I really do not ever want again especially now I have my little girl.
Pregnancy	• After pregnancy I have all the help in the world, but I am concerned about getting through the actual pregnancy drug-free. I may have to take lithium or some alternative if my mood deteriorates. This is likely as I have seen my mood affected with hormone changes since this illness. • If I stop taking this antidepressant to have another pregnancy, will this result in me being unable to look after my son properly? • Being as ill as I was in the last pregnancy.
Birth issues	• The delivery going wrong again. I have suffered panic attacks with anything medical (even having basic dental work done) since the birth so I would be scared that the birth would trigger a panic attack anyway. • Hard labour again, being ill again after birth, and getting another postnatal illness.
Effect on partner and children	• That I will suffer with PND again and be unable to cope. And this time there will be two children to look after which makes the prospect even more daunting. • Having mental health problems so severe as before and the effect it may have to my partner and I's relationship. • That I would be as ill as last time. That the effect on my children who are 4 and 5 would be too much if I were that ill again. • As a result of this should I leave a longer age gap, so that my son is less significantly affected if I become depressed again? • My son is clingy and anxious. Will having a brother or sister help him or cause problems?

(*continued*)

Area of concern	Comments from others
New baby	• Not bonding with baby. Really want to breast feed.
	• That I will fail my next baby the same as I did my son.
	• Is it unfair of me to have another baby given that I couldn't care well enough for my son to give him the best start?
	• What if this baby also has reflux/feeding problems/medical problems …? Could I put the baby or myself through that again?
	• Not being able to cope with a new born.
	• Can I cope with the stress of two young children?
Healthcare professionals	• I know I have been a drain on health visitor resources as well as the GP. Are they all going to curse me and think me highly irresponsible?

So what plans have others put in place or would consider doing so regarding this decision?

1. CONTRACEPTION

This is vitally important whilst you are still in the decision-making process. One couple were so sure that they did not want to conceive again that he had a vasectomy and she had a coil fitted. If you still have a shred of doubt, then possibly it is best to avoid permanent solutions for contraception until you are. In my case, having to have a hysterectomy solved that for me.

2. CONSULT WITH HEALTHCARE TEAM

This may involve
1. talking to your GP and local perinatal mental health team (ideally) to put an action plan in place, since they know your history intricately and will monitor you closely
2. making the professionals aware of previous history and treatment and being carefully monitored.

This is what one lady has put in place:

- I have briefly chatted about this to my CPN [community psychiatric nurse], although specific plans haven't been made yet I made it clear that I want to 'over prepare'. She suggested I might need a break at some point. There's a sanctuary place near me that offers respite for people with mental health problems. She said I might want respite there. I think it might be advisable to visit a mother and baby unit so I am familiar with it if I need to go there. My CPN said I will be very closely monitored.

3. PRIOR KNOWLEDGE

Many mothers have said that they feel that because they are aware of the symptoms and ways to help themselves, they would be able to recognise them, be more prepared and ask for help sooner.

4. MEDICATION NEEDS

Work closely with your GP or consultant to check that what you need and when is readily available. This will be very personal and always remember that what works for one person may not be the same for another, e.g.:

- I would request that I'm kept on antidepressants.
- Taking antidepressants earlier. Combination feeding my baby so that they will be able to eat if I need medication urgently.
- I will take a loading dose of lithium and possibly quetiapine following delivery and will not breastfeed.

A recent review was undertaken to evaluate the effectiveness of different anti-depressants for postnatal depression and to compare their effectiveness with other forms of treatment, placebo or treatment as usual.[1]

5. SUPPORT FROM PARTNER, FAMILY, FRIENDS AND OTHERS, E.G. SUPPORT GROUP

See Chapters 18, 20 and 21.

6. OTHER IDEAS

These were some additional comments about how mothers would manage next time:

- I am a lot happier in this relationship. Theoretically I wouldn't have the illnesses which resulted in the worry during my last one.
- Having more realistic expectations.
- Not work; be more open when feeling ill; rest when I can; be more organised with first child. Try de-cluttering.

I asked what parents felt would help to ease these concerns.

Method suggested to ease concern	Example
Talking	• To someone who has been through it again. • A support group. • Speak to people all the time throughout.
Taking action	• Following my own tips and advice as I have been through it once before.
Professional support and appropriate care	• Knowing that someone understands and knowing that I am doing okay. • Support through the pregnancy, very good antenatal care and possibly giving birth in a different hospital. • Help from the Mental Health team. • A support network put in place with midwife, health visitor, GP, hospital, possibly crisis team. Something in place to get medication quickly if needed. • If I knew there was a way I could be treated at home if I got ill again. • I would also plan to employ a doula for practical and emotional support – somebody there for both me and my husband. • Knowledge and information on chances of relapse as well as how best to prevent this. • I would prefer a home birth next time as I feel that having a midwife on a 1-1 basis will put me more at ease as I won't have to wait hours to get stitched up due to low staffing numbers at the hospital.
Partner, family and friend support	• A workable plan in place to avoid sleep deprivation in particular and generally to make immediate postnatal period as stress free as possible.
Money	• I feel I would need a one to one care mentally for myself and a nanny for the baby. If we won the lottery my husband and I agreed we would have another baby as we could afford to get this help.
Contraception	• I had to know that I would never have another baby. Even seeing a pregnant lady could bring on a panic attack, until my husband had a vasectomy.
Reassurance	• Knowing my child would not be taken away. Knowing that PP would only be short lived hopefully. • Nothing would ease them completely and therefore I can't risk it. • I don't think anything feasibly would.

I feel that there is much more awareness and support of perinatal mental illness now than when my son was born. I asked other parents if they had found any help, knowledge or support that has emerged since their first problematic experience. One mother sadly reports:

- No – I still feel this is a grey area. I feel let down. I almost took mine and my daughter's life and only didn't due to my family. I was almost sectioned and diagnosed correctly 9 months later. I feel very let down.

It is encouraging that most have found improvements though. Here are some of them:

1. CHARITIES EITHER LOCALLY OR INTERNET-BASED

- The House of Light[2] is a charity that helped me towards the end last time as I only found out about them later on and they were very helpful when I relapsed even though it wasn't postnatal.
- My local postnatal depression group has been really beneficial to me as it is reassuring to know that what I am feeling is somewhat normal and many other women are going through it too.
- The SMILE Group.[3] Peer support.

You can find local groups listed on the Netmums website.[4]

2. INTERNET, TECHNOLOGY AND SOCIAL MEDIA

- So much more such as Facebook support groups specifically for mums with PND. I always felt alone when I had PND and now I know how common it is! I also know that there is an end to this illness which when I was ill I didn't believe it would ever be possible to be normal again.
- The mental health resources out there, spiritual resources, friends and internet sources. Facebook was invaluable in reducing isolation, it didn't exist when I had my first.
- Knowing that there are others out there, that I wasn't alone. The information I was given about PND was minimal when I was pregnant.
- Also found apps to monitor and track mood useful, as well as the program mood tracker.
- I have made so good friends from the weekly perinatal mental health group. On Facebook I am part of a group for women suffering from mental health issues around this area.

3. PERSONAL KNOWLEDGE AND EXPERIENCE

- Just being through the illness before I think will help, as know I would get better and I and my family would be able to recognise the early signs of the illness and hopefully would get help and treatment earlier.
- I am a lot more aware of the early trigger symptoms to tell me when I am unwell and to take action.
- Have my experiences and coping skills I have already learnt.
- The biggest thing is knowing what I went through and knowing we have a plan to try to prevent it. If it does happen, I am well prepared and will notice sooner it is happening. I will also use a different service for the delivery – I will seek to have consistent midwifery support throughout pregnancy, labour, and postnatal, ensuring continuity of care and having a midwife who knows me will help.

4. GENERAL INFORMATION AND KNOWLEDGE

- In the last decade we have come a long way in the quest for knowledge and in learning about perinatal and postpartum mood disorders.
- I know a lot more now than I did from doing a lot of research on the subject.
- Feel more informed about bottle and combination feeding. Also we have more information about maternity nursing services. We also have a much better idea about how to regulate family visits and help from them.

5. HEALTHCARE SERVICES

- 1-1 CBT early after birth; better health visitor; health visitor home visits for up to 8 weeks.
- I have joined a postnatal depression support group, which helps a lot.
- The crisis team were brilliantly helpful and supportive and came to see me every day.
- A doula.

So what else would families find useful that currently appears to be unavailable?

Type of useful resource or support	Example
Information	• It is all there but it would be great to have all the options, charities, offers, treatment approaches, ideas under one roof, i.e. a book, the internet. • There needs to be pamphlets on the reality of all the postpartum illnesses that can occur and given to women during their pregnancy and at delivery.
Local support group	• I wish there were baby groups to go to if I ever had PND again that were specifically for mothers with PND. Going to normal baby groups was so hard and one specifically for PND Mums would be great so I could relax and feel less alone. • A PND group session. Aimed at women suffering with the illness. I know when I was suffering I felt like I was the only one. It would be nice to be reassured that it is actually quite common.
Contact	• Someone to talk to, to be honest and open with. Need a network of mums local to you to meet and talk to – that's what is needed.
Counselling	• Counselling during pregnancy and early stages of when baby born. • Mental help – me being able to talk to someone daily and them giving me support. • GPs that actually listen and act.
Practical help and support	• Practical help and support with someone being able to care for the baby and give me a break. I have not thought about breastfeeding as I know I will not have another baby but would imagine if I did then I may need help with this. Practical help with household things.
Partner and family support	• I would love to see better support for partners and families – during and follow up care. I still have regular psychiatric appointments (3 years down the track) but my husband had no follow up.
Services and funding	• More access to mum and baby units. More awareness of severe postnatal depression and puerperal psychosis. • System like 'Home-Start'.[5] More than 6 CBT sessions. Childcare support when breaks are needed. Some kind of respite care. All children from mental health households to receive childcare vouchers and attend preschool for a few hours from the age of 2 years. • I attended a very good support group run by 'Home-Start'. They had a crèche and focused on healing the mother. This was massively helpful but was shut as funding ended.

The one element that should be present in all of these is hope.

Without food man can survive for barely 30 days: without water for little more than three days; without air, hardly for more than three minutes; but without hope he may destroy himself in an even shorter time.[6]

We shall explore all of these areas in later chapters to enable parents to know what support they can have and professionals to work towards providing it.

REFERENCES

1. www.chimat.org.uk/resource/view.aspx?RID=212414&src=pimh
2. www.sheffieldlight.co.uk/
3. www.thesmilegroup.org/
4. www.netmums.com/local-to-you/local/index/support-groups/antenatal-postnatal-support
5. www.home-start.org.uk/
6. Mumford L. *The Conduct of Life*. New York: Harcourt, Brace and Co; 1951.

FURTHER READING AND RESOURCES

Links on the web

- www.panda.org.au/practical-information/about-postnatal-depression/32-prevention-of-postnatal-depression?start=1
- www.panda.org.au/images/stories/PDFs/PANDA_FS7_Having_another_baby.pdf
- www.bellybelly.com.au/post-natal/having-another-baby-after-depression#.UfJWWNKTj6U

Stories

- www.postpartumprogress.com/7-postpartum-depression-survivors-share-their-stories-of-having-more-children

CHAPTER 6

Relationship with the partner/ father and their wishes

There's a difference between who we love, who we settle for and who we're meant to be with.

Anon

Most new parents would probably be in agreement that no amount of knowledge or preparation for your first child completely makes you 'ready' for the realities, even if it all goes smoothly. The changes involved to you as individuals, as a couple, as a triad (or more) along with all the new adjustments in everyday living are massive. So to consider going through the process again, if there were additional challenges, clearly is a major decision.

Some men have that paternal instinct as a natural desire – like my dad, who was one of eight children and has always been a great father to my siblings and me. My mum is an only child and always wanted to have more than one child. Even though their finances were tight when they married, they knew they wanted a family. My brother was first, followed by me two and a half years later. My constant request for a younger brother or sister came true when I was 10. As a couple my parents both always knew they wanted several children. Likewise my plan was always for another baby, even after the very rocky road of the arrival of my son. I had the maternal instinct still as a strong, natural desire.

For my ex-husband it was a different matter altogether. He felt his age was a big factor. Also having experienced the very traumatic birth of our son and nearly losing me, followed by my spiral into and out of postnatal mental illness, it had understandably left him with a less than rosy image of fatherhood. On top of that the years of disturbed sleep was also a big factor. Once I began to get broody again, it left him cold. I can understand why. We needed to have communicated better about it. In time, from my perspective, it became a major part of our marriage breakdown. Other people have shared with me that their relationship did not survive the 'illness' because you do become a different person, even if only in the short term. Others say that their experience of parenthood made their relationship stronger and resulted in a deeper bond and determination to have another child. Perhaps if we had not had so many challenges we may have both been willing to have another baby. In the year or two that it took me to recover sufficiently to try again, the 'window' for my husband at the time had passed.

Some women may choose to go through the procedure again with the full intention of being a single parent. I do know of a situation where a mother had a second child knowing that in the longer term she would not stay with their father. She did not want her first child to be on their own. Planning for being a single parent would demand particular attention for as much support as possible from other sources, both personally and professionally, to minimise the risk of poor maternal mental health. www.lone-parents.org.uk/ is a useful resource. In some cases the pregnancy may start out as a couple, then due to relationship breakdown or bereavement there is a single parenthood. I will explore this later in Chapter 19.

For the vast majority of situations I am assuming that a couple will be involved. This may include same-sex parents. You will find a wealth of information at www.stonewall.org.uk/ For the purpose of writing this book, I will use the word 'partner' to be applicable to both genders, although some aspects may be more relevant to a male partner. We also need to consider that the couple may not be the same as a previous pregnancy – the poor mental health could have been with either the current or a past partner. For example, a man whose partner in a previous relationship had a perinatal illness may not be as willing to have a baby with a new partner. This will have further issues that will need to be considered, especially where a previous partner has died. Some parents-to-be feel far more confident with a new partner as they may feel their previous one added to their mental challenges.

Let's first look at the expectations of partners for the first pregnancy before we move on to considering the possible next one.

The mothers in my survey generally said that their partners were excited and happy about their first baby.

- He was very excited and thrilled at the prospect of being a father.
- We planned it so he was over the moon.

Some also expressed worries:

- Apprehensive, nervous, excited, worried about unborn baby and importantly his wife.
- Generally positive about having a baby but not particularly interested in talking about it either.
- He was very excited but also worried because we were a very tight couple.

A few were indifferent and some shocked and/or scared if the pregnancy was unexpected. Sometimes the initial apprehension turned into acceptance then excitement. For example:

- He was excited the baby was a boy and he was amazed at the birth. He was the most support I had.
- Happy about pregnancy, worried during the birth but delighted at safe delivery of son.
- My husband was more confused than unhappy. He was in two minds about the pregnancy. He came around to the idea about 2 weeks after I told him I was pregnant. He was excited about the birth. I feel he had a much better experience than most dads. He held our son first. He cut the cord. He was so happy he cried, something which I envied him for as I was just so tired I couldn't muster up any emotion.

If the actual reality of the early days of parenthood did not live up to expectations, then it may be one obstacle to a 'next time'. The perinatal period is the cruellest time to have a mental health challenge. No one likes to have their hopes crushed and it may be something they would rather avoid again. Hopefully by the time you are considering another baby, the other child will have developed into more delights than drudgery to help inspire you both! You may decide that the relatively short-term pain was worth the gain.

One common concern for partners was about the actual birth. Only since the 1960s has it become almost expected that the partner will be at the birth. Previously it was very much a 'woman's domain'. Since I had my son, the media has become far more open to showing in minute detail the births of babies. Gone are the days when all you saw was a sweaty lady, shouting for a few minutes (head only shot) and then, within seconds, the scene was one of the mother holding the baby and being kissed by the father when he was allowed in the room! Now we get blood, mess, swearing, 'warts and all'. I am fascinated by how different every birth seems to be. It is not surprising, because there are so many variable factors. The reaction of the father in the birthing room covers a range from 'incredible' to 'stupid' – one programme showed a husband locking his wife in a toilet whilst in labour 'for a laugh'. The expectation is that the man should always be present. I am not sure that is always a good idea!

Some of the descriptions of birthing partners were beautiful, however:

- He counted for me as I pushed and looked into my eyes, giving me confidence.
- Supportive, calm, perfect. Active and patient and helpful.
- He was amazing and kept me calm.
- He was with me through the labour and birth and was very supportive and protective.
- My support and advocate. He was fantastic.

- Support and a hand to hold!
- There for it all. Came on a partners and yoga day with me happily.
- My husband supported me, rubbing my back, playing music, making me comfortable, running a bath, organising snacks.
- He was wholly supportive. He was there at the birth and a great help to me.
- My husband was fantastic! He really threw himself into it. He was compassionate, entertaining (something I need when not happy or in pain). I was so proud of how much he went through and how well he dealt with the whole situation.

Some were less helpful!

- He was, I suppose, like any dad is. Confused, anxious and just rushed about shouting 'what shall I do?' But he did hold my hand throughout the birth.
- Not really interested or supportive at all during pregnancy. Helped a little during labour but also slept!!
- He was present, and more helpful than I expected, although he spent much of the time playing computer game, etc.
- Birth partner, albeit not a particularly hands on one!

Some did not know what to do:

- Present. Trying to be supportive but I didn't want to be touched particularly during active labour.
- Didn't know how to support me during labour and the birth but I wanted them to be there at the birth so they could meet the baby.

Where the birth was a less than perfect scenario, this resulted in some strong emotions:

- Absolutely livid with how I was treated in the birth.
- If anything, the birth was more traumatic for him, as he was not drugged and realised how very dicey it all was for a while.
- Excited about the pregnancy. Entirely traumatised by the birth.
- Distressed about what happened during and following labour.
- Very supportive, but did not enjoy seeing me so distressed giving birth.
- They felt helpless and insignificant.
- He was very active and sympathetic. A great comfort, although he felt helpless as the labour seemed to go awry.
- Was with me and wanted to help more but kept being told due to hygiene he needed to step away. He was upset that he did not cut the cord.

Two sad comments were:

- He wasn't there …
- Had been sent home.

Clearly, if you intend having another baby, 'the birth' needs to be discussed, if it was an issue the previous time. Talk to each other about what happened the last time. How did they feel? How did you feel about what he did or did not do? If you need a healthcare professional to talk through what happened and why, then ask for that. Very few partners like to feel the negative emotions as described above. Be candid and open. Would the partner want to be present next time? If not, would this matter to the mother? If this was the main reason for not wanting a baby, would this matter in the long run? We shall look at a better birthing experience later in the book. At this stage, acknowledge and deal with the past one.

Next we have the early days of parenthood. Discuss how that was for you both. I know my ex-husband would say that he felt he had 'lost' me. All my attention was focused on our son. All he could see was me working so hard to please this little 'thing' who gave nothing back in return. Some people struggle with the change to their sex life. A lactating women may not be a turn on for either party, along with the physical aspects and recovery needed in the postnatal period. This can be the cause of turmoil and stress for some, especially if the birth was traumatic. The NHS Choices website has advice on this.[1]

Once the baby was born I asked how much support their partner gave. The answers ranged from lots to a little. Those who considered that the support was the best included:

- He was very supportive. He took 2 weeks paternity leave and also helped me a lot in the evenings. He was keen to help. He took care of the practical things and helped around the house.
- Lots. Lots. Everything I needed. A lot – he was wonderful, still is :)
- He was very relaxed but supportive. He was always asking me how I felt and looking for signs I might be ill.
- He basically stopped working to support me, was amazing. He bonded to the baby in a way which I think is more usual for a new mum. He was endlessly patient, did the first half of the night every night, supported me in every way when I cried and cried and said I couldn't do it. He eventually came with me to the GP to make sure I told her how bad it was.
- My husband was brilliant and did all the house work; looked after my older children so I could be with baby.
- He was amazing and tried really hard to look after me.
- He was doing as much as he could, running around to visit us in hospital and look after a 17 month old.

Some expressed recognition of their partner doing their best – just not what was needed:

- He tried as much as he could to be fair.
- He was as good as he could be.
- A lot but maybe not the right type.
- Not enough. He just didn't know what to do.
- Not much, he said 'postnatal' applied only in the first few weeks. He was also depressed and had taken his paternity leave to visit me in hospital.
- Some support but he found it difficult to understand my perspective. Further complicated by ongoing issues with his family.

Some couples struggled together:

- Good but as a new parent it was difficult for my hubby to know what was normal. As I deteriorated he did not know if this was normal or not – no previous point of reference.
- We were both in shock so couldn't talk about it.
- Fully supportive, although he was baffled at the outset. Neither of us understood what was happening.

Some partners had their own challenges:

- Minimal help – he worked nights and slept for most of the day.
- Very little help as he was at work.
- Very little support as he was preoccupied with pending deployment to Iraq at 16 weeks.
- Not much help as we had moved in together, bought our first home, got married and had a baby in 1 year. He wasn't ready to mature.
- Not much, I had to ask for help.
- None emotionally – some practical with cooking and cleaning. He was not very nice to me at all.

The lack of sleep was an issue for some parents:

- None, he was exhausted and although he was excited he had no interest in helping out.
- My ex-partner didn't provide the support I needed. When I stated I was exhausted, the response was 'so am I', and it became a competition with him to show he was struggling as much as I was.
- Quite a bit, although when we first came home from hospital he tried to sleep when baby and I were up all night.

On reflection with these areas, review what went on the first or previous time. Commend each other for the support that you really appreciated and offer suggestions as to what might have eased the situation for you both. I recognise now that it would have been much better for us all if I had lowered my expectations. As a couple we should have relaxed our usual standards of household chores. We should have enjoyed the 'moments' much more. The need for sleep is a vital area that will be explored later.

The relationship that the partner has with the existing child or children may also have an impact upon their decision to have another baby. Some have an immediate and life-long bond that grows and stays throughout their life time. Others find it difficult to be close, especially if they perceive the child to be the cause of their partners' mental ill health. I will look at bonding for both parents in the next section of the book.

Then there is the crux of the issue of poor mental health that then pervades everything else.

Additional stresses were felt due to perinatal mental illness:

- He didn't really get it, he also struggled with the baby who screamed constantly from the second I handed him to Dad until the second I took him back. This meant I couldn't get a break more than about 1 hour, 3 times a week.
- He worked long hours so nothing for 4 days but then was quite good on the whole, initially. However it did ultimately cost us our marriage as he couldn't understand why I was as I was after so long and even told me once that I needed to get better or move out. A year later I moved out. He was very good with the baby, doing the household stuff etc., but found the mental illness bit hard. He wanted us to spend days together when I wanted to be in bed. He thought it was right that we spent time altogether rather than letting me have time on my own, in case I did anything.
- My partner was around for the first 2 weeks on paternity leave, and honestly I don't believe he bonded as well with my daughter as he did our son either so was quite distant from us. I generally felt he was avoiding helping and supporting me. This we had a lot of arguments about as I was on strict rest that I wasn't getting.

Mark Williams, who founded a support group for fathers whose partners had postnatal depression, describes some of the thoughts and feeling he experienced. These can be found on a DVD produced by PSS in Liverpool.[2] When his wife developed postnatal depression following the birth of their planned baby, he felt very lost and confused. Their previously happy relationship had changed beyond all recognition. 'Everything' appeared to be his fault. He could not understand why she was so unhappy and depressed – wasn't a baby all they wanted? He questioned if she actually wanted him any more. He did not want to talk to anyone about what they were going through due to the perceived stigma of mental illness and his wife's plea of 'don't tell anyone'. She was worried that Social Services would take the baby away. So much had happened to them as a couple in a short space of time and he found it all very challenging. One aspect that he found particularly hard was the unknown end to the illness. When would she get better? Would she ever get better? He had to take more and more time off work and then the financial pressures started too. He began to drown his sorrows in drink, which led to more problems.

Pauline McPartland, part of the team at PSS, says that 'something I feel strongly about is that dads really do matter too and their needs can be and often are overlooked in the postnatal period by professionals or indeed in the perinatal period when more education and awareness both of birth and beyond needs to be considered to prepare them for what lies ahead. Everything has generally been centred around mum and baby leaving dads feeling "what about me", almost grieving for the relationship and life they had BB (before baby) which in turn can leave them feeling isolated and even angry, as they struggle to understand this life transition and in turn this can and does affect relationships.'

Sometimes this can lead to their own mental health being affected. Sixty-seven per cent of the people who responded to my survey said that their partner's mental health had not been affected by their perinatal period. The remaining 23% reported a variety of impact. Some described the stress on their partner:

- No long term but the fact that I fainted after having had Emily really shook him. He had a very strong bond with her straight from birth.
- My postnatal depression ultimately had an impact on him. He felt he had to stay strong for me but he took too much on by himself (we moved house shortly after I gave birth, hc had job worries as well) and this led to him suffering with stress.
- Started drinking more.
- Not obviously but no doubt it was a very distressing and anxious time for my husband and family.
- Although he remained very strong and stalwart, he struggled with the worry and concern.
- He felt very stressed out with me and also had to cope with his mum dying around the same time.
- Not by the birth but by the subsequent pressure of having a wife with severe PND.

Some partners developed or relapsed with depression:

- I think he grew depressed as the postnatal year went on, and second year too. I was hospitalised two more times and this was extremely hard on him.
- He was also depressed but no one, even myself, noticed until much later.

- He suffered with mental illness in the past and after our first was born he went through a really tough time and had counselling and was put back on medication.
- He's always suffered from depression, but had to increase his dose of anti-depressants due to the stress. This lasted well after I was better.
- Now also suffers from high anxiety/panic attacks.

Mark Williams turned a corner in his life because of a chance remark by another man at a gym who commented he was on his way to a support group with his wife for her postnatal depression. The calm and 'matter-of–fact' attitude by this man was a revelation to Mark. With that simple connection and the popping of the belief that 'it's just me', he was able to acknowledge the situation. He has since formed an online support group for fathers at www. reachingoutpmh.co.uk and worked incredibly hard to increase the awareness that fathers also need support in caring for the mother of their child and their own mental health. The key is to find someone to open up to, as you will find a release by discussing your thoughts and feelings. Start with your GP and if they will not listen, move to one who does. Mark has found that men tend to communicate better with another man if they are side by side, rather than face to face, and engaged in a task, e.g. gym work-out, walking, digging. There is a comprehensive website based in Australia that has some great videos and information for fathers to support and guide about many aspects of the perinatal period at www.howisdadgoing.org.au/ There is an American site too at www.postpartummen.com/index.html

The other key area to consider is your actual relationship. Any new baby changes the dynamics of what 'was'. For some couples, a baby created through love enriches their relationship and lives, so adding to that family is an easier decision. Where pressures have caused that relationship to be challenged, it can have an impact. This is how some mothers described some changes in their partners, for example:

- He has changed though and I'm not sure we'll ever get back what we lost.
- I don't know – not mental health itself, but I know that when I did voice any of my thoughts he would get short-tempered with me and tell me to go and get sorted. Which made me clam up.
- I think afterwards as his wife suddenly wasn't his wife due to this baby and he was over the moon but I wasn't. Obviously when we separated he found it very difficult as baby was only 20 months old.
- He was in complete denial I was depressed. I left him 8 weeks on to live with my sister in England for a month while I decided if I wanted to be with him.
- He could not bear the thought of another pregnancy/birth/child, but mainly the thought of a natural birth. He can no longer watch programmes about childbirth.
- Maybe, I think my husband found it hard in respect to how much time I spent

with our son. As I was becoming manic, I insisted I was fine and that he should spend some of his 2 weeks off in the shed, doing man stuff. This gave me time to write my novel (part of the mania) and clean fastidiously when he wasn't in the house. I think he withdrew a little because I pushed him away. I also let him sleep overnight while I was gardening, cleaning, writing and lied that I slept on the couch so as not to disturb him … Am sure this was not good for his mental health. Due to the mania, I did think he was a little depressed – but this was likely due to my own heightened state of mind.

When a couple did go on to have another baby, I asked the mothers in my survey 'How did your partner's behaviour/feelings differ following another pregnancy in the light of your previous experience?' Some had a challenging time:

- He was no use at all, he even volunteered to take me to the viaduct to throw myself off and save everybody the hassle of having me around.
- He couldn't face it again – he was in denial to start with 'it can't be, you're just tired'. He found it very hard. He didn't bond as well with this baby. He was traumatised by seeing me nearly die after the birth. He had no proper support. He bottled it up and 3 years later it all came out when he had a breakdown, started an affair and destroyed his own life. Very sad.
- He was supportive but thinks that there were people much worse off than me with 'real mental health problems'. He thinks that if I can still look after the kids properly, which I did, it can't be that bad.
- They were really panicked.
- He was worried about it happening again.
- He was very anxious after the birth.
- He was more anxious, about me and about how he would cope with toddler and newborn if I was out of action in the same way as the first time around.

For others, the story was completely different:

- He was more supportive with baby chores and more affectionate, very good advocate for breastfeeding.
- He was amazing, supportive, loving, very understanding. He always made me feel safe and reassured me daily I would be fine.
- He was supportive and accepting of my moods.
- Just relieved it's all over, I think. And definitely more aware of when I'm having a bad day and tries to support me more.
- He was a lot more relaxed and helpful.
- He was more attentive and he went out of his way to ensure I was coping well.
- He was informed throughout and totally on top of the situation.
- He was more aware of the signs of me becoming unwell.

- My husband was overjoyed to find out I was pregnant. He adored our daughter as soon as she was born. He fussed over us both. I felt loved and cared for.
- He felt a great relief that we had decided to go through with it, because it was so much better than first time. Had we not done it, I believe we would have been forever tainted by the first experience. The second birth has healed some of the damage done by the first.

For some couples having another baby has proved to be the correct decision. They possibly worked their way through these questions. I have already covered some of these – I feel it is important to emphasis them again for the partner.

1. Love. Do you still love your partner enough to have that amazing desire to want to create another life together?
2. What is your relationship like with your partner? Do you hardly see each other due to pressures of work as it is? Have you achieved a good balance of life? Are you closer than ever?
3. Your age – mothers have a limited biological clock of course. With some men they are happy to have children way into what some would consider 'middle age'. Perhaps it comes to mindset, with the saying 'you are as old as you feel'.
4. Your health and energy levels – maybe if you have your own health issues they may have an impact on whether you feel you want another child or not. This is especially true if you are concerned about your partner also becoming ill as a result of having another baby.
5. Finances – are they in good or adequate shape for another child? Would this cause more pressure for you and therefore be a strain on both of you?
6. Career goals – if you are planning a promotion or move then maybe it is not a good time to consider another child.
7. Space at home – would you have room for another baby? Could you manage or would a bigger home be affordable and realistic? Remember that moving house whilst pregnant or postnatally may not be the best thing to do due to the potential extra stresses and strains that brings.
8. How do you feel when you see others with newborn babies? Envious? Relieved that those days are gone for you?
9. Age of the baby – how big a gap do you want? Some couples prefer their children close together, others with a few years apart. Perhaps if you have had a difficult time first time around, maybe waiting a few years is better. I would say that I felt ready when my son was about five.
10. What does your existing child/children say about the prospect of a sibling? Are they jealous? Excited? Horrified? Encouraging you?

If you do decide to have another baby then I strongly suggest that you also consider the previous chapters with your partner, so that you can plan together to minimise the chance of another difficult time. If you work on this as a couple, you both will feel more empowered, knowledgeable and able to deal with whatever comes your way.

REFERENCES

1. www.nhs.uk/conditions/pregnancy-and-baby/pages/sex-contraception-after-birth. aspx#close
2. PSS Parent and Baby Wellness Service, Liverpool. *Our Stories: postnatal depression* [DVD]. Available at: www.psspeople.com/whats-happening/news/stories-dvd-sale-now

FURTHER READING AND RESOURCES

- www.reachingoutpmh.co.uk/ a support group/network for men whose wives or partners are suffering from postnatal depression.
- http://postpartumdads.wordpress.com helping families overcome postpartum depression.
- www.fatherhoodinstitute.org/
- Barnes DL, Balber LG. *The Journey to Parenthood: myths, reality and what really matters.* Oxford: Radcliffe; 2007.
- Spencer O. *Sad Dad: an exploration of postnatal depression in fathers.* London: Free Association Books; 2014.

Research articles and information

- www.dad.info/
- www.netmums.com/parenting-support/postnatal-depression/partners-supporting-suffering-mums/fathers-who-suffer-from-pnd
- www.nct.org.uk/parenting/postnatal-depression-dads
- www.babycentre.co.uk/a1046187/postnatal-depression-in-dads
- www.app-network.org/partners-2/

CHAPTER 7

I want another baby but my partner does not!

The key to everything is patience. You get the chicken by hatching the egg not smashing it.

Arnold H Glasow

So you have considered all of the concerns, pros and cons of becoming pregnant again and one of you is willing to try for another baby – but the other partner does not! In my survey this applied to almost 20% of those who responded and was roughly half male and half female. As individuals we all have a right to make a choice based upon our knowledge and feelings. That choice will result in actions and behaviours that have consequences. What might those consequences be, and what can you do about it? Be aware that this is a scenario that many couples find themselves in, regardless of a previous pregnancy that resulted in poor perinatal mental health. It is a decision that cannot really be compromised on as you cannot be 'a bit' pregnant. You either have another child or you do not.

In the first instance (which may be like the proverbial 'locking the stable door when the horse has bolted'), it would have been better only to have started or continued a relationship in the first place knowing that you both shared a desire for a family. How many of us have let our hearts rule and quietened doubts with self-talk that 'I'll change his/her mind'? In a reply to a letter in the *Sunday Observer*, Mariella Frostrup[1] advised a lady wanting a child when her partner did not:

> You will struggle to live with a man who appears to care so little for what you desire most, and there can be little joy for him in a partnership where he'll forever be to blame for denying you the experience of parenthood.

Yet is this fair if at the centre of the partner's unwillingness to have another child is the huge impact a previous experience has had, when his biggest desire is to protect you and your existing children? The crucial aspect is to explore the reasons why one remains unconvinced of having another baby.

In my case, I was the one who wanted another one. I acknowledge now that maybe I did not make my perspective clear enough. That would be my main suggestion for anyone facing this dilemma – communicate. One way is possibly to write down how you feel in a letter to your partner. I found this online letter written anonymously:[2]

Dear Husband,

So you know how we had our two kids, and you know how great they are, and you know how we swore that we wouldn't have any more? Yeah, about that. I've changed my mind. Wanna make another baby?

I've been thinking about it a lot lately (translation: watching babies take baths on YouTube) and I really want another baby. My uterus has officially put out the welcome mat.

I'm fully aware I was the most vocal when it came to saying we weren't going to have any more children. I know I said things like 'over my dead body' and 'this womb is out of business.' For 5 years I've been saying that. I think I was even saying while I was still pregnant with our last child. 'Never again!'

I also know that I'm big enough to admit when I might have been wrong. All good reasoning and logic say that we probably shouldn't want another baby, yet here I am wanting one all the same.

I want to bring a little bundle of love home from the hospital and welcome it into our lives. I want the tiny fingernails and the curly toes. I want the warm smell of the top of the head.

I want the cute yawns, and the even cuter sneezes. I also want the sleepless nights. The unrelenting workload. The difficult juggling act. The screaming and crying (both mine and the baby's). I want the good and the bad. I want it all. I want a baby.

When our two boys came along we were so young (and so stupid). I didn't enjoy a single second of it. I was filled with panic and confusion, and an overwhelming sense of failure.

Never once did I feel like I was doing a good job raising our boys. I lurched from one disaster to the next, never taking a moment to stop and actually enjoy them.

You're right when you say that I can't live my life trying to make up for regrets of the past, especially when it comes to our kids. I agree. (If I did that I would still be back in high school trying to make up for making my best friend dump her first boyfriend for me.) But this doesn't feel like chasing down old stuff-ups and rectifying them. It feels like being given a chance to learn from the past.

I know you say that you're done. I get and respect that. Up until recently I was right there with you. Done with the nappies and the middle of the night feeds and the fog you seem to live in when there's a new-born in the house. I was done with all of that too. But all of a sudden, all of that is exactly what I want.

I've thought about the effect it will have on our boys. They've been the only two for a good while now, and are pretty comfortable with their lives. A new baby will change all of that, but I'm convinced that will be a good thing. They can learn new responsibilities (they're totally old enough to change a nappy right?) and learn a new type of love. They'll be the most awesome big brothers a kid could ask for.

It's not rational for me to want another baby though is it? I was so sick in my pregnancy with our other two children (yes, I vomited in our bed once, sorry about that). But despite the hospital trips due to debilitating sickness, I'm willing to go through all of that again to have another child. I know, call me cray-cray.

See, there's just something greater pushing this than logic. I feel like it's instinct. It's like being clucky, on steroids. I feel this desire so much so that I can practically see this little baby. It already exists (I know its sex and I've named it in my head).

My want for a baby is so real that I feel like someone is missing. To me our little family doesn't feel quite complete anymore. When we all sit down to dinner together at night I want to pull up a high chair and plop a fat little bundle into it and feed it mashed sweet potato.

I hate that I'm a smart, educated woman of the 21st century who is still pretty much just at the whim of her biological desires. I feel like an un-evolved dum-dum who wants a baby. A cute little button nosed, kissable, smoochable baby … oh god I think I just started lactating.

I know how hard it will be. We've done it all before remember, and how hard it was is pretty much burned into our psyche. But I feel like we are better equipped to deal with all of that now. We won't be so lost at sea, but instead will have a boat, life-jackets and supplies.

I know by asking you to have another baby puts you in a difficult position. All I'm asking it that you consider it again, and look at it with fresh eyes (preferably ones which don't focus too sharply on the lack of sleep or the baby poo).

So there you have it love, that's where I'm at. This is a joint venture of course, and what you want matters to me dearly. I can certainly promise a lot of fun making the little tyke. Will you think about it?

Much love,
     Your wife (+ the baby)

I think that this captures many of the thoughts and emotions that we can go through. Let's look at some of the issues further.

CHANGING YOUR MIND

As this lady expresses, she has changed her mind. Time can have this effect. If you do this admit that you were wrong and explain why you have reached your different decision. If you entered the relationship or continued it knowing that the partner did not want children or more of them (if they already had them), then it is not fair to then blame them because you have not 'convinced' them otherwise in the interim.

HAUNTED BY 'LAST TIME'

It may be that the passage of time does heal or cloud the memory of a poor, previous experience. Remember that you may have different memories of the former perinatal illness. I know that my ex-husband must have found the whole period very challenging. The mind has a great way of minimising or even deleting some memories and highlighting others well. I know he remembers the pain – I focused on the positives at the time and hopes for the future. Your timescale may be at different stages, so you may need to allow for that. If the birth experience, for example, was very difficult then perhaps some professional counselling would be useful to help come to terms with it. One of the reasons I wanted another baby was like the lady who wrote the letter above – I wanted the opportunity to do it all again with the knowledge and experience that would hopefully make it an enjoyable and happy time. I wanted to know what a 'successful' new mother felt like.

NOT NOW OR NEVER?

If the reluctant partner is saying no to another baby, clarify if this is a 'not now or never' decision. It may be that a career opportunity or house move would be better first. Find out the timescale and agree to discuss it again then. If you are both clear when this topic will be discussed, it can avoid the appearance of 'nagging' that can lead to resentment and bitterness. Allocate a comfortable, safe space and time to have the discussion.

BIOLOGICAL CLOCK AND AGE

If one of you is feeling that you are too old then perhaps point out that as an older parent you are probably going to be wiser and more patient than a younger person. If you feel that you are too young, put a timeframe onto it that you can both work towards and revisit then. Several couples from my survey expressed that by the time both of them felt completely ready to try again for another baby, it was too late.

FINANCES

Perhaps one of you is more concerned or cautious about money and feel that another child would put too much pressure on you. Discuss what is important to you both. If there is room for compromise or economic measures, then identify where these could be.

'STATUS QUO'

One of the couple may feel that you are all already happy and why put your current happiness at risk. They may not want to 'share' you any further. In this instance, like the lady above, point out the joy that a child has brought you, even after the difficult start. Reassure that you have enough love for everyone.

AM I BEING SELFISH?

If you are both in discord over the decision to have another baby, you may question if you are being selfish. As part of a loving relationship you usually want to please the other, and going against their wishes can make you feel bad. It can feel awful to be jealous of other people around you who are adding to their families. Wherever you go there seem to be pregnant ladies. The maternal/paternal instinct can be so consuming. Remember that 'other people' aren't you – their circumstances are relevant to them and comparison is just likely to add to your unhappiness. Talk to the other partner to explain how you feel.

VISION OF THE FUTURE

Clearly discuss what this is for you. Consider how you individually see the years ahead and 'paint the picture' with or without another child in it. Ultimately you both have to communicate well (*see* Chapter 9) in order to reach a mutual conclusion. You may need to have professional help to do this, e.g. www.relate.org.uk or www.bacp.co.uk. If you leave it to fester it can begin to undermine and unravel your relationship. There will be the rolling of the eyes and the comment made 'not that again'. There will be silent tears as you lay in bed facing away from each other and the chasm will widen. You may begin to drift apart because of the proverbial elephant in the room. Talk about it!

DO YOU STAY OR GO?

Ultimately you have the choice to stay in the relationship because you still love each other and have a good life otherwise. You will acknowledge that you have so much to appreciate and be positive about as it is and learn to accept that you will not be adding to your family. Perhaps instead you can work on different aspirations together, such as a new home. Many couples go on to have liberating and fulfilled lives without adding to their family, in the same way that childless couples do. My son got a new cat instead of a sibling!

The alternative is that you part company and seek a new partner to have more children with. As you already have a child/children together, that will involve more complications than if you are childless. There is no guarantee that you will find that other person. Every situation is unique and only you know what will be the right thing for you. You can choose to stay in the relationship and love them unconditionally or your desire for another child will become so big you will deliver an ultimatum. This will be to either let you have another baby or let you go. This is a huge step to take and once given it is very hard to go back on.

I do understand now that I have been through a grieving process for the additional child I will never have – for years I visualised her. It happened every time a piece of my son's baby equipment was given away or sold. Lauren Libbert wrote her story[3] about coming to terms with not having another baby in these words:

> Slowly, I am trying to become resigned to our tidy, tiny family. Instead of banging my head against a firmly shut door, I am filling our home with friends and their children, recreating the comforting, noisy atmosphere of my childhood, which, in some very small way, makes me feel better. But I can't deny it: there is a grieving process going on inside me for the third child I know I will probably never have.

I like the advice given by the Australian website, Belly Belly, on what to do if only one of you wants another baby:

> This can be a decisive topic, and may leave you feeling disappointed, hurt or even resentful towards your partner. Try not to dwell on it. Remember, your partner isn't trying to hurt you, he or she is just being honest about how he feels. If you feel you need to, spend some time repairing your relationship and building intimacy and connection. Remember why you fell in love with each other and spend some quality time as a family, as well as a couple. It is so important to remember that the kids are watching everything ... including relationship dynamics. They will one day walk in your footsteps as they enter relationships of their own and will draw on what they saw growing up. Seeing a relationship as something that requires its own special time to nurture, as well as a being a place of teamwork, love and great communication, will help them choose great partners who are capable of the same.[4]

REFERENCES

1. www.theguardian.com/lifeandstyle/2012/jul/15/mariella-frostrup-woman-wants-children-husband-does-not
2. www.mamamia.com.au/lifestyle/when-you-want-a-baby-and-your-husband-does-not/#OtuvwM2dZCMrkZe5.99)
3. www.dailymail.co.uk/femail/article-2385696/When-husband-dead-child-Its-issue-divides-countless-couples-But-Lauren-consuming-obsession-thats-exacting-terrible-emotional-toll.html#ixzz3IDgKDDVX
4. www.bellybelly.com.au/relationships/when-one-partner-wants-more-babies-and-the-other-does-not#.VFe4djSsXDU

CHAPTER 8

Unexpected pregnancy

Whether your pregnancy was meticulously planned, medically coaxed, or happened by surprise, one thing is certain – your life will never be the same.

Catherine Jones

Over the years the cry of 'Oh no! I'm pregnant again and I'm so worried' has been a regular one in my inbox and one of the motivational reasons behind this book. Several people have told me that in retrospect it was the best thing that could have happened because they were not feeling confident enough to make that decision consciously. Yet after they had accepted the surprise and made plans, it has been a welcome addition to their family. Twenty-eight per cent of the people who responded to my survey had an unexpected pregnancy. As one mum told me:

- If it didn't just happen as a surprise, I probably wouldn't have had any more because I was so worried about getting the postnatal illness again.

I am not suggesting that having a casual approach to contraception is the best way to have the decision made for you! The research indicates that having an unexpected pregnancy can be a risk factor for developing postnatal depression,[1] so if you know that you are already at higher risk, then it makes sense to avoid adding this factor too.

Here is one example that a couple were happy to share:

- My second pregnancy was unplanned. I was horrified and terrified. I continued with the pregnancy as it wasn't an option for me personally not to. I had fantastic care from the obstetric and mental health teams second time. My own psychiatrist consulted with a specialist perinatal psychiatrist and pharmacist to find out about whether I should continue to take antipsychotics during the pregnancy. I did, and my 20 week scan was done by a foetal medicine specialist to get as much info as possible about how she was doing due to taking the meds. They offered me a place in a MBU prior to delivery (I didn't take it up in the end as it was so far away from my husband and son). I saw my obstetrician consultant every antenatal visit. I saw CPN regularly throughout the pregnancy. I had a planned caesarean at 38 weeks on the dot. I had a single room in the hospital, they arranged for my husband or mum to be there 24 hours a day with me. They showed us round NICU beforehand so we knew what to expect if she was delivered struggling due to the meds or had withdrawal symptoms. Looking back, (she is now 6) I am SO glad it happened that way, i.e. by accident, because we would NEVER have planned another baby, we were so traumatised after the first time neither of us could face it again, so I am certain that we would never have had any more children and would have missed out on so much. I bonded really well with my little girl, and experienced lots of things in her babyhood that I thought I never would experience, because I had missed out on so much (being hospitalised for a long time) when my son was born. So having the decision taken out of our hands turned out in the end to be definitely for the best.

Here is another example:

- My third pregnancy was unplanned. I was still receiving support from the perinatal team. My baby was 16 weeks and I was a month pregnant with an unplanned baby on the way. Health professionals told me to have an abortion. I was disgusted they put that opinion out but they were horrified. I'd just spent 12 weeks in a Mother and Baby Unit. My teenage daughter fell out with me and went to stay with friends. My partner at the time said 'get rid of it', so we split up. I did the pregnancy on my own and had my neighbour at the birth instead of my partner. I made it clear I knew the warning signs. I made sure I had help everywhere. I got in touch with a doula and found that I qualified for funding for six weeks after baby was born. I was not ashamed. I had to do this on my own. I'm glad to say that it honestly was tough going having a baby who couldn't even walk and a new born but I got through it. Now they're 4 and 5 years old with birthdays 3 days 1 year apart. They share a strong bond. Nearly 5 years on now and I haven't been on any medication. I actually got back with my partner and had yet another baby with no problems and my older daughter was my birth partner. I would say while you're pregnant get as much support put in place, not just for 1–2 weeks but at least 6 onwards. It will make your life easier and if no one's listening – shout louder!

What can you do if you find yourself in this situation or are consulted by someone who is? Each situation is very personal and unique – these are some processes to consider. The pregnancy may not have been planned, yet by taking control and dealing with the situation you can take appropriate action. It cannot be ignored, nor can you be in denial for too long.

GET A PREGNANCY TEST DONE

If you do suspect that you are pregnant, find out for sure if you are! This may sound silly, yet I know that if I am choosing not to want to know the outcome of something, I will put avoidance techniques into place, e.g. refrain from opening a message or email in case I do not like the content! By delaying, I am simply making it worse because I may be getting over-anxious over something that is not definite. When you know for certain you are then in a position to get advice and make decisions. One mum commented:

- Don't assume that an 'accident' can't happen to you as it can! I have heard of several 'more mature' ladies who did not possibly think they were pregnant, and they were, including the lady who had 15 rounds of IVF and then got pregnant naturally 5 years later at 42! I think she went to the GP because she thought something was wrong – menopause, tumour etc. when the miracle of a baby had happened! The point is that the earlier you find out, the more time you have to adjust, plan, cope, make the right decision, talk it through, etc.

WILL YOU KEEP THE BABY?

In the UK you do have the choice to keep the baby, have a termination or have them adopted. The British Pregnancy Advisory Service[2] have a wealth of expertise and knowledge for women, men and healthcare professionals to help them through the process of making these decisions. The British Association for Adoption and Fostering (BAAF)[3] will advise over adoption and fostering. There may be many reasons why people feel that an abortion or adoption is the only way for them. To avoid years of regret, ensure that all possible options are explored, like this lady:

- I feel that I was at an extremely high risk of postnatal depression due to the previous pregnancy ending in termination. I was practically told that it was for the best. I went against my huge instincts and suffered regret and loss. I had no help with this and I was haunted by it. A risk assessment during pregnancy would have picked this up.

Where the reason is related to fear of relapse of a perinatal mental illness, look at all the avenues of help within the remainder of this book.

- I was strongly advised to have an abortion and in fact found it difficult for any-one to accept my decision to keep the baby. Even family members refused to support me.

YOUR MINDSET

Decide what your attitude to this is going to be. When you have considered all of your options, you can choose to consider it as a negative situation, in which case you are more likely to be depressed and anxious or you can make a plan of action and decide that you will accept the surprise with pleasure and positivity. One mum told me that after the initial shock she was actually delighted. Any pregnancy is a roller-coaster of emotions. In this instance, with the added concern about possibly suffering with a perinatal mental health challenge, this can potentially make it worse. Talk to people who you trust. Start with the father and be aware that their reaction may be extreme and/or not the same as yours. Allow them time to adjust and keep pathways of communication open. They will have concerns for you all.

You can also seek support from some other agencies who have particular support for anyone involved. Pregnancy Help[4] will offer support to the pregnant mother, partner or anyone connected to them who is not sure how to respond. They have a national helpline on 0808 802 5433 where 'experienced counsellors and skilled listeners provide confidential, non-directional support, to help clients explore their feelings and make choices that are right for them.' Brook[5] have support specifically for under-25-year-olds. The Family Planning Association (FPA)[6] will also offer advice and support.

PHYSICAL NEEDS

As in any pregnancy, it is vital to look after your health, both for yourself and for the baby you are carrying. Please *see* Chapter 11. Book yourself in with the GP and healthcare professionals as soon as possible to put a plan in place.

MAKE ANY NECESSARY CHANGES TO YOUR LIFESTYLE AND PLAN

The pregnancy may have come at a less than ideal time, e.g. just before a possible promotion or house move. You might have to re-evaluate and make adjustments, e.g. take a year off your studies and look at reducing stress on all of you involved.

TIMING

It may be that if you have an unexpected pregnancy without having experienced a mentally well perinatal period that you may feel more concerned than if it went 'well'. One mum shared her thoughts on this:

- I do know if I had had a second unplanned pregnancy … I doubt I would have coped. Key for me with my second baby was the absolute planning of everything – it was essential to my mental health that I had at least an illusion of control! Funnily enough, my husband and I talked quite a lot after no. 2 about what would have happened if there had been a 3rd unplanned pregnancy – and I knew that because my experience with no. 2 had been so positive, I would have embraced it … yes, been afraid at first but my 2nd experience made me very confident indeed that all would be well with a third.

IMPROVE YOUR KNOWLEDGE

After the initial shock and emotions of discovering that you are pregnant, empower yourself by learning as much as you can to minimise the risks of another perinatal mental illness.

BUILD YOUR SUPPORT NETWORK

This is important in any pregnancy and especially so in the scenario. Look at the further chapters for guidance on this.

REFERENCES

1. Mercier RJ, Garrett J, Thorp J, *et al.* Pregnancy intention and postpartum depression: secondary data analysis from a prospective cohort. *BJOG.* 2013; **120**(9): 1116–22.
2. www.bpas.org/bpaswoman
3. www.baaf.org.uk/
4. http://pregnancyhelp.org.uk/
5. www.brook.org.uk/
6. www.fpa.org.uk/

FURTHER READING AND RESOURCES

- www.babble.com/pregnancy/coping-unplanned-pregnancy/
- www.netdoctor.co.uk/health_advice/facts/unplannedpregnancy.htm
- www.mariestopes.org.uk/

PART 3

Ways to plan for and to have a healthier experience

CHAPTER 9

Communication, a positive attitude and knowledge

Hope doesn't come from calculating whether the good news is winning out over the bad. It's simply a choice to take action.

Anna Lappe

Looking back on my pregnancy, I had very high expectations of what the birth and new motherhood would be like. For some people those expectations may be met. So was I wrong to have had high hopes? Candidly, I was unlucky that the birth was traumatic. It was simply how my body responded. I was lucky that both my son and I survived. Maybe if that is where our challenges had stopped, the story would have been different. My spiral into puerperal psychosis was very significant for everyone involved and, not surprisingly, a factor that would have needed careful thought and planning if we had ever had another child. So have I learned any other ways that may have helped another time? I am aware that many of these techniques have their basis in cognitive behavioural therapy or CBT (a talking therapy that can help you manage your problems by changing the way you think and behave) and neurolinguistic programming or NLP (a connection between the neurological processes ('neuro'), language ('linguistic') and behavioural patterns learned through experience ('programming') and that these can be changed to achieve specific goals in life). This is how I have applied them.

In recent years I have realised the impact of positive words and thoughts. This can begin internally, then when speaking to others and in a group. I know when I was being trained as a teacher that if you told someone not do something, e.g. 'Don't spill your drink', they were far more likely to do so. By saying it in a way that outlines what you want them to do, e.g. 'Hold the cup carefully with two hands', the chances are that the drink will remain safely in the cup. In the same way, consider how you warn yourself about the possible consequences of an action. During pregnancy, for example, you may tell yourself not to feel tired. Simply the autosuggestion of the word 'tired' can make you feel lethargic. So, therefore, encourage yourself with the positive thought of: 'I want more energy'.

My suggestion is that in all the conversations to yourself and others about another pregnancy (and life in general), focus on what you want to happen as opposed to your fears. Some people like to write positive affirmations and stick them around their environment or write them in a journal. Remember to think that you want a healthy pregnancy/a straightforward birth/a baby who sleeps well. Avoid the 'Don't' list.

I am not saying that just because you think and speak positively it will guarantee a positive outcome – it could help, though. We all have come across 'mood-hoovers' – the kind of person who walks into a room and sucks the life out of it by being so negative. I know that when I attended antenatal classes there was one expectant mother who previously had suffered from postnatal depression. Every aspect that was covered, she would have a negative comment about it. I know I was not the only one who rolled their eyes every time she spoke, because she was always so disparaging about everything. Maybe at that stage I also had a closed mind to the very idea that the birth and becoming a mother might not be like all the books and films imply!

As a healthcare professional, if you arrive at work with the attitude and internal dialogue that you have a very tough day ahead of you, that you will have far too much to do and that no one will help you – guess what? That is probably what will happen. I know during my last couple of years as a teacher I allowed the school politics and paperwork to get to me. I would sit in the car park not wanting to go into the school, listing all the negatives reasons why I did not want to be there. My opening line to my team in the classroom would be: 'Don't worry – only three weeks, four days until half term.' Shocking!

I wish I knew then what I now know about the impact of positive thoughts upon myself and others. Often we allow ourselves to become bogged down by all the worst-case scenarios that could happen in life. I am not saying to ignore them and skip around like a character in a Disney film. I am suggesting that you acknowledge the worst-case scenarios and put a plan into place to minimise the risks. Then change your focus to the positives that may happen and allow yourself to dream of the future you would like.

I have heard people describe fear as 'False Evidence Appearing Real'. What scares you about having another baby? In Part One we have covered some of these. Go back through them and make a plan for being able to make them better next time. Every now and then I still get myself over-concerned about events that 'might' happen, then afterwards laugh at myself because I wasted so much negative energy on them unnecessarily. When I have my rational and sensible approach, I consider the scenario and possible outcomes and then I am ready to deal with them accordingly. A good friend of mine is an ex-soldier. He puts things into perspective by saying: 'Noone is trying to kill me, so everything else can be dealt with easily in comparison.'

Perspective is something that is likely to crop up in your thoughts and conversations around having another child. This can be difficult because we all have a tendency just to view situations from our own angle. As one mum suggests:

> You need to take a rounded view, looking at everybody's perspective – partner, impact on other children etc. It's tempting to be selfish and push for what you want, but nobody wants to live with a decision where you have browbeaten your partner into submission.

We covered this in Chapter 5 on decision making.

Communication and language can have a massive impact upon us. Here are some statements that the people who answered my survey have given me:

- I was called a stupid girl when I bled all over the hospital floor. A week after I was readmitted, as part of the placenta had not been removed, a senior midwife expressed concerns about me having postnatal depression. I never completed a questionnaire from HV. She kept telling me my marriage was falling apart. My mum and I begged for help from GP midwifes and HV only to be told I had baby blues.
- My best friend could not in any way empathise with my situation. I can remember someone telling me to pull myself together. I can't tell you how desperate this made me feel.
- My sister said, 'I don't want to know about it, I don't want to hear about it – you need to focus and show some positive mental attitude' … her words.

I will come back to comments from others in later chapters – here I want to remind you of how you speak to yourself. If you spoke to your best friend how you speak to yourself sometimes, would she still be your friend? Why are we so harsh on ourselves? I know when I was ill after having my baby I blamed myself for many aspects of it. When I had my hysterectomy a few years ago, again I blamed myself and somehow felt it was because of my broken marriage and therefore I deserved it. When you are feeling mentally vulnerable your mind can have a habit of being particularly nasty to itself. You have a choice to make because you are in charge of your own thoughts. You can choose to think differently.

You may find Paul McGee's book *S.U.M.O. (Shut Up, Move On)*[1] useful. 'Shut Up' means stop what you're doing, take time out to reflect, let go of baggage and beliefs that hinder your potential. 'Move On' means tomorrow can be different from today, look for new possibilities, instead of just thinking about it, take action.

I needed help after my puerperal psychosis to do this and my community psychiatric nurse really helped me to change my thoughts and beliefs that my illness was due to my own failings. Over time I also shifted my ideal of having another baby 'to do it properly' next time (still implied failure) to 'I want another one to enjoy it more next time'. This is where counselling can help. One couple who decided not to have another baby shared:

- Sometimes we have to let go of what might have been our previous 'perfect, idealised family' pre-PP. It might be that you always dreamt of 2.4 children, a chocolate Labrador and a conservatory but with time as we move through life's experiences, we have to be flexible and modify our expectations. Mental illness can change things. There is no need to religiously stick to previous ideals.

When you are mentally well it is easier to do this yourself and even better if you have a supportive partner who can reel you in at times and help you to focus on positive aspects and facts. One book I read recently that helped me to see how the emotional side of my brain has influenced me more than my rational side is by Steve Peters, called *The Chimp Paradox*.[2] This book has also helped me to understand others more. I went for a blood test a couple of months ago and the practice nurse had it on her desk – she highly recommended it too. If you feel that your thoughts and language could be better it is worth a read, as an individual and as a healthcare professional.

One exercise I recommend to healthcare professionals is to examine what they say to patients, because it literally can have life-changing implications. I have commented before about the psychiatrist who told us I would be more at risk next time round of poor maternal mental health and added that everyone would 'be on my case' next time round. I think that was a fair remark to say. Had my ex-husband been willing to try again I feel we would have taken comfort and action from that. Sometimes tactless remarks can cut deeply. Here are a few examples of comments from Katherine Stone's blog:[3]

- Here's some information on postpartum depression I'm supposed to give you. You're probably not going to get it, though, so I wouldn't pay too much attention to it.
- Women have been having babies for tens of thousands of years, and they got through new motherhood just fine. Toughen up.
- I know breastfeeding is really important to you, but you have to quit so you can be treated for PPD.

On the other hand these are taken from a list of '10 supportive things I'm glad someone said to me' by Charlotte Walker:[4]

- 'Here's my number. Call me any time. And I mean any time.'
- 'The times when you're unwell don't matter! I'd rather have one of you than ten other people with a clean sickness record.'
- 'I know you're taking your meds, but they're not working for you, are they?'

I recommend taking a look at both of these blog articles, regardless of your role. The tips can help us all support others better. Charlotte also covers '10 things not to say to a depressed person',[5] which is also worth a read. One activity I recommend to healthcare teams is to print these off and discuss each one in small groups as to how either they could be reworded better or not said at all. It helps to create a list of 'good' words and phrases. Looking at these lists can be useful to share with family and friends too, so they have a better insight into what to say regarding mental health.

One mum who suffered from postnatal depression said:

- We need to take the mystery and shame out of PND and empower women who may be greatly confused and traumatised, to seek assistance (note: not 'help' which implies helplessness).

If you start with yourself it is amazing how those around you will also begin to speak in similar ways. Think of it as the reverse of the *Jeremy Kyle Show* – the reality television programme where relationship problems are aired, often accompanied by insults, swearing and negativity! Have you noticed how the whole family tends to speak (shout) in the same pitch, volume and tone? It is like they taught us at college – a quietly spoken teacher tends to have a quiet class. A loud one will be noisy. My son has begun to pick up on my use of words much more. I admit that I can be the queen of hyperbole and exaggerate ridiculously. My partner often works away. My lip will come out as I wail, 'He's leaving me again'. My son's retort is now 'He's not leaving you, Mum – he is simply away on business.'

That puts it back into perspective!

I also think this is a useful guide to 'think' before you speak:

T – is it true?
H – is it helpful?
I – is it inspiring?
N – is it necessary?
K – is it kind?

So when will you begin to speak to yourself more positively and more kindly?

What you say is very important and we must also consider how it is communicated using the skill of building rapport. Do you ever read reviews of restaurants or hotels where it almost becomes a stream of abuse to the team who were serving? My thought on them now is to consider how the 'reviewer' behaved. I was in a hotel foyer recently during a heatwave. A red-faced man appeared and immediately launched into a verbal attack on the receptionist. He demanded to be changed to a room with air-conditioning and when he was told that none of the rooms had it, he went ballistic! She calmly told him that she could arrange for a fan to be sent to his room and offered a few more suggestions. As an onlooker I felt that the receptionist dealt with the situation very well. I also wanted to slap the man for being so very rude and hostile. Yes, he was hot. Yes, the rooms were hot. That was no excuse for being so nasty.

I have found that the best way to get good service is to be pleasant. If you bring out the best in people, then they are more likely to want to do their very best for you. One quality I admire in others is when I see them doing this. I now make a conscious effort to greet everyone I am in contact with in a warm and friendly manner. It is so easy to make eye contact and say something to make the other person also notice you. I am not meaning this in a flirtatious way – simply to acknowledge that the other person exists. Do we really want all shop tills to become self-service? I dislike those machines intensely! This is especially relevant in shops where the assistants can be simply ignored at the till or vice versa. Make the effort to say hello, smile and have a small conversation as they serve you. It makes them and you feel better.

If you learn these good habits in general, they will be natural to you when dealing with people with whom you wish to consult in the decision-making process and beyond, regarding another pregnancy.

As Thumper the rabbit in the film *Bambi* says, 'If you can't say something nice, don't say nothing at all.'

Likewise in a busy healthcare setting, the receptionists are often in the 'firing line' for delayed appointments. What purpose does it serve if you approach them 'on the attack'? Far better to be polite, calm and friendly. They are much more likely to respond the same way and do everything they can to help you.

Building rapport can help both parties to communicate better. It can also help to be aware of the mood of another person and match it accordingly. If two people are at opposite ends it can be hard to get that middle ground. For example, if you as a health professional are in an extremely 'high' and positive frame of mind, this can distance a patient who is feeling low. Consider as a midwife the first booking-in appointment when a lady sits in front of you. If you assume that she is deliriously happy about the pregnancy and you are immediately in a congratulatory mode, she is less likely to speak to you openly if she is really concerned about it. Similarly, if your communication is dulled because you are feeling stressed yourself, then the patient is not likely then to want to be joyful about her state. My suggestion is that you approach the initial moments of a meeting in neutral territory. That way you can easily adjust your emotional response according to the other person, for mutual benefit.

Having continuity of care and the opportunity to build relationship is important to some mothers, especially in the 'next time around' scenario, for example:

- Seeing same midwife at appointments would have been better. This may have help me in being able to disclose my fear/anxiety due to a termination that I regretted.

Being open, honest and candid is something that we all need to be aware of. As a patient, if we avoid being truthful, it makes the assistance from others much more difficult to ascertain. These mums commented:

- I would have preferred honesty from people who know how hard it can be, with or without PNI. All parents find it hard at times, but there seems to be an expectation that you should always be happy and enjoying it. In my case, had someone else talked about it I might have felt able to ask for help myself.
- I would have liked having truthful conversations about the implications of potential mental health issues after birth, rather than focusing on the 'perfect picture' of family life.

I also know that I feel far more at ease in talking to a health professional who not only asks questions about me yet also shares a little about themselves too, when relevant. I remember on the maternity ward a midwife mentioned that she was worried about her dog at the vets. I do not really like dogs yet I looked forward to her coming onto the ward, simply to ask about him as it took my anxious thoughts away from myself. It was only a snippet of conversation yet it made me feel like she was a genuine person and I could have told her anything. I also warmed to those who showed interest in a photo at my bedside as they took observations, asking who the people were. Small action – big difference. If you make others feel special, I strongly suggest that they will feel the same and feel far more comfortable about sharing their true concerns.

On the other hand, there were members of the team in the psychiatric hospital who terrified me due to their brusque and impatient words and manner. This led to me self-harming on occasion because I was too scared to ask for help. A mum told me:

- The NHS staff at hospital were lovely but I had a terrible midwife at our local village hospital who accused me of getting my money's worth out of the NHS as I wanted another Caesarean! I was very upset about it at the time. In the end I had to have a Caesarean as the placenta didn't move and I was hospitalised three weeks before the birth because of bleeding!

Think about the impact of your communication on others and how you can make it better.

So now that you and those nearest to you are making every effort to have a positive outlook and approach, what else may help? My suggestion is a better knowledge around the perinatal period and all it involves.

I would have argued with anyone during the last few weeks of my pregnancy that I was well-read and prepared for what was to come. I had read so many books and articles, attended classes and devoured pregnancy and birth magazines. I would not have arrogantly said that I 'knew it all', yet I did feel informed. In retrospect I read and absorbed what I wanted to happen and, without realising it, had mentally deleted any of the potential challenges I might have faced.

I know that I had unfairly judged the lady at my antenatal classes as being a 'mood-hoover' – now I realise that she was approaching her second pregnancy with experience! Incidentally, she was very well after her subsequent baby. One morning I was sitting in the doctor's surgery waiting to be seen about my postnatal depression and feeling every negative thought and emotion possible. This lady seemed to glide in, smiling broadly from ear to ear, pushing her new daughter in a pram with her son skipping at the side. He clearly adored his little sister. 'Oh Elaine,' she said, 'isn't motherhood wonderful?'

That was a lesson to me in being so judgemental!

I also realise that I was very concerned as a new mother about what I asked health professionals or told them for fear of being judged stupid or a bad mother. I remember on the maternity ward feeling very uncomfortable with big lumps under my armpits. I thought I had reacted badly to my travel-sized deodorant! It was only when a midwife noticed me putting antiseptic cream under my arms that she asked what was wrong. When I told her she replied, 'Oh, that's just your milk coming in – it will soon settle down.'

I felt stupid because I didn't know that and because I had 'read all the books' judged myself harshly that I should have known! Why should I? I had never had a baby before!

The learning here is for both parents and professionals. As a parent, simply ask a question about anything you are unsure of or concerned about. Once you know the answer it is more than likely your worry will reduce. When the midwife explained what these lumps were and that it was 'normal', my anxiety vanished. The healthcare professionals are used to dealing with pregnancy and birth on a daily basis so they know these 'little' things. Allow them to share their expertise as that is what they are there for, just as you would in any other service.

As a professional, continually reassure parents that you are there to help and that the chances are that any question they have, it is likely you have been asked it before, no matter how silly they may feel it is. If a thought is causing anxiety that can be eased by information, then that has to be a bonus.

Next time I feel I would have focused much less on knowledge about the birth. Yes, of course it is important to know what happens and to be aware of the possible procedures involved. I also would have been far more mindful of my mum's great advice that 'you know what the pain is and you know it will end by being rewarded with your baby.'

For me next time round my knowledge would have focused much more around what practical help I could have lined up and what services were around for us as a family to help our mental health. These days there is far more information available via the internet and social media. I am also pleased to say that this generally is improving as the desire grows to reduce the stigma around parental mental health and to increase services. The key is to find out what you need to know. This is what the basis of this section of the book is about.

During my role working for S+ The Real Leadership Company, I have recognised that there are many similarities between the excellent communication skills that they share with companies and individuals in the business world, that are also applicable lessons to us all. I invited their Global Director of Coaching, Mike Coote, to recommend those that he feels are most relevant to the topic of this book.

The world in which we live has increasingly become one that seems to find it particularly easy to focus on the negative first. We are faced with violent extremism at a number of levels, increased fear of personal safety, challenges of changing weather patterns and the resultant devastation … and the ongoing challenges of mental health.

Let's be candid about this – these are all real happenings and need a response from us. The challenge that I and others face is the reality of first and foremost looking at and for all of the negatives and, sometimes, completely ignoring the many positives that are also so much part of our lives.

Think of this illustration – a young child comes home excitedly from school proclaiming that she has scored 9 out of 10 on her spelling test. How many of us, with all the best will in the world, will ask them about the one that they got wrong first before congratulating them on the nine that they got right?

There is something very real about this and we need to understand the implications of what we are doing. If we focus almost entirely on the negative aspects of life and the challenges facing us, there is a resultant change in our neurological patterns and our very brain chemistry! That's always staggered me somewhat! We do have the capacity to think ourselves into increasingly negative patterns of response and behaviour.

And when we apply this to the world of mental health and specifically to the world of perinatal illness, it is vital that we begin to deliberately change some of our reactive negative patterns of speech, thought and behaviour into something tangibly more positive. Let me hasten to add that I am not mooting that we should simply start to think and say positive things and that the world will be a 'rosy glossy' place because of it.

What I am strongly suggesting is this: look to the positives that are in our lives, our children, our families, our health, the homes that we have and the (comparative) security of this wonderful country. Find the space and time in your life to point out the positives to others ... and to yourself. Start first with what is right and good before jumping into what is bad and going wrong.

Just as we can impact upon and alter our brain chemistry and response patterns with negatives, so we can also *really* impact upon them with hugely positive patterns. This is my heartfelt plea to business people, mums and dads across the world, children, aunties and uncles and all the other parts of the nuclear family – what you are and how you react or respond can and does have a huge impact on those around you. *Please* find the positives and focus first on them.

TOP TIPS FOR PARENTS

1. Think and speak using positive words – state what you want to happen.
2. Acknowledge your *fear* then put a plan in place to deal with it.
3. Choose to think differently.
4. Read some positive thinking books.
5. Consider your words and non-verbal communication to get the best from yourself and others.
6. Remember to ask for assistance with any of your concerns, as the acquired knowledge is likely to ease your anxiety.

TOP TIPS FOR HEALTHCARE PROFESSIONALS

1. Same as for parents!
2. Have a team meeting to examine the types of language that can best to use.
3. Apply 'THINK' to what you say.
4. Build rapport and match behaviour.
5. Reassure parents that you are there to assist, and answer questions about their health and situation to the best of your ability.

REFERENCES

1. McGee P. *S.U.M.O. (Shut Up, Move On): the straight-talking guide to creating and enjoying a brilliant life*. Chichester: Capstone Publishing; 2006.
2. Peters S. *The Chimp Paradox: the mind management programme to help you achieve success, confidence and happiness*. London: Vermilion; 2012.
3. www.postpartumprogress.com/20-things-i-never-want-hear-again-postpartum-depression-edition
4. *10 Supportive Things I'm Glad Someone Said To Me*. Available at: http://purplepersuasion.wordpress.com/2011/08/03/ten-supportive-things-im-glad-somebody-said-to-me/
5. http://purplepersuasion.wordpress.com/2011/07/31/ten-things-not-to-say-to-a-depressed-person/

FURTHER READING AND RESOURCES

- www.hanzak.com/2013/11/ten-top-tips-to-help-you-smile.html
- www.cheergiver.com/#axzz1nD4ZOORc
- Dalfen A. *When Baby Brings the Blues: solutions for postpartum depression.* Chichester: Wiley; 2009.
- Barnes DL, Balber LG. *The Journey to Parenthood: myths, reality and what really matters.* Oxford: Radcliffe; 2007.
- Hanley J. *Listening Visits in Perinatal Mental Health: a guide for health professionals and support workers.* 1st ed. Abingdon: Routledge; 2015.

CHAPTER 10

Pre-conception counselling

Planning is bringing the future into the present so that you can
do something about it now.

Alan Lakei

When my psychiatrist discharged me he said if I ever was pregnant again
'everyone would be on my case next time'. I never had the opportunity to
find out what that would have looked like. With the knowledge and experience of perinatal mental illness I know I would have researched the risks and
looked for solutions again. Getting the support and guidance from healthcare professionals even before conception would have certainly helped to ease
any concerns. The aim is to seek healthy, emotional wellbeing as opposed to
breakdown. I am aware that couples may seek pre-conception counselling for
genetic or medical conditions, but I asked if any in my survey had received
any for an insightful discussion around their mental health. Sadly the majority had nothing or very little, for example:

- No special counselling though I saw a therapist weekly.
- I had just started group CBT before I found I was pregnant. Even though I was
  ill the group stopped just after I had given birth due to funding.
- I had seen a professional in the community mental health team and asked
  about pregnancy and was told that they didn't see any problems. They said
  they would refer me to the perinatal mental health service. Unfortunately this
  never happened due to the referral being sent to the wrong place and no one
  willing to do anything about this.
- Yes. I brought the subject up myself with the midwife and I was in therapy during the month of conception so we concentrated on the issues I'd had. I was
  from there referred to another drop-in group. I was referred via my midwife to
  the highly over-stretched midwife with specialism for MH.

Some women were advised to change or stop medication, with a variety of
outcomes:

- The recommendation was to go off all medication except an antidepressant classified as safe. This sent me into psychotic mania in my second trimester.
- I was told to come off my antidepressants. Even though I was in hospital for a number of weeks prior to birth with pre-eclampsia, the hospital still ignored me when I said I was depressed. My mental health was awful and I would become hysterical and told to calm down because I was raising my blood pressure.
- Yes, advised to stop taking citalopram.
- Discussed but decided against. I was not pressured either way but I felt supported bordering on pressured to take antidepressants postnatally as a precaution.

I also asked if any provision had been made to pre-empt the likelihood of perinatal mental illness. Almost every reply was that there had been none or very little:

- My psychiatrist opposed breastfeeding but he didn't say this until after I was pregnant. I insisted on breastfeeding and he delayed creating a postnatal plan for medication. It was a mess and I went psychotic and was hospitalised for a month away from my baby. I maybe saw him for 15 minutes once a week.
- I remember having my booking in appointment at the hospital. Because the baby was unplanned and I lived with my parents the pregnancy was noted to be 'high risk' in my notes. It was never mentioned again and I still don't know what that meant to this day.
- Postnatal depression was never discussed until I saw my health visitor after my daughter was born.
- Minor – I sought help from the local hospital and had been assigned a psychiatrist.
- No. I told the midwife at the 'booking in' appointment about my previous mental health issues but she thought it was unlikely to be an issue and never mentioned it again. I told my health visitor when I met her just before my baby was due and she said she'd 'keep an eye on me'.
- No, even though I presented as very low during my pregnancy.
- I heard the standard 'You may experience the baby blues but it will pass' after the birth of my first and second child. I wasn't even sure what that was.
- No, leaflets were distributed after a NHS pre-natal course. Very little mention of PND.

Here are some examples where some pre-conception discussions took place:

- I was provided with a maternity support worker who visited me at home once I reached 20 weeks pregnant.
- I was in a state when I went to see a consultant. She referred me to a mental health midwife but the support was minimal and was discharged even though I said I was feeling low. I did have another mental health assessment and I am having CBT.

- Briefly, about the plan for accessing help quickly if I needed it.
- I discussed it but nothing was offered – I was just told I had a 50/50 chance of it happening again and it would 'probably be fine'. I felt terrified. During the pregnancy I saw my GP who wrote to the Community Mental Health team about my previous experience asking for advice. They said 'but she's currently well and not on medication so there are no concerns, re-refer if she becomes unwell afterwards'. When I did get ill again the Consultant at the mother and baby unit was disgusted by their treatment of me. She said they have no understanding of perinatal mental health in the general community teams. I should have been referred to her, had input during my pregnancy and been transferred to the mother and baby unit for assessment rest and recuperation immediately after the birth!
- Yes with my previous consultant and a new one.
- I told the midwife once I was pregnant. I was told I could not get an appointment with her unless I was pregnant, so ended up not talking to anyone before we conceived.
- Yes – I paid for a psychologist, who diagnosed me with post-traumatic stress, and I had a number of sessions to come to terms with everything that had happened. This left me feeling ready to have another baby. I continued to see her throughout pregnancy.
- I had a new amazing HV she was fantastic and my psychiatrist was a real help.
- Spoke to GP and changed to safer meds. Discussed recognising the signs.
- I was advised not to have another pregnancy due to medication I was on.
- I was referred to a psychiatrist at the nearest mother and baby unit to discuss the options if I managed to conceive again. We had IVF Frozen embryo replacement but it failed. We tried our best but it wasn't to be.

Others took their own actions:

- I made a very focused effort to prepare myself in a number of ways.
- No one offered to even take me seriously until my pregnancy was very far on then I decided to make myself heard and did a lot of hard work putting in a support plan myself. I got myself a doula for 6 weeks, etc.

Preconception care is a broad term that refers to the process of identifying social, behavioural, environmental, and biomedical risks to a woman's fertility and pregnancy outcome and then reducing these risks through education, counselling, and appropriate intervention, when possible, before conception.[1,2]

So what should ideally happen to help support couples who are considering another baby where the risk of perinatal mental illness is considered to be high? This is what as parents you should expect and what healthcare professionals should be aware of and provide regarding what to consider around risk, relapse and recovery.

The Clinical Knowledge Summaries provided by the National Institute for Health and Care Excellence (NICE) have published some Pre-conception Advice and Management Guidelines.[3] This include assessments and general advice for any woman considering pregnancy, such as diet, exercise, smoking cessation. There are more specific guidelines for some physical conditions, like asthma and diabetes along with genetic conditions, and also for the older mother. There is a defined set of guidelines for women with mental health issues. They particularly mention depression, bipolar and schizophrenia. You will find here advice around medication and where referral to a psychiatrist or specialist advice may be needed. There is guidance on the risks of taking antidepressants during pregnancy. Another source of information regarding medication is on a phone app called LactMed@NIH – it is geared to the healthcare practitioner and nursing mother, and contains over 450 drug records.

Another source of guidelines for healthcare professionals about pre-conception counselling (PCC) can be found at www.patient.co.uk/doctor/pre-pregnancy-counselling

Here is a summary[4] of what is recommended generally for women who are considering becoming pregnant:

Most pregnancies go well and without any major problems. But, it is wise to reduce any risks as much as possible. So, a reminder of things to consider before becoming pregnant, and as soon as you realise you are pregnant:

Things you should do:
- Take folic acid tablets before you get pregnant until 12 weeks of pregnancy.
- Take vitamin D supplements when you become pregnant.
- Have a blood test to check if you are immune against rubella, and to screen for hepatitis B, syphilis, and HIV. Ask your practice nurse to do this.
- Eat a healthy diet. Include foods rich in iron, calcium and folic acid; also, some oily fish.
- Have strict food hygiene. In particular, wash your hands after handling raw meat, or handling cats and kittens, and before you prepare food.
- Wear gloves when you are gardening.

Things you should avoid:
- Too much vitamin A – don't eat liver or liver products, or take vitamin A supplements.
- Listeriosis – don't eat undercooked meat or eggs, soft cheese, pâté, shellfish, raw fish, or unpasteurised milk.
- Fish which may contain a lot of mercury – shark, marlin, swordfish, or excess tuna.
- Sheep, lambs, cat poo (faeces), cat litters, and raw meat, which may carry certain infections.

Things you should stop or cut down on:

- Caffeine in tea, coffee, cola, etc. – have no more than 200 mg per day. For example, this is in about two mugs of instant coffee, or one mug of brewed coffee and a 50 g bar of plain chocolate, or two and a half mugs of tea.
- Alcohol – you are strongly advised not to drink at all.
- Smoking – you are strongly advised to stop completely.
- Street (illicit) drugs – you are strongly advised to stop completely.
- Liquorice – reduce your intake if you eat lots of it.

Other things to consider:

- Your iodine intake and perhaps discuss with your doctor about iodine supplements.
- Immunisation against hepatitis B if you are at increased risk of getting this infection.
- Immunisation against chickenpox if you are a healthcare worker and have not previously had chickenpox and so are not immune.
- Your medication – including herbal and 'over-the-counter' medicines. Are they safe?
- Your work environment – is it safe?
- Medical conditions in yourself, or conditions which run in your family.
- Screening tests for sickle cell disease and thalassaemia.

Research[5] states 'There is a great need for PCC as shown by the fact that almost all couples reported risk factors for which personal counselling was indicated. Pre-conception counselling may reduce the risk of adverse pregnancy outcome by enabling couples to avoid these risks. PCC can be provided by GPs, who have the necessary medical knowledge and background information to counsel couples who wish to have a baby.'

The BMJ have an online module for GPs on PCC.[6]

If you need further support about the funding aspects for the need for pre-conception counselling following a previous perinatal mental illness, refer to the economic report published in 2014.[7]

The majority of advice still is there for physical conditions – we need full parity of esteem in this area. Ideally as a couple, or individually, there should be this type of support for you. After all, you are doing a sensible thing by looking for ways to minimise and prevent perinatal mental illness that will be much cheaper in the long run for the NHS. Initially I would suggest that you see your GP and take along the following information in case they are not fully aware of what you may need to know.

Emphasise that the World Health Organization recognise this as a global concern and suggest it should consist of:

- assessing psychosocial problems
- providing educational and psychosocial counselling before and during pregnancy

- counselling, treating and managing depression in women planning pregnancy and other women of childbearing age
- strengthening community networks and promoting women's empowerment
- improving access to education for women of childbearing age
- reducing economic insecurity of women of childbearing age.

They have produced further details and documents.[8]

I have found a model for good practice by The Leeds Perinatal Mental Health Service[9] that could be useful as an outline for what you need to know.

> If you are planning a pregnancy, you may benefit from meeting with a member of our team to discuss the following:
> - Your individual risk of becoming unwell in the perinatal period
> - Whether treatment will be beneficial during pregnancy and postnatally
> - Risks and benefits of different medication during pregnancy and in breastfeeding; this may include meeting with a pharmacist and discussing the most recent information on medication
> - Relapse prevention strategies
> - Support and monitoring during pregnancy and post delivery
> - Early warning signs of illness
> - Care available should you become unwell.
>
> In most cases a single 90 minute appointment is sufficient, sometimes a follow up appointment is arranged to discuss things further. The preconception counselling clinic provides consultation, information and advice, not ongoing care. Referral to our service for treatment may be one of our recommendations should you become pregnant.

Action on Puerperal Psychosis has some specific advice for anyone who has bipolar disorder or at risk of puerperal psychosis.[10]

It may also be worth asking your surgery for an appointment or referral to a specialist perinatal mental health team or health visitor. It may be that a health visitor may already have a good relationship with a family and will certainly have a wider knowledge of the impact of poor perinatal mental health. They should have a generic public health awareness and role. Ask for referral via the GP or midwife. Melitta Walker, from the Institute of Health Visiting,[11] recommends that:

> Parents need the opportunity to talk and for support. They need encouraging that the experience next time may not be the same as previously. Give them the opportunity to reflect back on triggers and signs to look out for. Discuss and plan what to do if they become incapacitated again and put plans in place with a trusted healthcare provider. Ensure that their wishes are recorded when they are well for

what they would prefer to happen if they become unwell. Be aware that feelings and circumstances can change over time, so the plans may need to be revisited as appropriate. Consider ways in which 'losses' can be avoided next time, e.g. ensuring keepsakes are collected such as photographs and videos of the new baby, in case Mum has some memory loss. Generally parents find that if they do become unwell, recovery is quicker if their plan is met and they feel they have stayed in control of the situation.

In Chapter 26 on counselling and community support there will be more examples of what to ask for and/or set up if you are a healthcare provider. You may also find the websites http://beforeandbeyond.org and 'pre-conception health and health care'[12] extremely useful. They have pre-conception curriculum, tools, resources and articles for clinicians – aimed at the USA, yet the content is applicable to any parents. They also give ideas on ensuring that the father has optimum health too.

Another source of examples for 'Pregnancy relapse prevention plan' can be found in a presentation by Geerling and Stevens. In their clinic in the Netherlands they have devised 'Psycho-education, Psychosocial Interventions and Prevention Plan for Patients and Family Members'.[13] You may find some useful ideas here. They say that the main goals of this plan are to:
1. reduce stress by preparation and self-management techniques
2. prevent relapse during pregnancy and in the postpartum period
3. promote co-operation between all care providers.

In Hull, there is a very successful clinic for pre-conception counselling.[14] Their team leader, Katy Moss, shares one example of the positive outcome for one of their families and some of her key messages:

Anna was referred to the Hull and East Riding Perinatal Mental Health Liaison Team by her care coordinator from her local community mental health team. Anna was a 35 year old professional woman who had recently married and was planning her first child. Anna had a long history of involvement with mental health services and had been given a diagnosis of bipolar affective mood disorder. Anna had experienced more than one inpatient admission and had been detained under the mental health act. Anna was prescribed sodium valproate as her treatment and at the time of her preconception counselling was well on this. Anna attended to see the consultant psychiatrist and was given the opportunity to tell her story and an open and honest discussion took place regarding risk vs benefits of a number of medications both in pregnancy and breastfeeding. Literature was also provided which detailed this which allowed Anna and her husband time to go away and discuss their options and make an informed decision. The couple were then invited to return to have a further opportunity to discuss their wishes and decision making. Anna and her husband opted to change medication prior to conception and this was monitored closely by the team to ensure her mental health and emotional wellbeing remained good. Due to the severity of Anna's past history of relapse and the postnatal period being a known high risk period, it was decided with the couple that on the day of delivery she would recommence on the sodium valproate as a prophylactic treatment. This meant Anna would not be advised to breastfeed but she felt that the risk of relapse in her opinion outweighed that of relapsing. Anna went on to conceive and continued to receive support from the team. This included regular reviews, an arranged visit to the labour ward to familiarise with the environment and an individualised perinatal birth plan which included Anna's early warning signs, her current medication, the plan regarding the prophylactic treatment regime and that Anna was not able to breastfeed. The plan also provided the midwives and obstetricians with numbers for our service and the crisis resolution and home treatment team for out of hours support. I am delighted to inform you that Anna went on to deliver a healthy baby girl, she commenced her prophylactic treatment and her mental health remained good. Anna and her husband are currently thinking about a new addition to their family!

Katy also says:

The importance of having a preconception clinic within the perinatal service is difficult to put in to words, however the results and outcomes we have seen for women and their families speak for themselves. Preconception counselling has raised a whole host of issues for women that as a service we had not expected and as a service we have been able to listen to their views and develop a better understanding of the service users' dilemmas and concerns. By providing this service we have been able to work very closely with women and their families from an early stage which has helped with developing trusting therapeutic relationships.

A couple of notes I would like to make to professionals is that when prescribing to any woman for the first time we have discussions about family planning and the effects if any the prescribed medication would have in pregnancy and breastfeeding. Also when a lady is pregnant we think about what exposure the foetus has already had before abruptly stopping an effective medication increasing the risk of relapse and increased exposure of a further medication to the foetus.

As the expression goes, 'forewarned is forearmed'. Seek support at this stage so that it will hopefully help to nip some of your anxieties in the bud and enable you to feel secure with your plan for prevention and/or treatment.

TOP TIPS FOR PARENTS

1. If you feel that pre-conception counselling is something that would help you, shout until someone listens! Quote the references I have outlined to healthcare providers. Begin with your GP and ask to be seen by perinatal mental health specialists.
2. Go beyond the 'we can't see you unless you are pregnant' advice and insist that you need someone with whom to have an insightful discussion.
3. Do your own homework before that discussion, so that you can be prepared with your own anxieties to talk about and ways that you feel will make a difference to you and any possible future child.

TOP TIPS FOR HEALTHCARE PROVIDERS

1. If pre-conception counselling is not already part of your area's Perinatal Mental Healthcare Pathway, please investigate how this can be provided and ensure it is included.
2. Be mindful of excellent communication amongst healthcare providers involved in maternity and women of a childbearing age, to know who and where the patients in their care can access pre-conception counselling.
3. Use the examples and resources above to help formulate an individual care pathway for a couple.
4. Remember the importance of listening and then make a plan for the reasons listed above.

REFERENCES

1. Johnson K, Posner SF, Biermann J, *et al.* Recommendations to Improve Preconception Health and Health Care – United States. A report of the CDC/ATSDR Preconception Care Work Group and the Select Panel on Preconception Care. *MMWR Recomm Rep.* 2006; **55**: 1.
2. American College of Obstetricians and Gynecologists. *Preconceptional Care. ACOG Technical Bulletin 205.* Washington, DC: American College of Obstetricians and Gynecologists; 1995.
3. http://cks.nice.org.uk/pre-conception-advice-and-management
4. www.patient.co.uk/health/planning-to-become-pregnant
5. van der Pal-de Bruin KM, le Cessie S, Elsinga J, *et al.* Pre-conception counselling in primary care: prevalence of risk factors among couples contemplating pregnancy. *Paediatr Perinat Epidemiol.* 2008; **22**(3): 280–7.
6. http://learning.bmj.com/learning/module-intro/.html?moduleId=10032327
7. Bauer A, Parsonage M, Knapp M, *et al. The Costs of Perinatal Mental Health Problems.* London: Centre for Mental Health and London School of Economics; 2014. Available at: http://everyonesbusiness.org.uk/wp-content/uploads/2014/12/

Embargoed-20th-Oct-Final-Economic-Report-costs-of-perinatal-mental-health-problems.pdf

8. www.who.int/maternal_child_adolescent/documents/concensus_preconception_care/en/
9. www.leedspft.nhs.uk/our_services/Specialist-LD-Care/Perinatal_Mental_Health
10. www.app-network.org/what-is-pp/getting-help/bipolar-disorder-pregnancy/
11. www.ihv.org.uk/
12. www.cdc.gov/preconception/index.html
13. www.slideshare.net/ISBD/psychoeducation-psychosocial-interventions-and-prevention-plan-for-patients-and-family-members
14. www.humber.nhs.uk/services/perinatal-mental-health.htm

FURTHER READING AND RESOURCES

- www.uptodate.com/contents/the-preconception-office-visit has a list of many research papers relevant to this area
- http://babyworld.co.uk/2014/04/planning-conception-how-far-would-you-go/

CHAPTER 11

A healthy and happy pregnancy

Whether your pregnancy was meticulously planned, medically coaxed, or happened by surprise, one thing is certain – your life will never be the same.

Catherine Jones

I would hazard a guess that even the healthiest and happiest expectant mother and father feel some level of concern or feel stress to some degree during the pregnancy. Not only is there the responsibility of bringing a new life into this world with all the changes that will bring – your mind is full of so many thoughts and emotions too. My biggest desire in life was always to be a mother. Prior to having my son I had never been identified as suffering from any kind of mental ill health. I was thrilled and excited to be pregnant. I also had my concerns.

Like most mums-to-be my biggest worry was about the health of the baby. I was 32 years old yet the literature says that there are more risks the older you are. I pondered if my delay had potentially put higher challenges on my baby's development. Also, because I taught children with severe and profound learning difficulties, I knew families who had been changed forever due to having a child with disabilities, some who had been born that way and others who had been brain-damaged at birth.

Eighteen years ago the scans and tests were not perhaps as regular or detailed as they are now. Yet they also served as both a concern and then relief. You literally can feel your body respond whilst waiting for a scan – with a raised heart rate, fluttering tummy and generally feeling tense. As the scan is being done this is then matched with the excitement of seeing the outline of your child and attempting to work out which bit is which! When you are told that everything is normal and looking good, again you can identify the physical responses in your body as anxiety is replaced by excitement. Mentally then you allow yourself to indulge in making more plans. I think I would then feel inspired to go and buy something for the baby!

Particularly as a first time mother, the thought of the actual birth can be terrifying. I recall my mother telling me that labour is very painful. The difference is that you know what it is; it will end and you will be rewarded by holding your new baby and then forget it. She also reassured me that many others had gone through it and survived, plus many go on to have many more. Hence it could not be so bad. That was the mindset that I had. I also read the relevant books and attended antenatal classes. I felt that I knew the facts and also reassured myself that in hospital I would be well cared for by experts who had delivered babies for years. There was always that small voice tormenting me with a 'what if' scenario.

Concerns at work also bothered me when I was pregnant. In some ways I was over-excited and wanted to be very much acknowledged as being pregnant. For example, when we had a training day on lifting and handling techniques, I was thrilled to state my condition and be treated accordingly. At other times I would be hesitant because the erratic behaviour of some of my pupils could have put me physically at risk, so I had to be cautious. As my maternity leave approached I went into overdrive in wanting to leave everything perfect for the supply teacher and my class. In doing so I overdid it and finished early due to being ill with a urinary tract infection.

As a couple we had concerns over finances. I had wrongly assumed that maternity leave was on full pay. We had just got married and moved into a new house. We needed my salary and had decided that I would be a working mum. This was not my ideal at all, so I had the internal battle of dialogue between hoping that we would be okay and also not wanting to work and settling for less financially. I reassured myself with the belief that 'everybody else manages, so why couldn't we?'.

Some women worry about the new baby putting pressure on their relationship. In retrospect I did not see this as being a challenge. I did not realise the implications of all the changes being a mother would bring.

If I had been able to have another baby I feel my biggest stress would have been the anxiety associated with developing postnatal depression again. I also am aware that the people around me would have also been highly aware of this.

Stress is defined by NHS Choices as:

the feeling of being under too much mental or emotional pressure. Pressure turns into stress when you feel unable to cope. People have different ways of reacting to stress, so a situation that feels stressful to one person may be motivating to someone else.

Some signs of stress in pregnancy may include sleeplessness, loss or increased appetite, headaches, upset stomach and the inclination to want to take drugs that you know are not good during pregnancy, e.g. smoking, alcohol, caffeine.

So does being stressed in pregnancy matter? The research clearly identifies that it does have an effect on the foetus and the mother. I admit to being a little wary here of including a long list of these. If we are given medication and take the time to read the possible side-effects we could easily decide it is simply not worth taking! I do want to present a balanced perspective in order to help people be aware of those risks. The important lesson is then to be able to do something about preventing or minimising those risks rather than ignoring them.

Vivette Glover, Professor of Perinatal Psychobiology at Imperial College in London, said in an article in *World Medical News* that, 'Prenatal stress hugely grows the likelihood of a child having attention-deficit hyperactivity disorder, cognitive delay, anxiousness and depression. Stressed mothers also produce babies with lower birth weight, which can be an indicator for coronary heart condition in later life.'

I highly recommend a website that Professor Glover has designed specifically on this topic for medical professionals, policy makers and anyone interested about these issues.[1] It also has great links for parents, including suggestions for mothers as to how to reduce stress in pregnancy, by Harry Lerner.[2]

Studies have shown that when the mother is experiencing high levels of stress, her unborn child has been shown to respond and react to the increased level of the stress hormone cortisol, emotional anxiety and muscle tension. One excellent summary and explanation of the relevant research is by Graham Music, a consultant Child and Adolescent Psychotherapist.[3] He impresses that the purpose of this research is not to add further burden to already guilt-laden parents. It does mean that:

> armed with this information we can try to ensure that robust services and support structures are in place to minimise some of the worst risks to the developing foetus and the future child and adult.

Society generally considers stress to be negative, yet we do need a certain amount to help us become productive. Some research by scientists at Harvard's Department of Psychology[4] has changed health psychologist Kelly McGonical's thinking about it. She says:

> The harmful effects of stress on health are not inevitable, how you think and how you act can transform your experience of stress. When you choose to view your stress response as helpful, you create the biology of courage. And when you choose to connect with others under stress, you can create resilience.

So while she obviously wouldn't ask for more stressful experiences in her own life, she does have a new appreciation of the condition. 'When you choose to view stress in this way, you're not just getting better at stress, you're actually making a pretty profound statement,' she concludes. 'You can trust yourself to handle life's challenges. And you're remembering you don't have to face them alone.'

I recommend that you listen to her talk about this online.[5]

So what can you do to make another pregnancy a happier experience?

The ladies who responded to my survey shared some of their thoughts and actions during another pregnancy:

- We moved to a more accessible property. I was kinder to myself. I told the health visitor what had happened previously.
- Got a lot more help lined up. No building works!
- I had to seek help and be admitted to the mother and baby unit despite not wanting to, as I knew what I was suffering from. Previous to the birth I ensured everything was ready and organised for the birth.
- I saw a psychologist pre-birth and a psychiatrist. My husband took more time off work.
- I planned my self-care before, during and after the pregnancy in great detail. I readied everything I would need in advance. I made sure my husband knew what to look for in me, I confided in friends and gave them my 'what to do' file, and I made sure everyone knew what had happened before and what I needed this time. I accessed in advance all the holistic care I knew I would need. Finally I did many things I knew would help to relax and prepare me and the household for the baby's arrival.
- I took medication throughout pregnancy. Put things in to place to care for first child if I was admitted again.
- I prepared a checklist of who could help in what way – practical helpers, emotional helpers. Discussed my warning signs for others to look out for.
- I spoke to my GP. While pregnant I joined a children's centre.

Some of these ladies admitted that they had a range of negative emotions during another pregnancy, such as feeling extremely anxious, overwhelmed, low, very moody, argumentative, tired and worried. A common understanding was that they had been through pregnancy before, so they knew they could again. One mum described her emotional state as:

- Terrified … ambivalent about having the baby.

Others had a more positive state:

- Very well – felt attached to the baby from the moment I found out. Had a really good pregnancy. No depression but terrified of the PND coming back.
- Very happy but anxious. I started suffering awful arterial nose bleeds from 4 months pregnant, my father died, we had a car crash – so it was a very stressful time.
- Apprehensive but fully aware and I allowed myself to become empowered. I really investigated my options and felt strong. I think I did brilliantly actually!

Here are some of the ways that may help your thought processes during pregnancy.

At the simplest level there is the saying that if you are faced with a worry ask yourself the question: 'Can I do anything about it?' If the answer is yes, then do it; if it is no, why worry?

One key area about this is around the birth. No one can precisely predict how your body will respond during labour. What you can do is discuss, plan and prepare for a normal delivery, with an understanding and confidence about anything that could be considered a complication. I shall look at this is more detail in Chapter 12.

If I had been pregnant again, I would have made a bigger effort to rest and relax as much as possible. I would have been kinder to myself and either delegated tasks to others or simply allowed them not to be done. For a while it is possible to live without the need for straight cushions! I am sure my parents would have willingly done some ironing for me, for example – my responsibility was to ask for and accept offers of help. One approach to your daily chores could be to have a 'Do, Ditch, Delegate' approach. Decide what you have to do; what really can be left; and what you can ask others to do.

Of course I would have had another child around too, so the argument could be that they don't rest. I would have built into our days some quiet time. Rather than running around whilst he was playing, I would have sat down, with my feet up, watching him play. Children love being read to, so another opportunity to cuddle up on the sofa could have been for story reading. This perhaps is the time too to make the most of television and DVDs. I used to say that I would never allow a child of mine to sit watching programmes – how wrong I was! I would have gone to bed early on a regular basis. Even if you are unable to sleep, your body is still resting.

I feel it would have been important to talk about all my feelings and anxieties with my loved ones and health professionals. In view of my past illness I would have asked for a regular counselling session or at least explored where there was someone to listen. I have learned that nipping small worries in the bud can limit their growth. Everyone has day-to-day concerns – it is normal human behaviour. Where you feel that your negative thoughts are beginning to restrict your day-to-day functioning, then it is imperative to seek professional help.

Antenatal depression and anxiety can be just as common as postnatal. So ask for help with it. There are many sites to find more information on this – see the links at the end of this chapter. If you do begin to feel unwell, let your healthcare professionals know. If you get pushed back, persevere until someone will listen. These ladies shared these comments:

- When I was pregnant I requested to my GP that I be referred to the perinatal mental health service as I felt I was at risk of becoming mentally unwell. The GP refused and said I would be okay. I managed to find out that I could self-refer to the service. I feel that some GPs and other healthcare professionals have such a lack of knowledge in this area it is scary.
- I was relaxed at the beginning of the pregnancy but fearful in the background that my poor emotional health might happen again. I insisted that I wanted an elective C-section but that ended up not confirming this until around 36 weeks. This caused me considerable stress when I could have been relaxed.
- I became depressed during pregnancy, but I thought it was normal. It would have been useful to know that I could have seen my GP for antenatal checks, seeing the same person may have helped me spot my rapidly declining mood. Also information on what degree of anxiety about pregnancy and childbirth was normal and what you could do to overcome extreme anxiety.

One way to help may be to join a support group, either locally or online. *See* Chapter 21 on peer support.

Boots and Tommy's, along with other major organisations, have devised a five-point wellbeing plan for pregnancy – diet and nutrition; exercise; obesity; smoking; and mental health. They have a free booklet with hints and tips for a healthy pregnancy available.[6] They also offer a free support line for those affected by a miscarriage, premature baby or stillbirth and are anxious about their subsequent pregnancy. Their PregnancyLine midwives are trained to discuss this with women or their families.[7]

In pregnancy the importance of eating well is obvious. A healthy, well-balanced diet is vital to give you the energy both physically and mentally that are needed. The old belief that you are eating for two is not the green light to over-eating. There are many sources for advice on a good diet. Knowing that you are fuelling your body with the best nutrients can build your confidence that you are enabling your unborn child the best start and contributing to their development along with your own wellbeing.

Exercising is another well-documented way to a positive and healthy pregnancy. Having other children can be a bonus here as they are more than willing participants for a walk to the park or going for a swim. Many women find yoga and Pilates ideal exercise too as exercises can be adapted for expectant mothers. *See* Chapter 29 too.

Maternal obesity has become one of the most commonly occurring risk factors in obstetric practice as it can place greater risks to both the health of the baby and mother. The Royal College of Obstetricians and Gynaecologists offer guidelines on this area.[8]

It has been public health knowledge for years that smoking is not recommended during pregnancy; for example, babies tend to have lower birth weight. The NHS provide many guidelines and support to help with smoking cessation.[9]

Recreational drugs and alcohol are also not recommended during pregnancy due to known effects on the baby. Your GP and midwife should be able to offer local support and guidance. In addition you can find help at 'Talk to Frank'[10] and 'Turning Point'.[11]

Sadly domestic violence and abuse affects 15% of pregnant women. Have a look at Best Beginnings[12] for plenty of useful information and sources of help.

Preparation for your new family life can be helpful too. Knowing that you have all the baby equipment in place and sleeping arrangements sorted is useful. Painting a nursery whilst you have a newborn baby and other children is not ideal. Allow the rest of the family to contribute their ideas and help. I shall discuss this aspect more in Chapter 13.

You may find it useful to keep a journal of how you are feeling and ways that you find to make your mind feel more peaceful. Allow yourself the luxury of asking positive 'what if' questions – 'What if I am mentally well this time? What if the birth is a wonderful experience this time? What if I bond amazingly from the start with my newborn this time? What if I really enjoy early motherhood this time? Also consider a mobile phone app, such as 'Mind the Bump' to help your emotional wellbeing.

If you have to work during pregnancy, discuss with your employer the best ways to suit you both. Consider if you can work from home more or change your hours to avoid travelling in peak rush hour public transport or roads. You have a duty to your employer and yourself to remain fit and well during your pregnancy, so discuss how best you can do this. Surely it is better to plan and work at a sensible pace so that you can work until your maternity leave, rather than burn out and go off sick? When you have a day off, ensure that it is! Consider it being like plugging in your phone for a recharge of its battery. By taking regular rests you will have more energy to do what has to be done.

Begin to say 'no' – to yourself, loved ones and at work! There is no need to be a hero. It will be best for you and your baby if you begin to slow down and take the pressure off your usual to do list. If you use a phrase such as 'I would love to do that. My vital task today is XYZ. If you haven't done it by tomorrow, ask me again then.' The chances are that by then they will have done it or asked someone else to.

If finances are a concern, face up to them. Be aware of exactly what you have, what you spend and how much you need. If you have a clear picture and budget, you may find it is better than you thought. Burying your head or even hiding bills is not going to make them go away. Examine where you are able to make savings and apply it.

www.babycenter.com have the following suggestions for pregnancy:

> Limit 'information overload.' Reading pregnancy books, surfing pregnancy Web sites, and listening to your friends' pregnancy stories are fine – but don't delve into all the scary things that might (but probably won't) happen during your pregnancy. Focus instead on how you're feeling and what's happening to you now.

Pregnancy may be a great time to start or continue to use complementary therapies. I am always a big advocate of taking time out for being pampered and relaxing. Reflexology, massage, facials, manicures and pedicures are all excellent as boosts to your energy and confidence – especially as you can begin to feel like a beached whale! Look out for special offers or enquire at a local college about their student training sessions for cheaper treatments. Having your hair styled is wonderful too. One of my friends said that her top tip would be to ensure that you have your hair cut a couple of weeks before your due delivery date – a small detail that may help as it will be one less thing that needs doing when you then have another child!

Some of the ladies under the care of Staffordshire NHS trust have effectively used Emotional Freedom Techniques (EFT), also known as 'tapping' or 'acupuncture without needles'. This is a new and emerging psychological intervention.[13] It is a gentle therapy that has been used for a range of emotional issues related to pregnancy, childbirth and beyond, including tokophobia (fear of pregnancy and childbirth), needle phobia, smoking cessation, antenatal and postnatal depression and anxiety.

Dr Elizabeth Boath, an Academic Psychologist and Associate Professor in Health at Staffordshire University, has published widely in the field of antenatal and postnatal depression, including research at the Parent and Baby Day Unit in Staffordshire. Elizabeth is currently leading UK research into EFT and inspired by her experience in helping antenatal and postnatal women using EFT is seeking research funding to explore its use further. Elizabeth tells me that:

> With EFT, women gently tap with their fingertips on acupressure points (mainly on the head and hands) and relate this to the voicing of specific statements e.g. 'Even though I am scared of getting postnatal depression again …' EFT is simple to teach and easy to use and EFT's motto is 'Try it on anything', so once women have learned EFT it is literally at their fingertips, to use wherever and whenever they need it. So whether you are anxious in the first stages of labour, avoiding seeing the

midwife because you are scared of needles, suffering from morning sickness, trying to give up smoking during pregnancy, or have mastitis, EFT is well worth a try.

Decide to enjoy being pregnant! Remember Mike's comments in Chapter 9? As this will not be your first time, you know that the nine months pass quickly. Savour the situation. You have a choice to make. You can make your own life and all around you miserable if you are drowning in a sea of worry *or* you can choose to be proactive in making it a pleasant experience for all involved. Arrange for fun get-togethers with friends. Watch comedy films and programmes. Listen to uplifting music. Sing out loud (your other child will love this, depending on their age) or even hum in your head. Music helps control cortisol levels that affect our mood.[14]

We all have the internal dialogue of two contradicting voices. We have the negative one that screams all the nasty and glum aspects at us. Then we have the positive, more reassuring one that attempts to convince us that all will be well. Sally Gunnell, the Olympic athlete, says she calls her negative voice her duck. So when it quacks away she can simply tell it to 'Shut the duck up'!

Expect the positive and, just maybe, it will become reality.

TOP TIPS FOR A HAPPY AND HEALTHY PREGNANCY

1. Discuss your anxieties and concerns with others – they may not be able to fix the issues yet by exploring options they may be eased, e.g. your birth fears.
2. Build rest and relaxation into every day.
3. Eat well.
4. Exercise moderately.
5. Be proactive around concerns of obesity, smoking, drugs, alcohol.
6. If you are a victim of domestic abuse or violence, seek help.
7. Prepare for the new routine and practicalities of family life.
8. Keep a journal.
9. Discuss and arrange mutually beneficially work arrangements with your employer.
10. Limit information overload.
11. Tackle financial challenges and rearrange as needed.
12. Use complementary therapies.
13. Be kind to yourself and have fun including the use of music.
14. Silence the internal negative voice.

TOP TIPS FOR HEALTH PROFESSIONALS

1. Be aware of the significant risks to both mother and baby if stress, anxiety and depression are featuring strongly in pregnancy.
2. Know the signs to look out for and the correct questions to ask.
3. Find out what facilities, e.g. support groups or individual counselling, are available in your area.
4. Have a bank of resources for a healthy pregnancy – also be aware of the value of listening to a concerned mother-to-be.

REFERENCES

1. www.beginbeforebirth.org/
2. http://womenshealth.about.com/cs/pregnancy/a/mispregstress_3.htm
3. Music G. Stress pre-birth: how the fetus is affected by a mother's state of mind. *Int J Birth Parent Educ.* 2013; **1**. Available at: http://repository.tavistockandportman.ac.uk/602/1/Music.pdf
4. Jamieson JP, Mendes WB, Nock MK. Improving acute stress responses: the power of reappraisal. *Curr Dir Psychol Sci.* 2012; **22**: 51–6. Available at: http://wendyberrymendes.com/cms/uploads/CDPS_reappraisal-1.pdf
5. http://blog.ted.com/2013/06/11/the-upside-of-stress-kelly-mcgonigal-at-tedglobal-2013/
6. www.tommys.org/page.aspx?pid=1145
7. Freephone 0800 0147 800.
8. www.hqip.org.uk/assets/NCAPOP-Library/CMACE-Reports/15.-March-2010-Management-of-Women-with-Obesity-in-Pregnancy-Guidance.pdf
9. www.nhs.uk/conditions/pregnancy-and-baby/pages/smoking-pregnant.aspx#close
10. www.talktofrank.com/ Tel: 0800 77 66 00.
11. www.turning-point.co.uk/ Turning Point has many years' experience in helping people with drug problems. You can find information on the website, call them up or ask your questions online. Tel: 020 7481 7600.
12. www.bestbeginnings.org.uk/domestic-abuse
13. Craig G. *The EFT Manual.* 2nd ed. Fulton, CA: Energy Psychology Press; 2011.
14. www.expectantmothersguide.com/articles/the-benefits-of-prenatal-music/

FURTHER READING AND RESOURCES

- www.pndsupport.co.uk/what-is-antenatal-depression
- www.netmums.com/pregnancy/pregnancy-problems/stress-and-anxiety-during-pregnancy
- www.webmd.boots.com/pregnancy/guide/pregnancy-depression
- More information and links in my blog www.hanzak.com/2014/06/stress-in-pregnancy.html

- www.hanzak.com/2014/06/stress-in-pregnancy.html
- The National Parent Guide: http://nationalparentguide.co.uk/
- www.nutrimum.co.uk/ ideas and products for optimum nutrition in pregnancy and early motherhood

CHAPTER 12

A different birth experience

Nothing in life is to be feared. It is only to be understood.

Marie Curie

My first and only experience of giving birth began very well. I was so excited to be finally going into labour and knowing that within hours my baby would be born. The pains began on the evening before my due date and when we were advised to go to the hospital, all the boxes were ticked for me to have my baby in the water birth suite. My ideals were all going to plan with the music playing, and simply having gas and air as I laboured in the pool. Nature then took over – my baby was in distress so I had to get out of the pool; after a while he was born naturally although with the cord around his neck so they rushed him away. I had a retained placenta and a postpartum haemorrhage, needing to go to theatre to be repaired. I only held my baby for the first time when I awoke hours later. The full description is in my first book.[1]

I always felt that no one could have prevented what happened to me and that the team did all they could to ensure that we both survived, so I am grateful. The only thing I wish had happened was that at a later date someone had spoken to both of us as parents to explain clearly what had transpired. My ex-husband must have found the whole experience a very terrifying situation where he felt completely helpless. A doctor the following day simply told me that I was lucky to be alive and had the birth been a home one, or 20 years earlier, I would be dead! Regardless of the challenges we had later, this alone could have been the biggest contraception ever for not having another child. The birth experience would not have discouraged me trying for another baby, yet I can appreciate why it might be a huge impact for others.

For many parents who shared their stories with me, the birth was often a huge part of their journey. For some, it was a good experience:

- My delivery was a straightforward normal birth. She arrived quickly and safely.
- Exactly as I'd planned. Home birth, using a birth pool. Wonderful midwives.

- 5 hour active labour, using minimal Entonox. Basically the labour and birth I'd hoped for.
- I had an amazing birth experience, I laboured at home with a tens machine, went into hospital already at 10cm and within 30 minutes and 2 pushes had my baby.

I am sorry to say that the majority of the descriptions of births were not good experiences. I do not feel that it would serve any benefit to reproduce a long list of them here. If you are reading this to contemplate another baby, you know what happened at the previous birth for your child. Maybe it was something like this one:

- Terrible – requested birth pool or epidural, did NOT want to labour without pain relief. Instead, I had a midwife who could barely speak English who refused to check how well I was progressing on the basis that 'it was my first labour' until it was too late for pain relief. It was intense, incredibly painful and very frightening, and ended with my son having to be ventoused (VE) because his heart rate dropped. Post labour I went in to shock in the delivery suite and, instead of being reassured, was left alone on the delivery table not knowing why I was shaking and struggling to breathe and genuinely believing I was dying. No midwife came to reassure me at any point. I had to rely on my mum to hold my hand and put cold flannels on my face to try to bring my raging temperature down. It was the most traumatic experience of my life.

I recommend Kathleen Kendall-Tackett's article called 'Making peace with your birth experience'.[2] She writes, 'If you had a difficult birth experience, you cannot change that. There are, however, a number of positive steps that you can take to help you resolve your experience and heal from it.' These include getting support from others over it; learning and understanding what happened and being aware of the effect on your partner. She also suggests that some women blame themselves with a string of 'if only' scenarios. Kathleen recommends:

Recognise that you did the best you could under the circumstances and with the knowledge you had at the time, and let yourself off the hook!

She ends with:

Recognise that birth is only the beginning of a life-long relationship with your baby. Motherhood is a role you gradually grow in to. A difficult beginning does not need to be the blueprint for the rest of your mothering career. It is important to realise that a negative birth experience can affect your relationship with your baby, but it does not have to. This is why it is vital for you to get the support you need as soon as possible. I have seen mothers who have had difficult births try to make up for it by being 'Super-mom' – to everyone's detriment. It is difficult for anyone (even Super-mom) to be responsive and giving toward an infant or child when she is hurting inside.

Once you have processed what happened previously (we explored this in the earlier chapters), the key aspect is how to maximise the opportunity for what you would like to be a different experience next time. No two births are the same – what you ideally want is a better experience than previously. You no longer have the naivety of the first time. I have used the examples of birth stories shared with me to give me the main areas that parents-to-be can ask for, and for healthcare professionals to be aware of. Let's start by looking at the experiences of others who did go on to have another baby. These are the responses I received in reply to my question 'How did you feel about the birth experience in contrast to the previous time?':

- As planned and expected: 31.82%
- I felt more relaxed: 50.00%
- I knew more about what to expect: 72.73%
- I was more anxious: 9.09%
- I was less anxious: 22.73%
- I found it to be traumatic: 0
- **It was a good experience: 63.4%**

I asked mums what could have made their birth experience(s) better in retrospect. Some felt that there was nothing, as everything was as they expected and the care was good to excellent, whether at home or in a hospital. Another, like me, felt that:

- Doctors did their best and ultimately saved my life but the experience was not as I expected.

Communication was mentioned often. This includes direct interaction, where healthcare professionals listened to parents and offered support; compassion and reassurance including acknowledging that a woman knows her own body best and responding to her needs. Women appreciated midwives and doctors who gave the impression that they cared, gave them correct information and kept them well informed of what was happening. Parents often feel scared and worried about the birth procedures and really appreciate the team members who help to keep them calm. Remember that as a healthcare professional you are joining in with one of the most significant moments in the lives of the people there. It is one of the most intimate experiences a woman can have. I know many midwives who describe it as an honour and privilege to be there and they do get the emotional connection that can make it so much better.

- Friendly midwives that would have made me feel safe and not a burden. I just wanted to feel safe and looked after not terrified and abandoned.
- Having somebody with me through my labour – a midwife. Being looked after and being made to feel like I mattered.
- I feel that better communication from the staff that I came into contact with would have improved my experience. I felt that I was left alone the majority of the time, with contact when they wanted to check progress, or situations changed. As a first time mother, I feel staff should be more supportive and provide clear information.

Communication between the care team was also highlighted as important. This is very relevant where a mum has an existing mental health challenge and appropriate medication is vital.

- Overall the delivery was a good experience. However, my psychiatrist could have visited me instead of me visiting him five days post-delivery. Medication changes were not made until then. By then it was too late.
- Better communication – if mental health support had kept me on my medication even a smaller dose would have been better than nothing

For a birth 'next time round', parents especially feel that continuity of care is important. Where possible, you do not want to go through your history again during labour. It should be clear on your plan to allow you the freedom to relax and enjoy the wonder that giving birth can be.

Time was another area that women commented on. Although most of us would rather have a quick labour, some mothers felt their baby came too quickly! In some instances parents felt alone and scared during labour because staffing levels were so low. On occasion some women were unable to have their desired birthing plan because of problems with equipment or numbers of staff available. I know that I would have felt 'robbed' of the opportunity to use the water birth suite had it been unavailable for whatever reason. It isn't like you can say, 'Okay, we will pop back tomorrow.' You need it now! Others felt they would have preferred more time in hospital prior to discharge.

- Just being sent home was terrifying. Having never had a baby before, I had no idea what to expect.
- Someone to chat about first time mum concerns. I was overwhelmed, but happy to have my daughter.
- Not being left 2 weeks overdue and then to have to endure 37 hours of labour

to end with emergency Caesarean – no one was interested in delivering the baby any quicker.

Some women felt that their birth experience could have been improved if problems had been identified sooner, e.g. that the baby was breech. I remain grateful that my midwife appreciated that Plan A was not happening and immediately called for more members of the team.

Options and availability for pain relief was another area that made a difference to mothers, along with it being administered at the best time, e.g. an earlier epidural. Pain could be a whole book in itself. I admit that I am a wimp when it comes to pain! My brain tells me to say 'Ouch' even before a physical pain that I can see coming, e.g. if I am about to fall, hits my body! I have learned that I can control my pain level much more by keeping calm and, conversely, if I get myself emotionally worked up, it makes everything worse.

Although pain relief is very much wanted, several expressed their desire for the experience to be as natural as possible and therefore access to birthing pools and the use of hypnobirthing were valued, along with 'skin to skin' and a more mobile labour. Nineteen years on I still feel the loss of not having my baby put on me as soon as he was born. It was due to the concerns for his health yet I still am so sorry I missed that magical moment.

- I felt my son's birth was fine, so, although I would have loved a quicker, less medicalised birth, I was okay with what happened.

Some women who have a C-section feel an aspect of failure that they have not delivered their baby naturally, especially if they had a general anaesthetic and 'missed' it all. This is especially the case if it was not an elective section or the birth was traumatic in some way, even if it did not meet your expectations. There is a wealth of information on the website 'Emotional Healing after a Caesarean'.[3,4]

I know that exhaustion was a key impact upon my mental health and that started from labour. I missed a whole night's sleep, then had hours of labour followed by a general anaesthetic and a baby who hardly slept. When he did so, the rest of the ward was so noisy that after three days all I wanted to do was cry. Regardless of the physical trauma my body had endured, the exhaustion added to my vulnerability. I sometimes think that lack of sleep can be underestimated by many, yet it can be used as a form of torture. Whether or not you have a baby at home or in hospital, I feel that good sleep and opportunities to do so are vital. One aspect of hospital routine that has always amazed me is the number of ways to keep you awake or disturb a patient. Being woken up for a cup of tea when rest is so hard to come by; loud and thoughtless visitors; noisy ward bins; staff wearing heavy shoes on night duty and laughing and talking loudly. That's without the babies in the mix!

If I had been pregnant again I would have made every possible request to have a private room for the outset and rested as much as possible if I had to stay in hospital. If you give birth at home, also plan for as much rest as possible around the labour and birth. I would also have listened to advice when recommended to rest.

- Not letting me get so exhausted, making the decision to section earlier.
- Quicker diagnosis of problematic labour and much earlier C-section. Fewer nights of no sleep.

What qualifies as a normal delivery and what is a traumatic birth? Research by Cheryl Beck[5] says that 'Birth trauma lies in the eye of the beholder. Mothers perceived that their traumatic births often were viewed as routine by clinicians.' Most people would agree that my birth experience was traumatic. I agree with a comment made by another mother:

- I strongly believe that women who have experienced traumatic births should be offered a comprehensive, medical de-brief within a reasonable timescale and counselling if necessary.

I certainly felt that I would have appreciated that. I did not want to sue anybody – I simply wanted to know what had happened, and if I ever had another child was it likely to happen again and if so, what could be done to prevent it.

I was lucky that I did bond immediately with my son when I finally held him after I came round from the anaesthetic. I can appreciate why some mothers do not. In the physical detachment and shock of the whole experience I could have easily been convinced that he was not my baby or felt that he was the cause of it all or, as some mothers say, they feel numb to them. Healthcare professionals also need to empathise with these emotions. Remember how I wrote about the difference in states in the communication chapter? Be conscious of being too cheery and gushing about how much the new mother 'must be so thrilled'. If she is not feeling that way it can make her feel even more guilty because she perceives that is what she expected to be. It makes it very hard to admit if you are not experiencing that flood of maternal love. *See* Chapter 14 on bonding.

- To have been supported more to bond initially. I didn't hold Oliver properly for 24 hours and the times I was supported to hold him, it was to try breast feeding which was forced on you the minute you delivered.

Women also want good postnatal care, for example, in basic washing and self-care immediately after the birth and especially after a C-section. The day after the traumatic delivery I had, after all the tubes and monitors were taken off me, I was allowed to have a shower. The midwife who assisted me was amazing. She was so sensitive to the fact I felt my body had been battered. I shall always remember the gentle way she patted my back dry for me and then applied body lotion across my shoulders and down my back – wow! It was a magical, healing touch and so appreciated.

Apart from two people in my survey who had no support, all the other mothers had health professionals who had input into their birth plan based on their past experience. Some of the best examples of good practice included:

1. A team approach to the plan including specialist support, for example, including GP, CPN, psychiatrist, health visitor, social worker:

   - At my insistence I was allocated a specialist midwife and a CPN, and was under consultant care.

2. Empowering and enabling parents to make choices:

   - I had counselling on a regular basis and contact with a named obstetrician who promised me I could elect for a Caesarean at any time as long as I aimed for a natural birth.
   - I insisted on a C-section. This was because neither my partner nor I could face a repeat of the trauma. Instinctively I think I knew this would make the difference.
   - I chose a section – it was my choice and they said that it was fine.
   - I paid for a private obstetrician, who induced me and guaranteed me an epidural.

3. Extra physical care and observations:

   - I had a consultant due to my previous postpartum haemorrhage, and because my nosebleeds were so severe I was advised to have an epidural to reduce active pushing time. I was also being monitored for possible postpartum haemorrhage.
   - I was monitored more and monitored during and after labour.
   - I had to be monitored during labour and in high risk room due to problems with previous birth.

4. Generally concerned attitude and desire to make it a better experience:

   - People were very compassionate about my previous birth and I arranged a home birth so my fears of being abandoned and left couldn't happen again.
   - My consultant was excellent. He discussed hormone patches postnatally and also supported me in my water birth request.

5. Excellent communication is vital:

- One lady commented that healthcare professionals were involved in her birth plan the next time round although the labour ward refused to follow it. Another said she told them about her poor experience with a previous birth yet no one asked further questions. She had no handover from midwives to health visitors and the lady had to tell them herself. As parents be pro-active in expressing your needs.

For many years after the birth of my son I was unable to watch a birth scene on television or even in a film or drama. It used to upset me because I would feel so angry about the trauma of my experience. I have been impressed with some of the relatively new trend of 'fly-on-the-wall' programmes that now show real-life births, e.g. on Channel 4's *One Born Every Minute*. Yet in the majority of those shown it does perhaps appear that the labour and birth process should be in a hospital and that the main emphasis is around pain relief. I wonder if we are encouraging pregnant women to expect the birth to be painful, and therefore it will be? Are we setting them up to expect great vocal outbursts and potential panic over the 'threat' of a C-section?

I remember watching some births that were actually beautiful and calm, where the mother and her partner were so relaxed, and the baby did eventually just 'appear'. One that I especially remember was a stunningly beautifully lady who had even made her own 'birthing' bikini. The whole process was incredibly moving as she breathed and swayed in the dimly-lit water birth suite. That was how I would have wanted my experience next time round! I challenge you to focus on a good birth! One idea might be to buddy up with someone who has already been there. There is a website called 'Tell me a good birth story'[6] where you can read many examples of a lovely birth experience, in a hospital or home, and you can ask to have a buddy. Visualisation of the birth can help, provided the images are positive ones.[7]

Perhaps we also need to manage our expectations of a 'good birth'. I now realise that maybe mine were far too high! Yet that was based on my knowledge of being a first time mother. Had I been pregnant again I would have moderated what I expected to happen. The mothers that responded to my survey expressed a range of comments regarding whether their experiences have been met:

- No. Not what I wanted or expected. I think the staff did their best, though, I felt well cared for but just completely unlucky and cheated of the birth I wanted. And like a failure.
- Yes, everything I wanted and expected happened during my birth with my daughter.

- No not at all. Staff were unhelpful and unfriendly and nobody explained what they were doing and why.
- My expectations were greatly exceeded.
- Yes and no. I had deliberately had low expectations. I had feared I would end up having a Caesarean and was delighted that I didn't. However this was not my planned hypnobirthing experience. In reality I didn't care afterwards, my son was safe and alive, and so was I.

What else may help? You have given birth before so you are probably aware of these or may have dismissed them previously. It may be worth considering them the next time. I know at antenatal classes I was told about the importance of slow and deep breathing, yet that was as far as it went. There is a much bigger focus today on hypnobirthing, where mothers are taught the techniques for deep relaxation, leading to a reduction of pain. Some people find singing helps and also listening to certain music. TENS machines can be helpful where 'four electrode pads are stuck on your back and the machine transmits electrical pulses through your skin. The pulses are designed to stimulate the release of endorphins so your body can cope with the pain using its own hormones. These pulses also stimulate the nerves in your spine so the pain signals are blocked before they reach your brain.'[8]

Some woman hire a doula, who is specifically trained to help them through labour. See http://doula.org.uk/ for one local to you. Specific labour massage can help too.

Kaitlin Rose, in her blog 'Bring birth home',[9] recommends water as an aid to a peaceful birth.

> Using water as pain control during labor has been used for centuries. Immersing one's laboring body into water is amazingly effective in reducing pain. Warm water raises the body temperature causing blood cells to dilate, thus increasing circulation. This lowers a woman's blood pressure and eases inflammation. There are three unique benefits to laboring in water, specifically in a whirlpool tub – heat, buoyancy and massage.

I was extremely impressed when I read Debby Gould's book *Welcoming Baby*[10] as I believe her approach is one that I would have adhered to. I strongly encourage both practitioners and women to consider her suggestions. I am delighted that she agreed to share some in the following pages (pp. 131–5):

> Midwives need to be embracing their role as advocates and healers to support women, to deliver safe, compassionate care **and** actively seek to anticipate and work to alleviate maternal anxieties, including unstated anxieties. The role of the midwife is to help women recognise and access their own inner resources to help

with the physical, emotional and psychological challenges that childbirth and motherhood bring.[10]

According to Griffin and Tyrell[11] there are six emotional areas which must be met to create a sense of health and wellbeing. These are security; attention; connection; community; status; meaning and purpose. These are discussed in more detail in relation to maternity care in Debby Gould's *Welcoming Baby*.[10] However, here are some summarised thoughts on the first three, which seem to relate to the immediate birth environment for women.

1. SECURITY, OR RATHER A SENSE OF 'FEELING SAFE'

Feeling 'safe' during pregnancy and childbirth is paramount, and the midwives' role is to help keep mother and baby safe within a holistic compassionate caring model. Being 'safe' in labour and childbirth in the UK relies in the most part on the clinical competence and communication between the midwives and doctors caring for women. The importance of the role of the midwife linked to a wider multidisciplinary team is summarised by the saying 'Every woman needs a midwife and some need a doctor too.'[12]

Whilst 'feeling safe' is linked to a feeling of being in control, involving being listened to and having any concerns raised taken seriously, having evidence-based, understandable information is also a prerequisite to quality care. Good information is powerful, it can to help allay anxiety and enable women to make decisions appropriate to them. Women need access to information about care and what to expect in labour and birth, including what may happen to their body, mind and emotions during birth and an understanding of the different body sensations that women can expect to feel during birth. Midwives need to incorporate this into their daily practice and women need to be aware to ask about this to help prepare them for labour and early motherhood.

Websites like www.which.co.uk/birth-choice help women to find the right place for them to give birth and understand their birth options better. Here women can learn how they can shape their birth experience and find the best place for their needs. This website enables women to access evidence-based information on choice of place of birth, and submit information about them regarding what type of birth they would like and their previous birth experiences, and then it will give individualised suggestions for what might best suit them.

For many women childbirth is a time of heightened sensory experience. Information accessed through the senses bypasses conscious thinking and triggers fast-acting emotional responses. Therefore understanding personal emotional responses plays a crucial role in affording a greater sense of control.

One way to increase understanding and control of emotional responses, especially the fear-based responses of fright, flight and freeze, is to practise deep relaxation during the antenatal period. There are many ways to get deep relaxation training, it can be one to one face to face, in groups, or for personal use by listening with headphone to CDs and downloads. Even if women are planning an elective Caesarean section for their birth, these relaxation exercises will help them.

The three aspects of deep relaxation, understanding of physiology and body sensations and positive visualisation are fundamental to 'hypnobirthing' techniques and need to be a part of every midwife's skill set to share with women.

If you are a midwife reading this, try asking women: 'What matters to you?' and 'What would make you feel safe and secure?' If you are a woman reading this, relax and just let your mind drift and then ask yourself the same questions. What comes into your mind may surprise you but it may be a small thing that can make a big difference and it is worth a try.

These questions need to be explored in an open and non-judgemental way; it is important to withhold judgement as no one can know what is best for someone else. If you are a woman doing this exercise alone or with your planned birth partner or family, also be gentle with yourself and take time to let your deep subconscious percolate the answers gently to the surface. What you thought you wanted initially may not be what you discover you really want when you are deeply relaxed and just letting thoughts come and go, or alternatively it will confirm to you what you intended.

Another way to think about this is the metaphor of a birth library rather than a birth plan, which sounds so prescriptive and can lead to connotations of failure. Build a metaphorical library of things you might like to try. If what you choose first doesn't suit at the time, just let it go and try something else. This library metaphor helps to deal with the uncertainty that surrounds labour and childbirth by offering alternative options (and note that this list is just to get you thinking – it is by no means exhaustive):

- **Options to help coping in labour:** it is worth thinking about putting in your library deep breathing, relaxation, massage, music – different types, relaxation audio, singing, silence, bath, shower, birth pool, visualisation with and without pictures, medication and epidural (these may vary depending on individual circumstances, and choice and discussion around strategies for coping in labour should include the advantages, disadvantages and appropriateness of interventions for the individual woman).
- **Options for place of birth:** home, midwife-led and labour ward.
- **Options in relation to the 'golden hour' following birth, those precious early moments with your new baby:** skin to skin, getting to know your baby, making eye contact, friends and family involvement, photographs.

Thinking about these questions is a great starting point to help women explore what might be relaxing for them, what might make them feel more safe, secure and confident, which in turn will help the labour go well and adjustment to motherhood easier. It can also can open the door for greater individualised care, and foster honest conversations about personal anxieties and what can best be done to alleviate them.

2. ATTENTION: TO FEEL EMOTIONALLY CONNECTED TO OTHERS WE NEED TO GIVE AND RECEIVE ATTENTION

'Attention is an essential nutrient to wellbeing' (Gould, p 171).[10] By giving and receiving attention (genuine praise and flattery relating to what we are doing well), humans are able to emotionally connect. During such connection we suspend the critical consciousness of our minds. This suspension of critical consciousness enables us to receive new information deep into our subconscious, offering an opportunity to build confidence and self-esteem.

Midwives need to take time to talk and 'connect', i.e. the giving and receiving of attention, to maximise this power of reciprocity to build rapport rapidly with women and their birth partners.

Helping women and their partners to understand that their relationship with their newborn baby is also based on each other giving and receiving, is also likely to help this relationship develop better, irrespective of the circumstances of a complicated birth outcome.

3. CONNECTION

Building on the concept of reciprocal attention for bonding and confidence building, the wider sense of connection is important to human wellbeing. Fragmented care from multiple different healthcare providers serves to act as a disconnect between women and their families and healthcare professionals and can make some women feel more vulnerable. For women who already feel vulnerable after a difficult previous birth or for any other reason, it is worth exploring whether there is an opportunity to be cared for by a known midwife or group of midwives throughout pregnancy and childbirth, as there is evidence that women receiving this care have less chance of epidural, instrumental birth and episiotomy and greater satisfaction in the birth experience.[13]

Practical tips
Authentic self
Keep your own clothes on for as long as possible. Whilst it may seem attractive to use hospital-provided clothing because you will not have to 'wash' it afterwards, as many women say, keeping your own clothing preserves your identity and individuality within hospital environments. Maintaining your own identity increases the chances of you receiving individualised care, important for a sense of control and self-esteem.

Ditch the birth plan, but plan a birth journey

Think of your labour as a journey and part of the larger part of life, a sacred journey to becoming a mother, which may not take the exact route you planned, but plan anyway. Think of your birth plan as you would a birth library, with a whole host of things you can try to put back if they do not suit you, but with a list of what you might like to try first. Remember it is a woman's prerogative to change their mind. There is no such thing as failure in childbirth. Sometimes some women need more help than they or others originally anticipated, and that is okay. There certainly is no failure in asking and/or receiving help in childbirth.

Think of sensory elements (remember sensory elements are linked to the emotions and so can increase or reduce stress and this applies to everyone in the birth environment) that may help you relax, for instance water, music, singing and smells, and maximise the chance of that happening. Also think about what might irritate or make you feel anxious and do your best to minimise the chance of these things occurring.

Have a birth partner you trust. A woman is very helpful in the birth environment. You can have more than one.

Use of water in labour

Remember that the use of immersion in water is a great pain relief for labour but it may not suit all women. The use of birth pools for labour is endorsed for healthy women with uncomplicated pregnancies by the National Institute for Health and Care Excellence.[14] Birth pools are a really good option for women to try, and this is a mainstream possibility for women with uncomplicated pregnancies, not just for women committed to 'natural' childbirth. Once in it you do not need to stay in it, you can get in and out as you wish until the baby's head is visible. At this point if you raise the baby's head out of the water you must stay out.

Being flexible and realistic in your expectations and being aware that they will have been influenced by a previous birth will help you to manage them and the next birth. The saying 'hope for the best and be prepared for the worst' comes to mind, along with embracing different strategies to go through the process.

REFERENCES

1. Hanzak EA. *Eyes Without Sparkle: a journey through postnatal illness*. London: Radcliffe Publishing; 2005.
2. www.uppitysciencechick.com/making_peace.pdf
3. www.vbac.com/emotional-healing-after-a-cesarean/
4. www.plus-size-pregnancy.org/CSANDVBAC/csemotionalrecov.htm#The%20Import ance%20of%20Emotional%20Preparation%20for%20Birth%20After%20Cesarean

5. Beck CT. Birth trauma: in the eye of the beholder. *Nurs Res.* 2004; **53**(1): 28–35. Available at: www.ncbi.nlm.nih.gov/pubmed/14726774

6. http://tellmeagoodbirthstory.com/

7. www.givingbirthnaturally.com/women-giving-birth.html

8. www.dailymail.co.uk/health/article-1367240/How-I-remained-drug-free-labour--honestly-didnt-hurt-much.html

9. http://m.cafemom.com/groups/read_topic.php?group_id=14077&topic_id=13309546 (accessed 3 June 2015).

10. Gould, D. *Welcoming Baby: reflections on perinatal care.* Chester le Street: Fresh Heart Books; 2011.

11. Griffin J, Tyrrell I. *Human Givens: the new approach to emotional health and clear thinking.* Hailsham: Human Givens Publishing; 2003.

12. Shribman, S. *Making it Better: for mother and baby.* London: Department of Health; 2007.

13. Sandall J, Soltani H, Gates S, *et al.* Midwife-led continuity models versus other models of care for childbearing women. *Cochrane Database Syst Rev.* 2013; **8**: CD004667.

14. National Institute for Health and Care Excellence. *Intrapartum Care: care of healthy women and their babies during childbirth.* London: NICE; 2014.

FURTHER READING AND RESOURCES

- http://birthtalk.org have a look for their book due out in 2015.
- http://birthwithoutfearblog.com Birth Without Fear began as a simple passion to let women know they have choices in childbirth. It then evolved to become an inspiration and support to women and their families through their trying to conceive, pregnancy, birth and postpartum journeys.

CHAPTER 13

Early days with the new baby

Motherhood has taught me the meaning of living in the moment and being at peace. Children don't think about yesterday, and they don't think about tomorrow. They just exist in the moment.

Jessalyn Gilsig

On reflection, when I had my baby, I attempted far too much of everything in those early days of motherhood. I did not allow myself time to adjust to the physical demands that labour has on a body, especially the added complications I had. I subsequently discovered the research that implies that ladies who suffer postpartum haemorrhage,[1] as I had, could be at higher risk of developing postnatal depression. Complications from postpartum haemorrhage include orthostatic hypotension (a form of low blood pressure that happens when you stand up from sitting or lying down), anaemia and fatigue, which may make maternal care of the newborn more difficult. Postpartum anaemia increases the risk of postpartum depression.[2] They also should have extra rest due to the considerable blood loss and shock. I made no allowance for the extra demands of breastfeeding, the disturbed sleep and a whole new life! Looking back, I set myself a ridiculous schedule. Readers of my story tell me that at times they have shouted out loud 'Stop it!' as I recalled the endless list of activities I did. On rereading it myself, I can see exactly why.

In those early days of motherhood I felt various pressures. There was the time element because my maternity leave was shrinking with every second that passed. I was aware I had four months to be organised with my baby and our new family and then be ready to return to teaching full time. As an individual and as a couple we did like our surroundings to be organised. Neither of us made any allowance for a new baby in this. I also had wanted this baby so much that I was over-anxious to ensure that family life was the utopia I had always dreamed of. My childhood reading of Enid Blyton stories of 1950s, middle-class, English life was my blueprint. In all honesty I never wanted to be a working mum and I would have loved to have stayed at home. My personal high expectations of myself led to me feeling I was failing. Not an emotion I was used to or liked. Part of this too was to push away all offers of help instead of feeling that I had to do it all.

I felt the unnecessary need to impress all the visitors, who are an understandable part of a new addition to a family. They wouldn't have cared if the cushions weren't straight or that the baby's socks didn't match his T-shirt. I should have been more honest if I was tired or needed rest rather than being concerned with being a great hostess. I should have put a note on the doorbell when I was resting to explain the need for being undisturbed. It does concern me these days that new mothers are in and out of hospital within hours and then immediately have to face a stream of well-meaning visitors, when really their priority should be to themselves, their newborn baby, other children and partner. Next time round my key tip would be to be assertive to those around you and those caring for you to ensure what you feel will be best for your mental health is done. Those who love you will want to do their best to ensure your good health. I will say more on this in Chapter 20 on family and friends.

As a health professional, consider your role in the early days post-delivery. What support are you able to offer? Would you be able to set up extra practical support, e.g. by Home-Start?[3] How can you reassure the parents? How can you arrange for time for any post-birth debriefing? How quickly can you get appropriate treatment, if it is needed?

Had I gone on to have another baby I would have approached these early days differently. I asked other mothers if their prior experience of postnatal illness helped or hindered their understanding of their emotions the next time. Many commented that it had made them more aware of potential problems, a willingness to ask for help and to access treatment, if needed, sooner. Other comments included:

- I was very well prepared and everyone was looking out for me this time.
- I was far more aware of what I was feeling and was able to access treatment much earlier.
- I was paranoid I didn't have same emotions after birth and maybe I didn't bond so quickly. I do keep telling myself it's not as bad as last time and compare the last time with this time. I am more alert to the fact and I am able to spot the signs/behaviour sooner. Sometimes I can hold back my behaviour now and can see the triggers coming and avoid situations.
- To begin with, despite my very serious ill health, I was much, much better. I felt totally attached to my baby, loved him from the moment I saw him and didn't feel removed from reality like I had before. I was so happy to be alive and not be seriously depressed!
- My previous experience and knowledge hindered me, as I constantly worried about being ill again. I was so frightened about not sleeping that I couldn't sleep

but I did have a number of positive moments this time in the early days where I felt normal for a short period but this didn't last sadly.

- Helped, as I knew I had suffered with pre and postnatal depression with my previous pregnancy I was more able to recognise the symptoms and put a plan in place to cope. My husband was able to recognise this was out of my control and not due to his actions.
- I knew this one was how it was meant to be. I loved him from the moment I set eyes on him.
- I found it difficult to know the difference between 'normal' sad days and symptoms of the illness. As such, I overanalyse every emotion.
- Made me more vigilant.
- It made me more aware and more relaxed. I knew I had to leave housework etc. and not panic over silly things e.g. so what if the washing isn't done today – it'll be there tomorrow.
- I did not have this dark cloud feeling. I was elated, happy to hold and deal with my new baby – not frightened.
- I thought they helped – I realised quite how ill I had been and felt quite empowered that I wasn't making it up and was coping so well with two.
- I knew exactly what was going on, what to expect and how to look after myself. As a result, I was mostly absolutely fine. No, better – I was very happy as a new mum and a mum of two :)

These comments are understandable. Of course I love the positive ones. We must also learn from those who felt their prior experience influenced the next one in a less helpful way. There is the theory that you become what you think about. Therefore that if you are very sensitive to every slight dip in your mood, can you actually convince yourself that you are going to be ill again? I found in the years after postnatal depression that I could panic if I had an 'off' day, thinking it indicated the start of mental illness again. The approach is to keep emotions in perspective. Everyone has periods of feeling tired, flat and out of sorts. If that happens in the early days, go with the flow. Have your 'feel good' resources (*see* Chapters 29 and 30) and indulge in them. Nip the panic in the bud, and unless these feelings become regular or very severe, let them pass. Acknowledge the triggers then do something to avoid or stop them escalating. Perhaps the approach could be to:

Expect the best, prepare for the worst.

In my survey, one third of my respondents remained mentally well after having their next baby. That is great!

- Last pregnancy I got PND when my son was 8 weeks old. My daughter is now 11 weeks old and I am well!

One mum described her subsequent postnatal period:

- My mood began to become more labile over the next few weeks. I would cry a lot but also felt almost invincible – I was alive, I had two children, I WAS NOT DEPRESSED! I started cleaning a lot (I don't do that normally!) and walking MILES every day with the double buggy (despite having massively low iron levels even after 4 blood transfusions). I constantly asked people 'do you think I'm okay? This isn't like last time is it!?' I held a big 3rd birthday party for my first son in the house – I remember crying randomly and laughing and talking very fast. I was getting quite manic. Then BOOM I woke up one day and it was like I suddenly felt I was about to die. Filled with panic. The Perspex screen between me and reality was back. I could barely function. I was lying on the floor feeling like I was falling. I called the Samaritans and they said I needed to talk to someone! I was like 'err hello that's what I am doing!' It was the weekend and nothing else was open. On the Monday I saw my GP and was admitted to the Mother and Baby Unit where I spent October to December. I made a very good and full recovery but the guilt I felt about leaving my first son at home while I took my baby with me was horrific.

The others who were affected again generally felt that it was not as severe next time. They recognised the signs, took medication (if appropriate) and were treated. For example:

- It's not as bad – I think CBT is helping. It's hard for people to understand. One family member has even criticised and said it's all in my head. I worry maybe because it happened before I'm making myself ill again.
- A brief episode at 7 months postnatal – very quickly treated by CPN and GP – increased meds.
- It was similar but different. Sleeplessness but crushing sadness about my elder child. I felt like I was selfish for wanting another child and putting her through me being ill.
- To a lesser extent, as I had strategies to deal with the things I knew triggered negative feelings but still had lows, just less than in the first pregnancy.
- I had postnatal anxiety which would probably have led to depression if I hadn't taken antidepressants so soon.
- I did but I feel it was baby blues. And although I began to feel depressed again, I feel this was owing to external factors in my life at the time.

Several mothers have said that the next time round the change is not as massive as the first time as a new parent. The transition into becoming a family has already been made. You have got used to the fact a child is now a huge part of your life. Routines, behaviours and lifestyle adjustments have been reset accordingly. Also the realisation that the newborn stage is so short-lived. I never understood the well-meaning comment by a passer-by who looked in the pram at my newborn and said, 'Ooh, make the most of it. These days don't last long.' In many ways I was too concerned and watchful of the next stage of development rather than just relishing the here and now. I like to think that second time around I would have been far more relaxed about everything. One mum said that following her subsequent pregnancy her advice to new mums would be, 'Don't take the cards down until you are ready to dust!' Remember and acknowledge that you now have a new family structure and everyone involved has a whole range of changes to adjust to. We will look at these in later chapters, e.g. Chapter 17 about siblings.

First time round I had read all the books and felt I was well prepared. Had I been through another birth I may well have revisited all the advice from a new perspective of knowledge. There are some tips that are worth repeating, e.g. have the freezer well stocked; avoid other big changes in your life around the time of the birth. I mention them again as reminders. This time there will be the added organisation needed for childcare for your existing child or children. Identify areas that you know may be a trigger or area of concern and plan ways to reduce it. You may find some of the ideas at www.postpreg-nancywellness.com helpful.

I would like to mention again here about remembering to be grateful for what you do have in your life. In our modern, Western world we take so much for granted and 'expect' that good health is almost a human right. We perhaps need to remind ourselves that not so many decades ago (and still in some parts of the world) many women and babies did not survive childbirth. In the early days postnatally, if infection happened, they may not have survived either. So if you are feeling physically and/or emotionally unwell in the early days after delivery, please take comfort and strength in knowing that we have come a long way medically as a society. We may complain about too few resources yet we still have so much more than some nations. I say again to be kind, gentle and patient with yourself and those around you. You have every chance of making a full recovery (like the lady described above). Have faith and confidence that you will come through. You have, after all, been responsible for the miracle of nature in creating a new life. Focus on those special new 'moments' of being with your new family.

If for whatever reason you are away from your new baby, I would like to share this situation shared by a new mother as appreciation and as a tip for healthcare professionals:

- When I was admitted to the psychiatric unit (PU) it was for one night only. Our baby was taken away from me as there was no room in the MBU. That night, the health team wanted my husband to get some rest so suggested our daughter had a night on the nursery ward at the Women's hospital. The staff on the nursery ward started a lovely scrap book of our daughter – photos mainly. They didn't know how long we would be separated and it would provide me with an update, chance to 'keep in touch', see her progress etc. so I didn't feel I had missed out. It was a lovely touch and as I was only in the PU overnight, there wasn't much in it but I still cherish looking at those few photos and the write-up that the nurses, midwives etc. did for us in that little book. In summary, this 'memory scrap book' means a lot to any mum separated from her baby. Nice touch and very thoughtful.

Knowing the risk factors around postnatal illness, especially those identified by Kathleen Kendall-Tackett,[4] I would have done my best to minimise those applicable to the early days post-delivery and acted quickly in a subsequent one. First time round I allowed stress to build up, e.g. in my need to be perfect. I ignored the need for rest and sleep. I let pain, e.g. from mastitis, to build up. Some ladies do suffer from birth tears or effects to their continence.[5] If you are affected, tell someone. I never dealt with the trauma of the birth.

I would have considered the question 'What can I do differently and better?' next time and put a plan in place. What do you need to consider in your situation?

TOP TIPS FOR YOUR EARLY DAYS POST-DELIVERY

1. Expect the best, prepare for the worst. Consider what worked well last time, what helped, what did not.
2. Be kind to yourself. Remember that your body has been through a major experience, even if the birth was without complications. Adjust your personal expectations to a realistic level.
3. Remind family and friends that in those first few weeks you need time to adjust and to keep visits to a minimum.
4. Plan for easing day to day tasks as much as possible for this time when you are pregnant, e.g. fill the freezer with quick, easy and nutritious meals.
5. Live for the moment. Those newborn days pass so quickly. Spend time simply being with your new baby, other children and loved ones. The dusting will always be there – the precious early days will not.
6. The tendency will be to want to compare everything with 'last time'. Keep this in perspective. No two pregnancies, birth experience of child are the same. No matter what, it will be different this time.
7. If you have any pain, deal with it quickly, e.g. by contacting your GP or midwife.
8. Remember the importance of rest and sleep (*see* Chapter 16).
9. Seek advice and support with feeding (*see* Chapter 15).
10. If you have issues around the birth that were not dealt with immediately post-delivery, ensure that you ask for the opportunity to talk it over with a health professional to understand what happened and how you felt.

TOP TIPS FOR HEALTH PROFESSIONALS EARLY DAYS POST-DELIVERY

1. Reassure, support and respect the concerns of the mother and her family.
2. Ask questions regarding any aspects of pain and take appropriate action.
3. Refer for additional support, e.g. Home-Start.
4. Check that any anxieties are taken seriously and listen to what the mother tells you, taking appropriate steps where needed.
5. Ensure that any challenges around feeding are dealt with (*see* Chapter 15).
6. Check that any remaining issues around the birth experience have been covered.

REFERENCES

1. Anderson JM, Etches D. Prevention and management of postpartum hemorrhage. *Am Fam Physician.* 2007; **75**(6): 875–82. Available at: www.aafp.org/afp/2007/0315/p875.html
2. Corwin EJ, Murray-Kolb LE, Beard JL. Low haemoglobin level is a risk factor for postpartum depression. *J Nutr.* 2003; **133**: 4139–42. Available at: www.ncbi.nlm.nih.gov/pubmed/14652362
3. www.home-start.org.uk/
4. Kendall-Tackett K. (2007) The central role of inflammation and how breastfeeding and anti-inflammatory treatments protect maternal mental health. *LEAVEN.* 2007; **3**: 50–53. Available at: www.lalecheleague.org/llleaderweb/lv/lvjulaugsep07p50.html
5. Williams A, Herron-Marx S, Carolyn H. The prevalence of enduring postnatal perineal morbidity and its relationship to perineal trauma. *Midwifery.* 2007; **23**(4): 392–403. Available at: www.sciencedirect.com/science/article/pii/S0266613806000179

CHAPTER 14

Bonding with your baby

Parents have the glorious opportunity of being the most power-ful influence, above and beyond any other, on the new lives that bless their homes.

L Tom Perry

Pregnancy, birth and early parenthood are often a roller-coaster of emotions. I remember going through a whole range of feelings – sometimes two extremes at the same time. When I finally held my newborn son, after I came round from surgery, I felt so relieved that I was alive and then to finally have him in my arms was like every single Christmas and birthday present had come at once. As I explored his tiny fingers and toes I did feel that rush of maternal love that I expected. He was *my* baby – the one I had always wanted and loved, before he was even conceived. I did feel like the lady in this quote:

Before you were conceived I wanted you; Before you were born I loved you, Before you were here an hour I would die for you. This is the miracle of life.

Maureen Hawkins

By the time he was four months old and he was so ill in hospital, I thought my heart would break and would have done anything to suffer his pain for him, if I could have done. Three months later I was a gnat's whisker away from seriously hurting him, or worse, finally yelling 'get that thing out of my house'. On his first Christmas Day my son was referred to Social Services as a child 'at risk' because I had shaken him 'to shut that bag of bones up'. It is a fair comment to say that although I bonded initially, that bond was severed. I shall mention more on child protection issues in due course.

Being admitted to a psychiatric hospital without him was initially a relief because I was so exhausted and had crumbled into puerperal psychosis – I could not look after my own needs, let alone a baby. For a few weeks I had to focus on myself in order to function again. Increasingly I wanted to be with him and it wasn't long before the bond was rebuilt. The most amazing method of bonding that happens with breastfeeding had been forced to stop due to our separation. That could never be restored and has always left a sadness in me. My experience did show me how it is possible to feel a distance from your own child and therefore I can empathise with those who do not feel that initial surge of love. Very often this is part of perinatal mental illness, as the guilt that this may also bring adds to all the negative thoughts and feelings. I know how ashamed I felt of my awful emotions about my son for that period.

Had I become a mother again, I would not have taken for granted that I would have felt that initial attachment next time. Of course I would have hoped for it, yet now I know ways that can help if needed.

The mothers in my survey also shared myriad emotions in those initial days of motherhood, following either their first or subsequent delivery. Again, I present these so that you will be able to recognise that your experience is likely to have been shared by others:

- I was elated but also in shock and overwhelmed. I was so exhausted it was difficult to feel anything other than tired.
- I was excited but also very nervous as I already had a 3 year old and no family or friends around to help.
- I was already a mum and loving it. This time it felt somewhat different although I loved her I didn't feel like she was mine … it was a very strange feeling.
- I hated it and felt I had made the biggest mistake of my life. As soon as she was delivered I felt repulsed by her and wanted someone to take her away.
- Felt bad that I didn't feel the urge of love that others spoke about but thought I must be tired and it would come in time – just didn't expect it to be 2 years later!
- I was nervous about how I would cope with 2 children, terrified that I would get ill again. But I felt close to the baby immediately.
- I felt very overwhelmed at having 2 children under 2. I was worried my other children would think I didn't love them anymore.
- Like many mums I expected that rush of love when I first had my baby and to look at her with everything feeling perfect. But I didn't and I think mums should be more prepared that it doesn't always happen.
- Deflated – I didn't feel the overwhelming bond/love I expected.
- I hated it. I felt like my whole life had been taken from me, with no benefit. I felt nothing for my baby and hoped he would die so that I could return to normal.
- Good – excited – pleased he was here.
- I felt panicked, overwhelmed and lost. It felt like I had been given an alien to look after, with no instructions, help, support or assistance – a bit like being chucked into the ocean without a life aid.
- I felt very anxious and could not relax – or sleep. I was constantly questioning my abilities and had no confidence.
- Surprised – expected a huge gush of emotions but didn't have that. Was slower, more gradual.

- Elation, total and utter happiness and a feeling of completeness.
- Great, I never had any problems. I'm a natural mother.
- At first stressful, then blessed.
- Loved my baby. Delighted to have her with me. Felt well and elated in spite of difficult labour.
- I felt no bond with my son, but I had been warned that many women didn't. I was handed my son, and my husband was crying, and all I just kept thinking was that my stitches were killing me and I wanted to sleep. I looked at my son and felt nothing.
- I felt I had completely ruined my life at the same time as feeling an overwhelming respect and responsibility for my baby. I was terrified.
- A little overwhelmed to assume the responsibility but generally confident and easy going.
- Awesome.
- I was excited as I had waited 10 years to have a 2nd baby.

Fifty-five per cent of the mothers who responded to my survey felt that they bonded initially with their baby, the others did not. Some felt a connection at the first scan; first kick; first gaze with their child – or much later. Sometimes their feelings changed over time.

- At first but then grew to not like him.
- I felt emotionally dead – I felt no connection at all. I couldn't believe he wasn't dead. He was 5 months when I saw him and thought 'OH MY GOD YOU ARE MY BABY! WOW!'
- To be honest, I'm not sure, I guess I just felt kind of in shock.
- It's strange to try and explain, I never got this rush of love like people say. I didn't hate this baby I just didn't really want this baby but didn't want to harm or anything bad to happen to it. I just felt numb.
- I loved him but I didn't feel anything positive at all. I felt very respectful and seen by him, if that is bonding.
- In part, I did feel damaged and resentful although I love her from the outset.
- I don't think I had the chance as I was still recovering from birth when she ended up in incubator and then couldn't hold her for a few days. Then I was too scared to pick her up after what happened.
- I breastfed him every 4 hours on the dot in hospital then put him back in the crib and turned to face the other way.
- I definitely loved him, but I was so tired and so afraid of doing something wrong that I couldn't enjoy him at all.
- Struggled to breastfeed and I was physically unwell and felt unable to look after her.
- I was waiting for a bond, for some sort of connection and it just wasn't there.
- I distinctly remember (despite being so tired that I fell asleep while they stitched

me up) thinking 'kiss him, that's how you are meant to react' but really not caring about him at all.

Increasingly the media are raising awareness around bonding and hopefully will begin to reduce the stigma that is often felt by those affected.[1] As a healthcare professional you are in a position to reassure parents that if they do not feel that initial bond with their baby, there are ways to help. It does not mean they are bad parents.

Attachment and bonding were described by psychiatrist John Bowlby as a 'lasting psychological connectedness between human beings'.[2] There is a great deal of research that illustrates that a secure bond between a child and their caregiver impacts upon the child's development. Likewise, if a baby appears not to respond in a way that a depressed mother may want them to, this can add to mutual distress.[3] For example, a baby may be fretful because they can pick up on their mother's anxiety and/or lack or response – this in turn can be interpreted by the mother as meaning that they are ineffective or unloved.

The good news is that even if the initial bond is not created and develops over time with the mother, as long as the child is getting its needs met by other caregivers, their attachment learning processes will not be affected in the long term. They will know that if they respond in a certain way, e.g. crying, their needs will be met promptly and they will learn to trust and feel confident and secure – key elements of secure attachment. As time goes by, the mother may begin to feel a heightened level of commitment to their child and take greater joy in being with them. The crucial aspect is for the baby to be in a safe environment where its needs are consistently gratified by adults.

Bonding is important because children with secure early attachments are more likely in later years to be better at solving problems and conflicts; be more self-reliant, adaptable and form good friendships; have a more empathetic nature and have higher self-confidence and self-esteem. The opposite is more likely to be true for those children with anxious attachments, for example, less emotionally healthy, be socially withdrawn from peers. Studies suggest that the usual emotional upsets and quickly resolved anxieties that occur in all pregnancies do not harm the baby emotionally, but major emotional disturbances and unresolved crises throughout the pregnancy may lead to emotionally troubled children.

So let's explore some ways that can help you to bond with your baby – this can actually start when you are pregnant. I know that this can be especially difficult if the baby was not planned for or if you had difficulties previously.

WHAT CAN YOU DO PRENATALLY TO BOND WITH YOUR BABY?

We now know that babies can feel, hear, see, remember and think before birth, so it therefore makes sense to strengthen the bond you share as early as you can. Research shows that a growing foetus has the emotional and intuitive capabilities to sense their parents' love.[4]

I was aware of some of these ideas when I was pregnant yet I confess I felt silly even talking to my unborn son! Now I am wiser, it is something I would actively encourage – even if just in your own, private times. I include these ideas in case, like me, it did not occur to you in a previous pregnancy that they could help the emotional wellbeing of all concerned. We know that when a mother is upset and her heart rate is changed, the baby responds accordingly. Likewise, if you can find time and space to relax together, this is great to build the emotional bond. If you are aware of the developmental milestones of your growing child you will be able to adapt the sensory stimuli accordingly – www. beginbeforebirth.org/ is a useful resource for this.

1. Create a special bonding time on a daily basis – this could involve the father, siblings and any significant others too (*see* later Chapters 18, 20, 21). Put your feet up, breathe slowly and deeply and talk to your baby about what you may be going on to share with them, either now or in the future. Your bath time may also be ideal to really relax. Reassure them that they are loved and how excited you will be to meet. Think positive thoughts – Navajo women are not even allowed to speak of bad things when they are pregnant because of the direct negative impact it has on the baby. It is also important to put your emotions into perspective. I am not naively saying that you should become the image of a 'New Earth' mother who floats through life – we all have off days! Acknowledge that and find ways to make the next one better.

2. Music is an excellent way to stimulate your baby. The best music is that which mimics the 60 beats a minute of the mother's heart rate. Classical music such as Mozart and Vivaldi are ideal and most lullabies are at this beat. Sing yourself too and when your baby is born they are likely to feel soothed and relaxed by the same songs. Look out for the new CD by Jennie Muskett, *With You in the World*.[5]

3. Perhaps keep a journal of your positive hopes and dreams for the life with your future child. One day you will be able to share it with them so that they know they were loved even at this stage.

4. Read to your baby. I confess I used to think that this sounded daft! Yet they can hear you and it can help you relax. As you listen or read, add movement such as patting, stroking, rocking, swaying, or any other rhythmic response. Have a look for some suggestions at http://belly-books.com/ and their blog at The Reading Womb.[6] An older child will enjoy this too (depending on how old they are).

5. Talk to your baby throughout the day to tell them what you are doing, for example. Wish them good morning and say goodnight. It is your voice they will respond and turn to more when they are born.

6. Have a 3D ultrasound scan. These are now amazing images that will help

you appreciate that you have a new little being inside you. Often seeing the actual facial features can really help.

7. You can play a game with a torch for your baby to 'see' and follow the light. This is like the images you see if you close your eyes and look to a light source. www.disneybaby.com/blog/fun-ways-to-interact-with-unborn-baby/

8. Touch and massage are excellent ways to connect. Play games by pressing on your abdomen gently and feeling the baby kick back. Touch your stomach as much as you can, gently massage oil over your lower abdomen. This will help to form a connection to your baby by feeling her move in your tummy and also help to prevent possible stretch marks!

9. Pregnancy yoga, swimming and Pilates may all be great ways to encourage bonding.

10. You may find a phone app that helps guide you, e.g. www.bestbeginnings. org.uk/phone-apps Mind the Bump, www.mindthebump.org.au/

PREMATURE BABY

Tommy's charity have produced a guide for parents who have been told they are at risk of having a premature baby or those who have already had a premature baby. It explains premature birth, giving causes and risk factors as well as information on everything parents can do to avoid it and how medical teams will try to help avoid it. It also covers the baby's time in hospital and what parents need to know going home with their new baby.[7] They have also produced an app.[8] Healthcare professionals can find resources to assist them with parents who have a sick or premature baby at www.bestbeginnings.org. uk/supporting-parents-of-premature-and-sick-babies

WHAT CAN YOU DO POSTNATALLY TO BOND WITH YOUR BABY?

Ideally you will experience the immediate skin-on-skin contact as soon as your baby is born. If this is not possible, remember that you have a lifetime to make up for this. I love the warm hugs my son, now 19, gives me when he is home from college! The key to good bonding is to provide a relaxed, loving, caring environment that will promote trust and feelings of security. Here are some ways that may help facilitate this:

1. Be aware of how your baby will grow and learn and what stage their sensory development is at. This will help you to provide the correct sensory stimulation, e.g. being aware that newborns have fully developed hearing, yet can only see light and dark without detail. Each experience of the five senses will help to build connections that lay excellent foundations for learning. Be aware of over-stimulating as this can make a baby very grumpy!

2. Play simple games with your baby, such as 'peek-a-boo'. Find out if there are local groups for you to attend.
3. Be familiar with the cues that your baby gives so that you can be attentive and respond to them quickly. Lynne Murray's work in her book *The Social Baby*[9] gives some great ways to help with this. In her latest book, *The Psychology of Babies: how relationships support development from birth to two*,[10] she includes advice for dads and 'managing a bad day'.
4. Breastfeeding is a wonderful way to build a strong attachment as not only does the skin-to-skin warmth and eye contact add to a feeling of security, the baby is also getting its needs met and should be comfortable. Breastfeeding also produces two hormones, prolactin and oxytocin, that are believed to enhance feelings of bonding, nurturing and contentment. Nikki Lee[11] suggests:

   Bathe together – when Mum and Baby experience skin-to-skin contact in a warm bath, the mother's levels of oxytocin are raised. Her nipples then become more erect and it is easier for the baby to attach to the breast.

5. Where breastfeeding is replaced by bottle-feeding, remember that closeness and good eye contact are still possible.
6. Continue the talking and reading that you began during pregnancy. The responses of your baby back to you will help you feel more connected. You now can show pictures too.
7. Use the music you played whilst they were still in the womb to relax and calm them. Have your 'quiet time' space again.
8. Touch is very important for you both as hugs and kisses from parents produce natural chemicals in the baby's brain, opioids, that reduce pain awareness and induce feelings of joy that encourage bonding. Some parents find keeping their baby close, in a sling, is a good way to keep that togetherness. Bathing together and massage is also good. Find out if there are baby massage sessions in your locality.

It is also important to give your baby and yourself 'time out'. In retrospect I was overbearing with my son because I tried too hard to bond with him. Possibly he was often attempting to tell me 'enough Mum' and I misinterpreted his clues. This in turn made him cross and made me feel useless as a mother.

We also have to be aware that each baby, even from the same parents, has a different temperament. Just because your first baby was a certain way does not mean a subsequent one will respond in the same way to you. Although we are primarily concerned with parental mental health, we also have to be mindful of the babies' too.

I asked the parents in my survey to describe the temperament of their baby in the early days and weeks. This could impact upon how easy or otherwise it is to bond with them. Some described the model child who slept well, ate well and was generally calm, content and relaxed. I liked these comments:

- Much better temperament than mine which was a blessing!
- I called him my gourmet eater and my little thinker.

Some described challenges around colic and feeding:

- Very bright and alert overall but she had terrible colic the first few days and screamed constantly.
- Very colicky and cried a lot as though in pain.
- Immediately quite settled but as the weeks went on she became very unsettled and lots of colic/crying.
- A very unsettled baby, made sounds like a dog's squeaky toy, had lots of problems breastfeeding.

It was with sadness that I read of the different perceptions of their baby if the mother had a perinatal mental health problem:

- In hospital he was fine – sleepy. After a couple of weeks it felt like he was crying constantly although my family said he wasn't.
- Restless, hungry, didn't sleep, fretful (whilst in my care). When he was in the care of others he was more restful and less fretful.
- I am sorry I have lost this memory of my baby – lots of missing moments in my baby's life. I have been since told was due to PND.

Sleep and crying were also areas of concern:

- Very, very distressed. High maintenance, as the health visitors called him. He cried almost non-stop, he did not sleep, he was inconsolable. My abiding memory was of walking up and down almost 24/7 exhausted, and in so much pain and so scared that I could not calm him at all. In fact he stopped crying so infrequently that I could soon hear him crying even when he actually was not.
- My daughter never slept for more than 2 hours at a time day or night.
- Very high needs. Inconsolable crying. Only calmed (mostly) when walked in a sling, or walked and held. Never self-settled. At night, often cried from 5 p.m. until the early hours of the morning.
- He was horrendous. He cried what felt like constantly from the day he was given back to me. He continued to be difficult and not sleep very well either.

It was evident that some of the bonding techniques described above did work:

- Very relaxed but also very hungry. He liked to be close to Mum and seemed to need lots of skin to skin for comfort.
- He was fairly calm but would not sleep at all during the day and cried if he was not being held constantly.
- Very calm, relaxed. Slept well. Almost as if he sensed his mummy was unwell.
- Very easy going. By the 4th day, baby was sleeping and eating extremely well. Slept very well overnight. Fed almost exactly 4 hourly all day and night. Cheerful and interactive when awake.

I am covering these areas of concern in later chapters. Healthcare professionals may be interested in some additional resources and information to include in their approach and services. Tameside and Glossop NHS Trust have produced the *Getting It Right from the Start* DVD.[12] There is also the 'Getting to know your baby' (website and app),[13] which includes a section on supporting parents in challenging circumstances. Also have a look at Viv Bennett's blog post, which discusses the tools and opportunities available to help health visitors get messages on infant mental health to parents.[14] Some areas have been using approaches involving 'Watch, wait and wonder' techniques.[15] Please take inspiration from Monika Celebi at OxPip,[16] who run training on parent–infant interaction groups. I strongly recommend that you subscribe to the mailing list at Public Health England, Perinatal and Infant Mental website.[17] Some areas run baby massage groups. What have you got in your area and what could you introduce?

It would be remiss of me to avoid the area of child protection and safe guarding. It is necessary in some instances, yet remains an area of stigma, concern and fear. One of the reasons that parents are unwilling to say that they are facing challenges is because they fear they will be labelled as 'bad' or 'unfit' and Social Services will take their child away. I know that I felt ashamed that my son was put on the Child Protection Register when I was ill. I felt embarrassed to be 'on the other side' at case conferences. In my professional role I had been involved with cases at school. I never thought 'it would happen to me'. It did. At the time I did have thoughts of harming my precious baby. I did shake him to attempt to stop him crying. I did need to be watched. It was a process. The professionals who were caring for me at the time recognised that we needed support. Sometimes we might have to accept it even if it challenges our previous expectations and judgements. As a teacher I have been given head lice by a pupil more than once! Snobbery just needs to disappear. I could also argue that if I had known and applied some of the actions and behaviours I now have, I may not have become so ill and the involvement of Social Services not necessary. That is what we need to aim for.

As a healthcare professional, there should be safeguarding policies and protocol in your area. If they do become necessary to put into action, please always remind parents that the main aim is to the keep the family together.

It is only in extreme cases that this does not happen. This is usually due to criminal actions as opposed to illness.

At this stage I simply wanted to encourage and reassure you that there are ways to help build that amazing maternal and paternal bond with your child. You may be blessed that it comes and grows naturally. If not, I hope there are some ways above that you will find useful to apply – and have fun!

TOP TIPS FOR PARENTS

1. Remember that the feeling of attachment with your child may take time to grow – that is okay.
2. During pregnancy, discover ways that help you to bond with your baby, such as talking, reading, touching and playing music to them.
3. Find activities that help you in pregnancy such as yoga, Pilates and swimming, which also help you feel closer to your unborn child.
4. Have a 3D ultrasound so that you can 'see' your baby prior to their birth.
5. When you have your baby use feeding as a great time for closeness and eye contact.
6. Continue and develop all of the sensory stimulation you did in pregnancy along with an awareness of how your baby is developing.
7. Learn to recognise and respond to your baby's cues so that you can meet their needs appropriately and confidently.

TOP TIPS FOR HEALTHCARE PROFESSIONALS

1. Be familiar with the available resources and research around infant mental health and bonding.
2. Reassure parents that they may not feel a bond with their baby in pregnancy and help identify strategies that they can use to help.
3. Be aware that new parents may not feel a deep level of attachment to their new baby – reassure them and find tools to help them.
4. Identify, or create, opportunities for parents to bond more effectively with their baby, e.g. baby massage groups.

REFERENCES

1. www.dailymail.co.uk/femail/article-2098475/We-didnt-love-babies-What-happens-maternal-instinct-just-doesnt-kick-Three-women-break-motherhood-s-greatest-taboo-.html
2. Bowlby J. *Attachment. Attachment and Loss: Vol. 1. Loss.* New York: Basic Books; 1969.
3. Murray L, Cooper P. Effects of postnatal depression on infant development. *Arch Dis Child.* 1997; 77: 99–101. Available at: http://adc.bmj.com/content/77/2/99.full

4. Carista Luminare-Rosen, PhD. *Parenting Begins Before Conception: a guide to preparing body, mind, and spirit for you and your future child.* Vermont: Healing Arts Press; 2000.
5. www.withyouintheworld.com/album.html
6. https://thereadingwomb.wordpress.com/.
7. www.tommys.org/sslpage.aspx?pid=602&nccsm=21&__nccspID=991
8. www.tommys.org/new-free-app-to-support-parents-of-premature-babies
9. www.socialbaby.com/social-baby-pb.html
10. Murray L. *The Psychology of Babies.* London: Constable & Robinson; 2014.
11. Trotter S. Nursing in practice: breastfeeding basics: advice for new mums. *Nursing in Practice.* 2008; **44**(Sep/Oct): 23–5.
12. *Getting It Right from the Start* [DVD]. All orders to be sent to: Jakki Minton, Tameside and Glossop Community Healthcare, Selbourne House, Union Street, Hyde SK14 1NG. Tel: 0161 366 2331. Fax: 061 366 2385. Orders can also be e-mailed to j.minton@nhs. net For more information about the evaluation of the DVD/booklet, *see*: Lee P, Foley S, Mee C. Getting it right from the start: evaluation of a DVD and booklet for new parents. *Community Pract.* 2013; **86**(11): 32–6.
13. www.chimat.org.uk/resource/view.aspx?RID=197711&src=pimh
14. www.chimat.org.uk/resource/view.aspx?RID=220151&src=pimh
15. Chen H, Lee T. The maternal infant dyadic relationship: looking beyond postpartum depression. *ASEAN J Psychiat.* 2013; **14**(2): 161–9.
16. Celebi M. Babywatching: facilitating parent-infant interaction groups. *J Health Visit.* 2014; **2**(7): 362–7.
17. www.chimat.org.uk/pimh

ADDITIONAL RESOURCES
Bonding with your baby in pregnancy
- www.webmd.com/baby/guide/bonding-with-baby-before-birth
- www.babycentre.co.uk/a1049630/10-ways-to-bond-with-your-baby--bump
- www.scottishbooktrust.com/blog/bookbug/2014/08/reading-to-my-unborn-baby
- www.parentmap.com/article/11-books-to-read-aloud-to-your-unborn-baby

Bonding with your baby
- http://video.about.com/babyparenting/Ways-to-bond-with-your-baby.htm
- www.helpguide.org/mental/parenting_attachment.htm
- www.whattoexpect.com/first-year/ask-heidi/week-1/postpartum-bonding.aspx
- www.iol.co.za/lifestyle/family/baby-toddler/got-the-baby-but-not-the-feelings-1.1306286#.VLPpptKsXDU
- www.socialbaby.com This has resources for both parents and professionals, including some in different languages
- www.iaimbabymassage.co.uk Information about baby massage
- https://drewstarr.wordpress.com/page/2/ Baby bonding blog

Infant Mental Health Resources
- www.aimh.org.uk/
- www.waimh.org/i4a/pages/index.cfm?pageid=1

Good practice

- Baby Steps is a perinatal educational programme by NSPCC designed to help pre-pare people for becoming parents, not just for the birth itself. www.nspcc.org.uk/fighting-for-childhood/our-services/services-for-children-and-families/baby-steps/
- 'Parenting Ladder' – in South Warwickshire, health visiting teams are using this system to offer bespoke support to parents so they can focus on their child's needs. It was designed to support a young couple with children, where serious concerns around their care had been identified. https://vivbennett.blog.gov.uk/2015/02/03/south-warwickshire-ft/

CHAPTER 15

Feeding your baby

Breastfeeding should not be attempted by fathers with hairy chests, since they can make the baby sneeze and give it wind.

Mike Harding

Of all the essential parenting routines, most people would agree that how you feed your baby (breast or bottle) and how baby responds can be a major factor in determining the quality of life for all involved. So if you had a troublesome or wonderful experience with a previous baby, it does not follow that this will be the case with a subsequent baby. I feel it is important to acknowledge this subject, share experiences of others and give you some ideas to maximise success.

When I was pregnant I firmly believed I wanted to breastfeed my baby when he was born. Some of my friends were doing so and made it look easy and convenient. Being an avid reader of all the baby care information, I was convinced that 'breast is best'. In reality, this was true, most of the time. I persevered through painful mastitis (a condition that causes a woman's breast tissue to become painful and inflamed) and even as I spiralled down into puerperal psychosis, the one thing I still could do well was breastfeed. It gave me joy, opportunity to bond with my son and made me sit down! After being hospitalised without him, breastfeeding was literally stopped overnight. Eighteen years later I still feel that sense of loss and sadness at being forced to cease an action that was beneficial to us both. Even now I can feel emotional if I see a mother breastfeeding her child. It is the eye contact and delightful suckling noise that tweaks my heart strings. Had I ever had another child I would have chosen to breastfeed again because I still believe this would be best for me and my baby.

From the mothers who replied to my survey, 62.5% breastfed; 19.5% bottle-fed: 25% did combination feeding. The fact that 94% had said that they initially wanted to breastfeed indicates that their best intention and expectation were not met. These are some of the reasons they gave and indicate how it is linked to maternal mental feelings:

- I went on asking for help. Due to my size on both pregnancies it was difficult. It did not help to have people drumming into me that every mother could do it and basically no such word as 'can't'. I felt it was my duty as a mother and felt quite suicidal that I couldn't do it. No one seemed to understand why I felt it was so important.
- I did but after a few weeks I hated it. I didn't want to sit and hold my child. I remember thinking of him as a parasite.
- I had researched and was excited to try and breastfeed but didn't realise how painful it would be or how drained I would be following the birth.
- I desperately wanted to feed but he wouldn't latch and I was unable to carry on and was left feeling like a failure especially with the comments of a midwife.
- I felt pressured by midwives. I wasn't very good at it and was on antibiotics which I was told would not affect my milk, but my daughter refused feeds. I switched to bottle and felt I had failed.
- Yes originally, but I felt under huge pressure to continue once I wanted to stop.
- There was no medical reason why I couldn't breastfeed. I just felt bullied by the medical profession and refused to be railroaded.
- Unable to after 14 days due to medication and severe decline in mental health.
- I had it in my head that he had to have exactly the same as my first baby, and I had breastfed her for a year.
- Initially but struggled and felt pressured by healthcare professionals to keep trying to breastfeed.

Just over half of the mothers in my survey felt that they had sufficient help with their choice of feeding.

- I suppose in some ways I did and other ways I didn't – whilst in hospital some workers kept offering me a bottle saying I wouldn't be a failure if I didn't breastfeed. When I got home I was having to ring up constantly through struggling but only really got a visit twice a week if that.
- Yes, I got a lot of support from breastfeeding support workers and health visitor. I was having lots of problems with feeding. My milk was coming out too fast which meant that although baby would latch on correctly he would then yank his head back constantly. This led to me having lots of blisters and eventually getting mastitis.
- Almost overloaded by a breastfeeding advisor who visited at home. I wanted to give up but felt like I would let everyone down.
- I now believe he may have been tongue tied and nobody noticed as I was in terrible pain for quite some time.
- The support in hospital was very poor – I had a breastfeeding 'consultant' demonstrate it to me, and that was it. It wasn't until my son cried all night and I was in tears that a senior midwife realised he wasn't latching on at all.
- The health visitor was great. The midwives in hospital were telling me it hurt

because I was doing it wrong. In retrospect, it would have helped if they just admitted breastfeeding does hurt!

- Later on the breastfeeding clinic were amazing, but early on I was given no help at all.
- From the midwives and neonatal unit I did get sufficient help.
- The only 'help' was a health visitor telling me that I was feeding him wrongly when he was a few days old!
- I struggled to get help in hospital. Midwifes at home were well meaning, but I was still very worried about the feeding.

Pressure around choice of feeding and support varied for the mothers who shared their experiences. In a handful of scenarios, there was no pressure and good support from others, for example:

- There was no pressure, it was my decision to breastfeed. However, in hindsight I should have stopped breastfeeding earlier and switched to bottles. I think the health visitor realised this but she never brought up bottle-feeding except to say that it was my choice and they would support me whatever I decided to do.
- I was supported – I presumed I'd breastfeed as my mum did but I found it made me so panicky that I chose to stop. My professionals supported me totally in whatever I did.
- I took to breastfeeding very well. I had no issues with that. I was always encouraged to breastfeed but I went in with an open mind and would have done whichever suited my son and I. Breastfeeding was fully a personal choice although if I ever had more children I wouldn't do it again.
- I was fairly well supported in bottle-feeding but the hospital could have done more to help me breastfeed.

Sadly other mothers shared sorrowful events:

- I was not supported in breastfeeding. Because I was crying all the time and obviously not right, some professionals did say maybe I shouldn't breastfeed as they felt it was making me worse. When my baby was 4 days old I rang the postnatal ward in the middle of the night as my nipples were so painful, cracked and bleeding. I explained the problems and said how I really wanted to breastfeed but that I was struggling and asked for help. They left some formula at reception for my husband to collect. I really didn't want to do this so had to breastfeed my baby whilst in so much pain, crying and squeezing a pillow. I started developing a phobia of breastfeeding my baby. I had to look up things on the internet and managed to hire a breast pump so I was able to give my baby breast milk.
- I had lots of problems and asked for help on numerous occasions but didn't get the appropriate help. I felt really angry and annoyed when I was in the bed

struggling and being ignored and then midwives pressuring other women to breastfeed who were insisting on formula feeding.
- No proper support, wasn't mentioned much at antenatal classes or in hospital. Emily didn't latch on correctly and it caused excruciating pain, soreness and bleeding. I almost gave up and was devastated.

Choice of feeding was often affected by either problems with the mother or baby:

- I knew I wanted to breastfeed but due to my mental and physical condition was unable to.
- Fortunately I never felt guilty that I was unable to breastfeed as I was just happy that my baby was content. However, I am very disappointed that my condition deteriorated so that I was unable to breastfeed. This deterioration in my condition could have been avoided and, if so, I am sure I would have been successful in breastfeeding.
- I was definitely not supported. It was a big issue for me. Having to switch to formula. I even tried pumping while in the psychiatric ward.
- While my daughter was in PICU [paediatric intensive care unit] – very little support. Needed information and expressing whilst baby was on ventilator, there was no info in the breastfeeding room at all at the hospital.
- I wanted to breastfeed so much but it wasn't possible. He then had problems with bottles.
- Yes, felt pressure to continue breastfeeding when I was struggling with massive sleep deprivation.
- After 10 weeks I was so ill that I bottle-fed, however I then felt so guilty so combination fed for a month and they were all supportive.
- No one explained what drugs were safe for breastfeeding. I can't even talk about it. It was like no one knew or healthcare professionals were afraid of lawsuits.
- It was very difficult as milk did not come until about 4 days after birth but I was still supposed to try and force out what I could. No option was given for baby to be bottle-fed during this period.
- No one told me or explained that bottle or combination feeding was an option. Finally the option to BF was taken away from me, due to the antipsychotic medication.

Many mothers commented that it was their own personal belief, knowledge or desire that caused an internal pressure, often leading to a sense of failure:

- I put myself under pressure to breastfeed. It felt like the only thing I was doing right, having 'failed' at the natural hypnobirth I had planned and wanted.
- I did feel pressure to continue but mainly I had created this myself. Also by 5 weeks my baby refused a bottle.

- Breast is best and all that crap!! I wanted to breastfeed anyway, however when I started it became obvious I couldn't provide enough milk for Thomas causing him to lose too much weight!
- I wanted to breastfeed but looking back I feel a lot of the reason for this was that as a mother you are almost railroaded to thinking that not doing it is bad and you have failed.
- I put myself under pressure to breastfeed. As soon as I was sectioned they put me on drugs that meant I couldn't and I felt that decision had been taken away from me. The reason they had to section me as I refused to take the drugs they were saying I needed because they couldn't say they were okay to take whilst breastfeeding.

Where personal thoughts and feelings were added to by pressure, procedures or policy from healthcare professionals, family and friends, this made it worse:

- People often have strong feelings about breast vs bottle and they let you know how they feel in no uncertain terms. I felt pressure no matter what my decision was.
- I put a lot of pressure on myself to do it and felt very upset when I couldn't continue. I had to stop because my son was ventilated in intensive care for such a long period of time that my milk dried up, despite hours of relentless pumping. When I did finally stop, the midwives in the hospital were so pleased because my son had lost so much weight that he needed a high calorie formula – yet they weren't allowed to tell me to stop torturing myself with it. Ridiculous!
- I felt under pressure from the midwife to breastfeed, she made me feel formula was a poor choice.
- I did feel pressured due to all the medical staff, posters, 'Sure Start' centres all going on about it.
- As my little girlie was a little early and born by C-section my milk didn't come in for a few days, they tried to pressure me but after my first I already thought I won't feel guilty if it doesn't work out! After my first they made me feel like a bit of a failure.
- I was put under pressure to bottle-feed. This was by the hospital who considered my baby premature and told me he would end up in SCBU if I refused and insisted on breastfeeding. I later found out the hospital policy was that babies born at 37 weeks were considered 'term' and placed on a bottle-feeding regime as standard, whereas in surrounding Trusts, babies born at 36 weeks were considered 'term'. My baby was born at 36 weeks and 2 days.
- Some family members didn't approve of breastfeeding but my partner did, commenting constantly that his friends' wives or girlfriends managed it!
- My partner and his family were pressurising me into giving up breastfeeding.

Information was also a concern for some:

- I believe I wasn't given enough info on breastfeeding, I was just told it's best for you and baby. I had to do a lot of the research myself to make sure I was prepared to do so.
- Yes bombarded with leaflets, too many posters and what felt like propaganda.

I asked mothers if they felt their choice of feeding, personal or forced, had helped or hindered their mental state. Only a few said that it was not affected. Many said it hindered:

- I think not breastfeeding and his problem bottle-feeding led to my mental state declining …
- I think if I had breastfed on demand, it would have made matters worse because the lack of support and rest would have made breastfeeding impossible. However, the fact that I thought breast was best made me paranoid that my son was ill due to bottle-feeding (he ended up lactose intolerant but I thought he was seriously ill). I needed support to believe it was okay not to breastfeed.
- Yes it made me worse as I couldn't stand my baby being anywhere near me so breastfeeding was awful. I only lasted 3 weeks and 3 days feeding her and then moved onto bottle-feeding which was a massive relief.
- I wanted to breastfeed but was not given the support. I felt guilty that I didn't breastfeed him.
- It definitely contributed to my PND. By about 3 months I was constantly in agony from breastfeeding and couldn't stop crying. I was clearly depressed by this point. I wanted to stop breastfeeding but because of the PND I could not make the decision to stop. My brain was not functioning and I did not understand how to bottle-feed. However much I stared at the instructions I couldn't take it in! My GP did in fact eventually suggest I should switch to bottle-feeding and she told me to ask the health visitor to advise me on how to gradually make the switch and to give me clear instructions in the form of a timetable. However, when I asked the health visitor to write down how I should reduce my feeds she refused and said she wasn't allowed to give me specific instructions! In the end my mum made the decision and just made up a bottle one day and gave it to the baby. I really wish someone had done that weeks before!
- Definitely hindered. Breastfeeding meant no other person could care for my daughter, particularly at night. The pressure I felt as sole carer was overwhelming.
- Hindered. Once we had realised how little milk I was producing I felt awful as I was the reason he had lost so much weight! I was the one that got frustrated with him for constantly wanting to feed, now I know why, the poor mite!
- Probably hindered a little as I was 'tied' to him. However, I felt positive that it was one thing I could do for him that nobody else could.

- Probably didn't help when I was breastfeeding because the sleep deprivation made my anxiety levels go through the roof!
- Hindered. His heart condition meant he wasn't feeding well, so was feeding constantly. I complained to the midwife every time and she had me join a breastfeeding group. No one picked up on the fact that his medical records stated that he had a heart problem, so didn't have the breath to feed properly. This should have been picked up.
- I felt that the problems I experience hindered my mental state and that if I had been offered appropriate and useful support, this would have made a big difference. I also felt like a freak and that I didn't fit into a category of breastfeeding or formula-feeding as everyone seems to only recognise these two options. I feel that more should be known about expressing, informing women of this option and supporting them with this. I felt a failure as I had all the problems I did with breastfeeding and that everyone else had no problems with it.
- I strongly believe that trying and failing to breastfeed was a strong trigger for my puerperal psychosis.
- My sense of self-worth was completely dependent on my ability to breastfeed. I felt under huge pressure to admit defeat and give up. If I had failed, I think I would have killed myself. I still feel that I failed my son, despite the fact that he was exclusively breastfed from 3 months and I continued until he was 14 months old, because he had some bottles in the early weeks.
- Yes – felt exhausted and stressed doubting my body's ability to produce milk. I didn't understand my baby was possibly unsettled due to growth spurt. Felt like even my body was taken over. My mind was elsewhere and hubby slept elsewhere. Led to relationship issues.
- Hindered – undiagnosed thrush and mastitis despite me asking the Health Visitor and Midwife and GP!
- Hindered as I was putting pressure on myself and had to express milk as baby in neonatal unit and wouldn't take the drugs as I thought more important to breastfeed than look after myself.
- Hindered. As horrible as it sounds, I felt like I was glued to a child/baby that I didn't even like or want.
- Hindered. I had no idea how all-consuming it is to start with and couldn't get him to combination feed which drove me mad. He was also slow to solids so felt I'd been conned.
- Feeling forced to breastfeed massively hindered my mental state. I was exhausted and no one could give me a break. My son had a tongue tie and couldn't latch on (he was 6 weeks old before I was told this) and combined with his reflux, his inability to feed caused the constant crying. He lost a lot of weight. I became so panicky about him choking that I was scared to be alone with him. I cried every time he needed feeding for weeks.
- I felt extremely guilty and that I'd let everyone down by bottle-feeding. I knew it was the wrong thing to do but I was also unable to breastfeed because I had

thought it would be easy and I did not know you have to stick at it and practise for it to work. I was too exhausted to try and make it work. I mix fed for three months but for me it was something to be ashamed of. I had strongly received this message and I believed it myself.

- Hindered. I was so, so tired and if I had bottle-fed him at the start I could have had more sleep, which would really have helped.
- Breastfeeding was very hard for me – as I didn't want to be near my baby!!!
- Hindered to a certain extent as I had a hungry baby and was really draining me feeding him.
- I think I was overwhelmed and had I been well, switching to bottle would not have affected me.

Others explained how it helped:

- Helped. I felt I am doing the best for Emily. Feeding time was resting time for me and Emily together.
- I think it helped in the sense that I was so unwell I didn't even want to hold my baby and being bottle-fed meant my husband could do the feeds.
- I think that breastfeeding was hard because Jack was a big baby but it also gave me alone time with him. We bonded through this. I was of the mind that if it didn't work out then that was okay.
- Once I changed from breast to bottle-feeding I felt so much better. My baby slept for longer periods and I was released from the relentless 24 hour merry-go-round of feeding my baby every 2–3 hours. Breastfeeding was draining, both mentally and physically, particularly as the milk I was producing didn't satisfy my baby and the process wasn't calming for either myself or the baby.
- Helped, as it kept me close to my baby and I was able to bond with him.
- Going with bottle-feeding helped – one less pressure/drain on me physically and at least my baby was content and not hungry.

Then there were some who felt their mental state was helped, hindered or both by their choice of feeding or were not sure.

- Both – I hated the pain and being tied to the baby, and desperately wanted to give her to someone else. But also I felt it was the only good thing I was doing with/for her, as I was so sad and felt so incompetent and she screamed so much all the rest of the time.
- A bit of both. I needed a break badly, but I felt I was good at something.
- I'm not sure really. Either way I have felt like I have failed. If I didn't breastfeed I would have felt like I never tried, and because I did breastfeed for 14 weeks and then couldn't continue after a long struggle to feed my baby I still felt like I failed and could've done better. I feel like I should have been able to feed her. I struggled to supply her with milk after being ill. But I still feel like that was

maybe my fault for having her at home? Could I have been treated better if I had her in hospital?

Hindsight can be useful:

- Looking back I can say that it may have been beneficial if I had been bottle-feeding. It may have enabled me to have more time. Sleep more. But then again, it may have been exactly the same.
- In hindsight I should have considered mixed feeding, as I fed him every hour and a half, day and night for 7 months. He was a big baby and was 20 pounds by 12 weeks old, so just hungry all the time.

I admit that I found some of the experiences described to me above very distressing. If you are reading this as a parent, did you recognise your situation here? If you are reading this as a healthcare professional, can you identify any of your practices here? I am sure that we will all agree that feeding a baby can have a huge impact upon the mental health of mothers. So now let's look at the myths and facts surrounding the ways to feed a baby and lay the foundations to help make an informed, non-judgemental choice.

MYTH 1: POSTNATAL DEPRESSION IS CAUSED BY BREASTFEEDING

In Chapter 2 we looked at the causes and risk factors for postnatal depression, for example, 'Stress, sleep disturbance, pain, psychological trauma, history of abuse with inflammation as underlying risk factor'.[1] Research in the field of psychoneuroimmunology (PNI) has revealed that depression is associated with inflammation manifested by increased levels of proinflammatory cytokines.[1] I encourage healthcare professionals again to look at the 'identifying women at risk' film for the evidence and examples.[2] I have not found any evidence to suggest that this myth is true. The research says that:

Breastfeeding may protect against negative moods and perceived stress. Breastfeeding mothers had more positive moods, reported more positive events, and perceived less stress than formula-feeders.[3]

Sometimes postnatal depression can be confused with D-MER:

Dysphoric Milk Ejection Reflex is a condition affecting lactating women that is characterized by an abrupt dysphoria, or negative emotions, that occur just before milk release and continuing not more than a few minutes. D-MER is not postnatal depression or a postpartum mood disorder.[4]

MYTH 2: IF YOU HAVE POSTNATAL DEPRESSION YOU SHOULD STOP BREASTFEEDING

> Current research … indicates that if mothers want to continue breastfeeding (whilst being treated for postnatal depression), sound medical rationale supports their decision.[5]

There does appear to be a connection though as regards cessation of breast-feeding by mothers who may have postnatal mental health issues, as identified by Watkins *et al.*:[6]

> Depressed mothers are less likely to breastfeed, nurse for shorter durations, and have more negative emotions and experiences toward breastfeeding. New moth-ers experiencing breastfeeding difficulties may be more likely to be suffering from PPD, highlighting the importance of screening.

I have put more references for this area at the end of the chapter.

MYTH 3: IF YOU TAKE MEDICATION FOR POSTNATAL DEPRESSION YOU SHOULD STOP BREASTFEEDING

This depends on the type of medication, e.g.:

> The selective serotonin reuptake inhibitors (SSRI) types of antidepressants are usually recommended for women who are breastfeeding. Tests have shown the amount of these types of antidepressants found in breast milk is so small it is unlikely to be harmful.[7]

I have listed several sources for information on suitable medication at the end of the chapter. I also recommend that you visit www.breastfeedingnetwork. org.uk/detailed-information/drugs-in-breastmilk/ and www.medsmilk.com/ pages/introduction. There is also an excellent book By Dr Thomas W Hale and Dr Hilary E Rowe: *Medications and Mothers' Milk*.[8]

University of Adelaide researchers have found that women on antide-pressant medication are more successful at breastfeeding their babies if they keep taking the medication, compared with women who quit antidepressants because of concerns about their babies' health. http://medicalxpress.com/ news/2014-04-proof-antidepressants-breastfeeding.html

Some of the choices that need to be considered around taking medication whilst breastfeeding include individual decision; severity of illness; health of baby; benefits of breastfeeding; side-effects; current information; impact of no treatment and other helpful treatments.

One very important supplement to take is vitamin D to prevent your child

developing rickets. You can use the simple checker at www.vitamindmission.co.uk/take-the-test. For further details look at www.rcpch.ac.uk/news-campaigns/campaigns/vitamin-d/vitamin-d-rcpch-campaign

MYTH 4: YOU GET MORE SLEEP IF YOU BOTTLE-FEED YOUR BABY

I used to think that this was true – it is not.

> Efforts to encourage women to breastfeed should include information about sleep. Specifically, women should be told that choosing to formula feed does not equate with improved sleep. The risks of not breastfeeding should be weighed against the cumulative lack of evidence indicating any benefit of formula feeding on maternal sleep.[9]

Another study by Dorhiem[10] states:

> Poor sleep may increase the risk of depression in some women, but as previously known risk factors were also associated, mothers diagnosed with postpartum depression are not merely reporting symptoms of chronic sleep deprivation.

I have put more examples of research at the end of the chapter. You may find the articles at www.uppitysciencechick.com/PPD-Sleep.html to be useful too.

MYTH 5: YOU ARE A BAD MOTHER IF YOU STOP BREASTFEEDING

This is clearly not true, although as many of the mothers who shared their story with me testify, they believe it is. The crucial learning point here is that:

> Postnatal depression has a significant negative impact on breastfeeding duration. Assistance with breastfeeding issues should be included in the management of postnatal depression.[11]

There are many sources of information concerning the positive effects of breastfeeding, e.g.:

- www.breastfeedingnetwork.org.uk/ an independent source of support and information for breastfeeding women and those involved in their care
- www.laleche.org.uk/ for friendly mother-to-mother breastfeeding support from pregnancy through to weaning
- http://abm.me.uk/ the Association of Breastfeeding Mothers (ABM).

I want to suggest that it has both positive and negative effects on women who are suffering from a mental health issue postnatally.

Certainly in my case, I felt it was one of the few things as a mother I was successful at. It made me feel important as 'Mum' and I was pleased I was able to do something that is widely recognised as being best for my baby. It could be a calming and relaxing experience that definitely increased the bond between us. It was easy (mainly) and convenient and something I felt was very special and precious. A short-lived joy in life. Breastfeeding was the only thing I felt I had any control over at that time and it gave me a sense of confidence whilst it appeared the rest of my world was crumbling. I enjoyed the whole sensory stimulation of it, so any form of pleasure during mental distress has to be good.

Breastfeeding can also have possible detrimental feelings if you have a postnatal mental illness. Feelings include it as being pointless; can make you feel self-conscious and embarrassed in public; demanding and tying; too invasive and overwhelming. If the mother perceives it is the cause of her postnatal illness, this can build fear and resentment. If the baby struggles to feed and/or the mother misinterprets their clues, they can feel inadequate. It may be too painful to deal with. They may feel pressured by others and persevere through feelings of guilt or shame, which then can affect their bond with their baby.

I have found two great resources to help in this area:

1. for parents: www.panda.org.au/9-our-services/printed-material/77-postnatal-depression-and-breastfeeding-booklet
2. for healthcare professionals: www.nhbreastfeedingtaskforce.org/
3. www.rcm.org.uk/college/about/alliance/philips-avent – developed using the latest evidence and in consultation with breastfeeding experts, this resource has information and illustrations to help midwives to support women to establish and continue breastfeeding.

Both the research and the voices from mothers would strongly indicate that **whatever suits the mother regarding feeding is best for the baby**.

- Yes, there was always pressure to breastfeed, stating 'breast is best', and pointing out the advantages breastfeeding brings. I felt like a bad mother when I chose to change from breast to bottle. I know the medical staff frowned on my decision to change, but for my mental health I had to make this choice. At no point did any medical staff address what was best for the mother, which would automatically make things better for the baby.

Based on the clinical-evidenced based research and the voices of many other parents, my message to healthcare professionals would be along the lines of this:

> We need to listen to the individual mother in front of us, without judgment. We need to ask her what her goals are for her relationship with her baby, and find out how we can help her accomplish them.[12]

To mothers I would recommend that you are kind to yourselves. If you really want to breastfeed, ensure that you have the support that is needed. Find out during pregnancy where and who can offer help as soon as you have the baby. If you decide that you would rather bottle-feed, or combine breastfeeding with bottle-feeding, then make arrangements accordingly. I include links to resources at the end of the chapter. If your own needs or those of your baby change, then allow yourself to be at peace with the decision. Make sure that you find out if there have been any new products or changes in equipment since your previous days of feeding a baby. I only discovered breast shells late into that stage – they are brilliant to pop over one nipple as baby feeds from the other. I was able to collect enough milk for someone else to give him a feed.

Take strength from the words of Rachel Remen, who writes in her article 'Mothering the mother':[13]

> Healing may not be so much about getting better, as about letting go of everything that isn't you – all of the expectations, all of the beliefs – and becoming who you are.

Next time around you also have the experience and knowledge that whichever way you feed your baby, you know that it is a relatively short-lived period. Before long they will be communicating well what they wish to eat or not and emptying the fridge within hours of it being restocked!

Here are some more ideas for you to consider.

TIPS® Toolkit for Breastfeeding (reproduced with kind permission of TIPS Ltd)
This breastfeeding factsheet is written by Sharon Trotter BSc – Breastfeeding Consultant and Neonatal Skincare Advisor. Sharon is a midwife with over 30 years' experience of helping new mums and seven years' personal experience breastfeeding her own five babies. Author of the best-selling breastfeeding book *Breastfeeding: the essential guide*, Sharon works independently as a breastfeeding consultant and baby skincare advisor. She is founder of TIPS Ltd which is well respected for the quality of its assessment of mother and baby related products reviewed through the TIPS® Award Scheme.

Congratulations on your pregnancy!
Whether you're a first time or an experienced mum, you're bound to have a few questions about breastfeeding. I am delighted to share with you my common sense breastfeeding tips – they will hopefully help dispel any myths you may have heard.

At this very special time, I want to give you the encouragement you deserve and help boost your confidence.

Most of us agree that breastfeeding is best for mum and baby (and dad too) but that's not enough to guarantee success. Lack of support, conflicting advice, poor information and negative attitudes are all too common. Learning to breastfeed takes time. It is much easier if you have had the chance to watch other mums feed and if you give yourself plenty of time to find the most comfortable position for you and your baby. To succeed, you will need constant support, plenty of encouragement and lots of practical tips. There are simple and effective solutions to any problem you may encounter when learning to breastfeed.

How long should I breastfeed for?

The World Health Organization (Baby Friendly Initiative) recommends that mothers breastfeed exclusively (no other food or drink) for six months. Once mixed feeding is introduced, breastfeeding should be encouraged for up to two years and beyond. Like breastfeeding, mixed feeding should always be baby-led.

Getting help ...

Peer support groups are ideal for ongoing support. Speaking to a mum who is an experienced breast feeder (whether a friend or breastfeeding counsellor) is a great help. To find your nearest peer support group contact a breastfeeding association, for example the Association of Breastfeeding Mothers, the Breast Feeding Network, Lactation Consultants of Great Britain or La Leche League.

My breastfeeding top tips ...

Surround yourself with positive support from family, friends and people who really know about breastfeeding and *always* include your partner.

Positioning and attachment

- Get help with positioning and attachment from the start – this isn't 'hands on' manipulation but one-to-one explanation and reassurance.
- Be creative! There are 360° of attachment so finding the perfect position for you and your baby may involve quite a bit of trial and error. You'll know when you've succeeded because feeding will be comfortable.

Breastfeeding should not hurt – if you're in pain get help from someone who really understands breastfeeding. To have a friend or a breastfeeding counsellor who is experienced in breastfeeding would be a great help at this time.

- If your nipples are sore:
  - correct your positioning and attachment to prevent any further damage
  - rule out tongue-tie as this could be the cause (see the TIPS® factsheet about tongue tie for advice)

- once baby is well attached the nipples should heal but you might like to express small amounts of breast milk, smoothing it into any sore bits, as your milk contains its own healing properties. Seek help if the soreness persists.
- Biological nurturing – this approach has been shown to make the most of the mother's and baby's own instincts. It suggests new ways to hold and cuddle babies and aims to increase the enjoyment of breastfeeding. This can greatly help with positioning and attachment. You can visit www.biologicalnurturing.com for more information.

Milk supply – listen to your baby's cues: breastfeeding can only work when it's baby-led.

- Stimulate your breasts – the smell, sight and touch of your baby will help your milk supply.
- Having a bath with your baby can really help with attachment problems. Skin-to-skin contact with your baby in a warm bath will raise the levels of circulating hormones. The laid-back position also seems to aid attachment.
- Feed your baby whenever they want to be fed, especially during the night when your hormone levels are higher. This helps promote and maintain a steady milk supply.
- It takes around 6 to 8 weeks for the delicate balance of milk supply and demand to become established, so don't be tempted to introduce bottles or formula feeds. Your breasts will produce enough if your baby is feeding well. Expressing too soon can actually upset your milk supply. Once breastfeeding is fully established you can consider expressing occasionally, if you need to be away from your baby for short periods.
- Try to be with your baby as much as possible – close contact (not necessarily skin-to-skin) really helps to stimulate milk-producing hormones. Baby-wearing (using slings or carriers) has the same effect.

Baby's weight – growth charts used in the UK are based on bottle-fed babies so weight gain for your breastfed baby may appear to be slow. These charts are being replaced with World Health Organization breastfeeding growth charts.

- As long as your baby is waking up for feeds, taking feeds well and having wet and dirty nappies, you can be reassured that they are getting enough milk.
- It's not unusual for a baby to feed between 12 and 20 times a day in the first few weeks. But this will settle down I promise!

Including Dad – always include your partner so they can share the feeding process.

- Skin-to-skin contact is good for dads too, and should be encouraged. This will help promote a closer bond as you all settle into your new family unit.

Breastfeeding is so much more than just a way of feeding your baby milk …

- Breastfeeding will help you lose the extra weight your body gained during pregnancy.
- Breastfeeding gives baby the emotional and psychological stability they need to become self-confident, relaxed, independent and secure.

Above all enjoy breastfeeding – with each feed you will get a rush of endorphins, which are basically 'happy hormones'. This makes you and your baby feel good and is nature's own stress-buster.

For more information and advice about breastfeeding, see the Breastfeeding FAQs on the TIPS website (www.tipslimited.co.uk) TIPS Ltd © 2015.

REFERENCES

1. Kathleen Kendall-Tackett. (2007) www.internationalbreastfeedingjournal.com/content/2/1/6
2. Identifying Women at risk – a learning programme for midwives www.beatingbipolar.org/perinataltraining/
3. Groër, Breastfeeding and Maternal Stress, (2005) http://brn.sagepub.com/content/7/2/106.abstract?ct
4. www.d-mer.org/
5. Journal of Perinatal Education. (Fall 2010) www.ncbi.nlm.nih.gov/pmc/articles/PMC2981185
6. Watkins S, *et al.* (2011). www.ncbi.nlm.nih.gov/pubmed/21734617
7. www.nhs.uk/Conditions/Postnataldepression/Pages/Treatment.aspx
8. Hale TW, Rowe HE. *Medications and Mothers' Milk*. 16th ed. Plano, TX: Hale Publishing; 2014. Available at: www.ibreastfeeding.com/books/2014-medications-and-mothers39-milk-345.html
9. Montgomery-Downs HE, *et al.* Infant feeding methods and maternal sleep and daytime functioning. *Pediatrics*. 2010; **126**(6): 1562–8. Available at: http://pediatrics.aappublications.org/content/early/2010/11/08/peds.2010-1269.abstract
10. Dorheim SK, *et al.* Sleep and depression in postpartum women: a population-based study. *Sleep*. 2009; **32**(7): 842–55. Available at: http://highwire.stanford.edu/cgi/medline/pmid;19639747
11. BIRTH **30**:3 September 2003. Available at: http://onlinelibrary.wiley.com/doi/10.1046/j.1523-536X.2003.00242.x/abstract;jsessionid=286DB88E12531750CED70634B3610B28.d02t04?deniedAccessCustomisedMessage=&userIsAuthenticated=false
12. Stuebe A. Is breastfeeding promotion bad for mothers? Available at: http://bfmed.wordpress.com/2011/02/21/is-breastfeeding-promotion-bad-for-mothers/
13. Remen RN. Mothering the mother: understanding and healing postnatal depression. Available at: www.goodreads.com/quotes/491458-healing-may-not-be-so-much-about-getting-better-as (accessed 3 June 2015).

FURTHER READING AND RESOURCES
Research
- www.unicef.org.uk/BabyFriendly/News-and-Research/Research/Mental-health/

Common breastfeeding myths
- www.llli.org/nb/lvaprmay98p21nb.html

Plenty of research articles
- www.chimat.org.uk Child and Maternal Health Observatory and Public Health
- www.gov.uk/search?q=breastfeeding
- www.marcesociety.com an international society for the understanding, prevention and treatment of mental illness related to childbearing

Current guidelines on breastfeeding
- www.bestbeginnings.org.uk/News/pathways
- www.unicef.org.uk/BabyFriendly/ Baby Friendly Initiative – enabling health professionals to support mothers and babies
- www.ouh.nhs.uk/women/maternity/postnatal/infant-feeding/documents/care-pathway.pdf NHS Breastfeeding Care Pathway
- www.nice.org.uk/guidance/ph11

Promotion of breastfeeding initiation and duration
- www.nhs.uk/start4life/documents/pdfs/introducing_solid_foods.pdf Start4Life – feeding your baby leaflet

Tips for bottle-feeding
- www.netmums.com/baby/feeding-your-new-baby/feeding-baby-bottle-feeding
- www.nhs.uk/conditions/pregnancy-and-baby/pages/bottle-feeding-advice.aspx#close
- www.whattoexpect.com/first-year/photo-gallery/tips-for-bottle-feeding-problems.aspx#/slide-1
- www.aptaclub.co.uk/article/preparing-a-bottlefeed
- www.smamums.co.uk/baby

Cessation of breastfeeding rates
- Groër MW. Differences between exclusive breastfeeders, formula-feeders, and controls: a study of stress, mood, and endocrine variables. *Biol Res Nurs*. 2005; **7**(2): 106–17. Available at: http://brn.sagepub.com/content/7/2/106.abstract?ct
- www.postpartumprogress.com/postpartum-depression-and-breastfeeding-challenges-the-connection
- www.nctba.org/breastfeeding/postpartum-depression-and-difficulty-breast-feeding-may-go-hand-in-hand/
- Odom EC, *et al*. Reasons for earlier than desired cessation of breastfeeding. *Pediatrics*. 2013; **131**(3): 726–32. Available at: http://pediatrics.aappublications.org/content/early/2013/02/13/peds.2012-1295.abstract

Medication and breastfeeding

- www.nice.org.uk/guidance/cg192: professional guidelines
- www.ppmis.org.au/

Public information

- www.breastfeeding-and-medication.co.uk
- www.sign.ac.uk/pdf/PAT127.pdf Management of perinatal mood disorders – useful medication advice
- www.rcpsych.ac.uk/members/sections/perinatal.aspx Royal College of Psychiatrists
- www.app-network.org/ Action on postpartum psychosis
- www.motherisk.org: Mother risk – protecting the unborn
- www.womensmentalhealth.org/ Massachusetts General Hospital Center for Women's Mental Health, a perinatal and reproductive psychiatry information centre
- www.medsmilk.com/pages/introduction Excellent resource regarding medication and breastfeeding

Sleep and choice of feeding

- www.unicef.org.uk/BabyFriendly/Parents/Resources/Resources-for-parents/Caring-for-your-baby-at-night/
- www.nhs.uk/conditions/pregnancy-and-baby/pages/getting-baby-to-sleep.aspx
- www.cheshirebabywhisperer.com/ A multi-sensory approach

Books

- Finigan V. *Saggy Boobs and Other Breastfeeding Myths*. London: Pinter & Martin; 2009.
- Trotter A. *Breastfeeding: the essential guide*. Prestwick: TIPS Ltd; 2004.
- Blenkinsop A. *Fit to Bust*. Lonely Scribe; 2011.

Films

- www.youtube.com/watch?v=j4-N2roKmHo
- www.nhs.uk/conditions/pregnancy-and-baby/pages/breastfeeding-help-support.aspx#close NHS Choices Breastfeeding Challenges
- http://youtu.be/tuV8WiVKfGw Family members
- http://youtu.be/FjqOqJLkyFs Behind the mask

CHAPTER 16

The importance of sleep

Sleep is that golden chain that ties health and our bodies together.

Thomas Dekker

I am often asked if there was anything I felt could have been done to prevent my spiral into severe postnatal illness and then puerperal psychosis. My immediate reply is 'sleep'. Kathleen Kendall-Tackett[1] believes that sleep disturbance is one of the key risk factors of postnatal illness. I would agree. Make it a priority to ensure that you find ways to enable both mother and baby to sleep as much as possible.

I now can see that I was in a vicious circle – I was always anxious and therefore my baby was. That affected our sleep as I only cat-napped, expecting him to wake – and he did! The more tired I was, the worse everything else was and I crashed – big time. Instead of resting I would be busy. When my baby and I were separated due to me going into hospital I remember feeling really guilty that his father had got him to sleep through the night much better. It added to my belief at the time that everything I did as a mother was wrong and useless. I blamed myself for his poor sleep. On reflection that was true to an extent, because a restless mother means a restless baby. What we needed was guidance to help us. During those early months, at every interaction I had with health professionals, I mentioned how little we were sleeping. I appeared to be fobbed off time after time until it was too late and I reached crisis point. Being offered a place at the sleep clinic in 'four months' is not a solution. Neither is being told by many that 'You have a new baby, what do you expect?'

I often use the analogy of the extreme sleep deprivation and inability to relax as the common feelings we all have prior to the need for an early start the next day. Perhaps you have an early journey or momentous occasion. The chances are that you will have selected the clothes you will wear; set a couple of alarms; double-checked travel arrangements and sorted as many risk aversions as possible. You may have a camomile tea, a lavender bath and watch the news and weather for any possible changes to your plan or clothing. You switch the light off at 22:37. In a restless state and fidgeting you then see the clock at 01:47, 02:53, 04:19 … by which time you are drowning in a sea of panic and self-doubt as to your arrangements or rehearsing events in your mind. Each time you look at the clock you tell yourself that you must sleep or you will be so tired. Then just before you do need to get up, you fall blissfully asleep. Do you know that kind of night? That was how my brain was constantly after being a mother for seven months. I lost the ability to switch off. I also began to feel that it was pointless sleeping because my son would soon be awake to need feeding. Looking back I was my own worst enemy and pushed away all offers of help 'because I was the only one who could feed him'.

My most recent night like that was prior to being interviewed on *BBC Breakfast*. I was at the hotel next to the studio so there were no travel concerns and my outfit was ironed and ready on the hanger. I went to sleep quickly only to wake at 03:11. Try as I might, I could not get back to sleep. On the sofa next to me on the programme later was Lucie Malangone who told of how her sister Emma[2] had taken her life whilst suffering from postnatal illness. The description of her sleep deprivation especially reminded me of how near I had been to taking my own life and my heart went out to Emma's suffering and the consequent unnecessary loss to her child and family. I felt the effects of that one disturbed night for several days. It reminded me of the frustration and exhaustion you can feel.

One mother described lack of sleep like this:

- I was in a bubble. I could hear, see but could not feel. I was numb to emotion. Nothing seemed real and every hour and day I would wait for that bubble to pop. Then one day it popped so loud I think the whole street had wondered what had happened to that former beauty queen. It was then I realised I was asking too much of myself: trying to be that perfect mum when it clearly didn't exist. So I reached out, got some help so I could catch up on sleep and slowly I began to feel and laugh once again.

Another explained how lack of sleep affected her:

- I had insomnia through most of my pregnancy. I think this was because I was excited about the baby, and nervous, and because I was made redundant in the second month of pregnancy so had lots of things occupying my mind with this too. Because I wasn't working, I could allow my sleep routine to drift – if I didn't get to sleep until 5 a.m. (this was quite usual), I would lie in until 11 a.m. as I didn't have the pressure of work to get up for. In hindsight, I should have stuck to a normal routine and got up at 7 a.m. Then I think my body clock would have adjusted itself back into a more normal pattern.

Tips from other mothers include:

- My top tips to pass on especially with another baby – in hindsight, I should have spoken to my GP and maybe used sleeping tablets to help me through this period. Of course, we all want to avoid drugs during pregnancy but there is a time and place to reach out for help and I missed the chance of getting help for my insomnia. Had I had a crystal ball, I would definitely have sought help. By the time I went into labour, I was seriously sleep deprived. Combining this with a long and difficult labour, C-section, haemorrhage, etc. and probably 3 nights with little or no sleep around my baby's birth, it was all a step too far for my body. Getting the sleep during pregnancy could have perhaps prevented this spiral and decline postnatally. **In summary, if you are not sleeping, do something about it. Don't leave it to catch up with you after your baby is born!**
- In hindsight I should have gone to my GP to discuss the insomnia I experienced in pregnancy. I should have got on top of it so that when I went into labour I was better equipped physically to cope with a 32 hour labour + emergency C-section!! Maybe they could have prescribed something safely for me to help? Engage with your GP and discuss any problems in pregnancy. Don't ignore things. If not, you may not be aware that you are storing up problems for later, e.g. in labour or afterwards.
- I have a special alarm clock that wakes you up with gradual increase in light (great for SAD sufferers). It also has a great function where it gradually lowers light at night too to help get off to sleep. On their web page they claim it can help perinatal depression www.lumie.com/collections/light-therapy-womens-health

Had I had a second child, establishing a good sleep routine for us all would have been top of my list for the whole family. In those early days and weeks especially, I feel I would have either delegated or simply allowed the general household tasks just to be left undone. When baby rested, I would have done – even if was sitting with my feet up on the sofa watching daytime television. This may not have been as easy, having a toddler around. Kellymom[3] suggests:

If you need a nap and your toddler doesn't – childproof a room of the house that has:
- a door or a baby gate (so your toddler can't 'escape' and play in the toilet while you're resting)
- a bed or comfortable spot on the floor where you can lie down and nurse
- interesting toys that your toddler is likely to play with without much interaction – some moms also put on a favourite video
- a snack and a drink for toddler

When you want to nap (or at least rest) while baby naps, close off the door so you can lie down with baby without worrying about what your toddler is getting into. A friend says she would lie on the floor with baby and let her toddlers use mom as a 'road' for their matchbox cars – rest and a massage all 'rolled' into one!

I would have chosen to breastfeed again, if possible, and made better arrangements for night feeds, such as saving up enough milk with breast shells to let someone else do one in the night.

When my partner died, it was sleep deprivation that became my biggest challenge again. I found this symptom of grief hardest and the one I knew had a profound effect on the following day. It was my main worry that if I did not sleep on a regular and sound basis then I could be very prone to suffer from depression again.

Some of the ways I use to get a better sleep pattern have been:

1. Ensuring my bedroom is comfortable and a place I enjoy being.
2. Having a relaxing, candlelit bath with restful music.
3. Writing a list of things I need to remember or do the next day to save myself from keeping thinking of them.
4. A relaxation CD or app, e.g. from Hampshire Hypnotherapy Centre.[4]
5. Getting up and having a milky drink downstairs for a while.
6. Playing Scrabble on my iPad! Some sleep experts say that a screen is bad before you go to sleep – this works for me as it switches my mind off from 'to do' things.
7. If I cannot sleep, then I allow myself to accept that my body is resting whilst I am lying down – that is better than scurrying around.
8. Try breathing in for 4 seconds, hold breath for 7, then exhale in 8 seconds – repeat.[5]

The Mental Health Foundation say that:

> Sleep is as important to our health as eating, drinking and breathing. It allows our bodies to repair themselves and our brains to consolidate our memories and process information. Poor sleep is linked to physical problems such as a weakened immune system and mental health problems such as anxiety and depression.

They produce a pocket guide including simple ways to improve your 'sleep hygiene', such as adjusting the light, noise and temperature in the bedroom and changing your eating, drinking and exercise routines.[6]

As time passed with my son, he did begin to sleep better. I remember going to see a new health visitor for his pre-school assessment. I told her that we now had undisturbed nights because just before we went to bed we would lift him out of his bed to empty his bladder. The new health visitor was horrified and told me that was completely the wrong thing today and was against current guidelines. By then I was well enough and had the confidence to tell her that it worked for us and was better than us all being disturbed by having to strip and change beds in the early hours! Sometimes as a parent you have to do what works for you.

Also look out for what soothes your child. One bedtime I found Marius with his head in our laundry basket searching frantically. He told me he wanted one of my 'dirty' nighties, 'because it smells of you'. I hasten to say he meant worn as opposed to dirty! I found him one and he settled to sleep snuggling my worn nightie and sucking his thumb! It then became one of our routines that as I changed my nightdress he would have it first for a few nights before it was washed and the process started again. He clearly got comfort from my scent and the feel of a cosy item of clothing.

One day I spoke to a group of mums at a support group. One explained that her biggest problem since having her new baby was getting her toddler to sleep alone. Apparently he idolised his new sibling and wanted to sleep with him. I suggested to the mum that when she undressed the baby to put the clothes on the toddler's treasured teddy bear as he was going to bed. It worked a treat!

Here are some other comments and suggestions from other mothers:

- I'd say that perinatally, I remember having the best night's sleep I've had in 8 years the night before I (prematurely) gave birth to my son. I often wonder if nature was preparing me in some way because in every other way I was totally unprepared! I was unable to sleep – unable to give myself permission to sleep – once I'd had him, and that undoubtedly affected how I viewed my new life as a mum. From the moment I had him I was terrified of the responsibility and that set the scene for PND. I felt constantly on 'red alert' and when I had a breakdown about 3 years afterwards, I still had that feeling :(Yuck.
- I would say this quote helped me enormously unfortunately I can't remember who said it but it is not my own – I saw it online somewhere: 'Do not stand up when you could be sitting down; do not sit down when you could be lying down; do not be awake when you could be asleep.' This phrase became the best advice, permission and my watchwords for dealing with life with two children. My other top tip is … be prepared. Really take time to experience as best you can what life will be like with a new baby; think about how your life will change: be *prepared*.

This is the experience of another family:

- My anxiety was so severe after the birth of my first son that I was unable to sleep, despite being exhausted. Of course, this made my depression and overall inability to cope even more pronounced. I struggled to go to sleep, and once I had woken for a night feed, I couldn't go back to sleep. I know now that this was a symptom of the illness.

Second time around, I recognised that sleep was going to be key to my mental wellbeing. Thankfully, although I did suffer from anxiety in my second pregnancy, I was better prepared for the birth, so I was less anxious going home, and I was also already on antidepressants. However, although I was breastfeeding, I chose to introduce a bottle of formula at night from day one. I used to go to bed at 7.30/8 p.m. and my husband would do the next feed. This meant that, most nights, I usually got 4 or 5 uninterrupted hours of sleep, which was vital to help me cope – particularly because, with older children to look after, I was unable to nap during the day. I also believe that an hour of sleep before midnight is worth two hours of sleep after midnight!

I really think women are let down when it comes to options for feeding – there's a lot of pressure to breastfeed but no information about combination feeding, when in fact choosing combination feeding kept me breastfeeding for six months. Knowing that I could have that break when I needed it was key to my mental health this time.

Another controversial thing which I did this time but would not have dared to do with my first child was to co sleep. Night time breastfeeding was significantly easier co sleeping. I chose to share a room with my baby this time (to avoid having to get out of bed and wake myself up too much!) and, although my son would start the night in his cot, more often than not, we'd end up co sleeping after feeds, and I often went back to sleep when I was feeding. I followed safe co sleeping practice (no covers on the baby, lying on my side with my arm out and knee up) and my husband slept in the spare bed, so I never felt that there was a risk. In fact, I was so in tune with my baby that I only woke when he needed feeding, whereas my husband heard every murmur and whimper. Having separate beds isn't the best for intimacy with your husband, but our priorities were all about sleep in those first few months! Husband was also on duty if my older child ever woke in the night.

My baby was a bad day sleeper, but pretty good at night once we were past those first few weeks. I could cope well during the day because I was getting a decent amount of sleep altogether, and that solid block of 5 hours or so was the key. I was also significantly more relaxed with baby number 2 – whether he picked up on that, I don't know, but he definitely felt like he was an 'easier' baby, even though, objectively, I think he was more demanding than my first son!

I have included links to other resources for settling a new baby and a toddler at the end of the chapter. This is what another mother recommends:

- I am one of those very rare parents that have fantastic children who sleep and have done since about 6 weeks! People often ask me what my trick is … and to be honest I'm not sure … I think I have been very blessed. One tip I would give though is not to pander to a baby. My children learnt to sleep in all levels of light and noise. Especially with 2nd babies, they need to be able to sleep with a certain amount of noise in the house.

I have been delighted to meet Evelyn Burdon, a former health visitor, who now specialises in helping parents to settle their baby into a good sleep routine, sooner rather than later. I wish I had known some of the techniques that she suggests, although the nightie idea that my son used was one (much later on). Evelyn met many depressed, sleep-deprived mothers during her 30-year career. She now works in private practice as the 'Cheshire Baby Whisperer' and makes home visits in Cheshire and supports mothers all over the UK with her email and telephone support package. Evelyn advises parents how to use a multi-sensory approach to sleep that is based on the five senses of smell, sound, sight, touch and taste. All babies use their senses when they drift off to sleep and Evelyn advises parents how to implement the techniques for their baby and how to create a multi-sensory nursery. For more information, Evelyn has written a book, *The Ultimate Sleep Guide for Babies and Toddlers*,[7,8] that gives parents a step-by-step approach to changing negative sleep patterns into positive ones and a detailed plan of action to encourage their baby to sleep to natural sleep potential.

> Remember the importance of sleep for all the family. Whatever works for you is fine (provided it is safe).

TOP TIPS FOR PARENTS

1. Acknowledge that lack of sleep can be a key risk factor for poor perinatal mental help so prioritise it.
2. Discuss insomnia with your GP and follow advice to overcome it.
3. Put plans in place to maximise rest for all the family – if this means delegating tasks or relaxing your usual routines for a while, so be it.
4. Experiment with a range of techniques that help you sleep until you find one, or a combination that is effective.
5. Have confidence in what works for you and your family.
6. 'Do not stand up when you could be sitting down; do not sit down when you could be lying down; do not be awake when you could be asleep.'
7. Apply a sensory approach to teach your baby to settle and sleep.

TOP TIPS FOR HEALTHCARE PROFESSIONALS

1. Take comments about lack of sleep extremely seriously and offer immediate and practical solutions to help.
2. Even if you disagree with a system that is working for the family, support their instinct.
3. Be aware of the many techniques that can help both mother and baby to sleep.

REFERENCES

1. www.internationalbreastfeedingjournal.com/content/2/1/6 A new paradigm for depression in new mothers: the central role of inflammation and how breastfeeding and anti-inflammatory treatments protect maternal mental health. Kathleen Kendall-Tackett.
2. www.dailymail.co.uk/news/article-2424496/Post-natal-depression-Wife-Army-major-threw-train.html
3. http://kellymom.com/parenting/parenting-faq/tips-newborn-toddler/
4. Easysleep App for iPhone and iPad https://itunes.apple.com/au/app/easysleep-hypnosis-insomnia/id953858719?mt=8 and for Android https://play.google.com/store/apps/details?id=uk.co.hantshypno.easysleep
5. www.drweil.com/drw/u/VDR00112/The-4-7-8-Breath-Benefits-and-Demonstration.html
6. http://mentalhealth.org.uk/publications/sleep-pocket-guide/
7. www.cheshirebabywhisperer.com/
8. www.amazon.co.uk/Cheshire-Whisperer-Ultimate-babies-toddlers/dp/1500453749

OTHER RESOURCES

- http://sleeplady.com/toddler-sleep-problems/getting-toddler-to-sleep/
- www.thesleepstore.com.au/sleep-information/toddlers/facebook-threads/toddler-sleep-after-baby-no-2-arrives
- www.babysleepsite.com/tag/new-baby-and-toddler/

CHAPTER 17

Older siblings: new relationships and routines

> Like branches on a tree we grow in different directions yet our roots remain as one. Each of our lives will always be a special part of the other.
>
> *Anonymous*

I mentioned earlier that when I give my presentations, I always include a wide range of my family photographs to illustrate that all the messages I aim to convey involve real people. As my son loves photography and has always been skilled at information technology, I asked for his help to put some photographs together, when he was about 9 years old. We came across one of him on his first Christmas morning looking very sad and bewildered. I explained that it was taken at his grandparents as it was when I was very ill in hospital. I have explained my illness to him a little bit like you do the facts of life with a child – appropriate to their stage of development. He had some knowledge at that point about mental illness. For a while he looked thoughtful and then proclaimed:

> I've just thought – if I was the age I am now and all this had happened to you if I'd had a baby brother or sister, I'd be a traumatised child!

At the time I smiled, and explained to him that we would have done everything we could to avoid it next time. It was a comment that struck me as very perceptive and therefore I can fully appreciate why others may be reluctant to consider a subsequent pregnancy.

A review of the literature does indicate that the children of depressed parents can develop their own issues, for example, in their social-emotional and cognitive development.[1] The good news is that:

Other sources of resilience in children include social and cognitive skills that help them receive positive attention from adults other than their depressed parents and help reduce their depressed parent's feeling of non-competence and rejection. It seems that an understanding of the parent's illness and recognition by the child that he or she is not to blame for the parent's illness-related behaviour is very important to the development of resiliency in a child.[2]

I asked the women who replied to my survey, 'Before the pregnancy when you were postnatally depressed did you have any other children in your care? If so, how did they respond when you were ill?'

Sadly, some reported negative impact:

- My eldest was three at the time and although they said she won't know what's happening, she's been very clingy since. She's 7 now and still can't sleep on her own without me.
- My 3 year old got very demanding and had some challenging behaviour.
- My eldest was very concerned and upset that Mummy was poorly.
- He tried really hard not to get upset in front of me.
- She was only 17 months old. I can remember she just looked lost.
- My daughter ended up being separated from me and that really took a toll on her.

Others appeared to have no change or effect, e.g.:

- I tried to hide it from her, she was 4 at the time and I don't think she knew anything.
- No change.
- He was only 6 – it didn't affect him, thank God.

I also asked if they received any support for the existing children. Some had none. Others described that their husband, partner, other family members and friends helped. One child went to stay with her father for a few months; another said her 7-year-old daughter was a great help to her and with the new baby. A couple of mothers told me that they appreciated help from volunteers, e.g. Home-Start:

- An early years visitor came once a week for 6 months after I was diagnosed. She played with my daughter and did fun stuff that I wasn't able to at the time. She also helped me take the children out to the park or for a picnic.

I also asked how the mothers coped emotionally and physically with caring for and loving another child in relation to their existing sibling. Several of the mothers replied that they had no problems with this and were fine. In comparison to the previous pregnancy, some said it was better:

- Much easier than the previous time.
- Good, actively tried to include my first child to help his relationship with the baby and tried to make time for both children.
- It was magic – after 2 boys I had a girl – very exciting.
- It was really fine. My husband was ill so I had to do a lot of the running about for my first child and I coped well.
- I tried my best not to leave eldest out. My husband was out of work at the time and he was a tremendous help. I slept when baby slept.

Guilt was mentioned too by some around sharing their love or in comparison to the previous early postnatal stage:

- I felt as though I grieved a little because my love was being split into two instead of focusing on one.
- I'm finding it hard to spread the love which is causing overwhelming guilt. I ache a lot and I still have bad days and strugle with everyday life.
- I feel guilt that my first son didn't receive the love and care that my second one will. I suspect that my relationship with my second son will be stronger and more stable and I hate that it should be that way.
- It was hard, a lot of guilt as to dividing attention.
- I struggle with the fact that I bonded calmly but definitely with the 2nd baby when I didn't for a long time with 1st.
- This was really hard – my positive thoughts around my new baby and how different it was to last time made me feel awful once again about what happened the first time around. I was riddled with guilt about what had happened last time. I wanted to run away with my new baby and start again how it was now – all the horror of the early days last time around came back to me.
- Found it both lovely and really hard when I bonded so easily with my second daughter, when I had found it so hard with my first daughter.

Some mothers expressed that they judged themselves harshly:

- I was so hard on myself as I did love my new baby but I was terrified of the illness striking again and the fear of being separated from my elder daughter if I was ill again.
- That was the hardest part and the part I am still having issues about today. Caring for my son came natural, even though he didn't sleep through but I felt I had no energy and caring left for Emily. I often sat by her bed after she had gone to sleep, crying because I felt so bad for shouting at her all day, that's what I felt I did. I worry that it damaged my relationship with her long term.

At each stage of the decisions and outcome, you may want to include your older children. The level of conversation will vary depending on their age and if any subsequent pregnancy is unplanned.

PRE-CONCEPTION

Your existing child/children may well go through a period of asking if they are going to have a baby brother or sister. They may also have strong opinions either way. I know my son reached a certain age when he felt a baby in the house would spoil his Lego creations, so he wasn't fussed about having one! You may have family discussions casually about what it might mean if you were to add to the family or not. Or you may decide that as adults and parents it is your decision alone. Perhaps in view of your previous challenges, this may be the best idea. Children will only be able to process the idea of a new sibling according to their level of development and age. If they have strong opinions either way, this potentially could add to your concerns at a later date. If you do have another child and your existing child was against it, and then you are ill, this could add to your feelings of guilt. If they are very keen to have a sibling and you decide not to, it opens the potential flood gate for them to criticise and blame you as the years go by for denying them something they wanted.

DURING PREGNANCY

This is the stage that potentially could add big excitement and anticipation for your existing children of any age. There are many resources and suggestions for preparing children for a new baby in the family that are easily available. For example, I include a list of picture books below, appropriate for younger children that may help prepare them for the changes ahead. You also might include imaginative play with dolls to show how the baby will have to be fed, changed, etc. As you brush up on current knowledge, trends and resources in newborn babies, involve the children. The ideas for bonding in pregnancy are ideal for including the existing children, especially in quiet time and reading together. The key aspect in the dilemma that you are facing is to remain as positive as you can as regards warning your child about the possibility that you may become mentally and/or physically unwell. It may be more sensible to tackle any challenges if and when they actually arise. If you give your child 'a list' of all the possible scenarios, then you are simply going to sow the seeds for them to worry about things that may not happen. Put your effort into making plans for them in case they are needed, e.g. additional childcare arrangements if you were to become unwell.

Focus on aspects of their personal life that will stay the same; reassure them that they will still be loved just as much and that you will all have a new person to join the family. Be realistic in telling them that new babies can do little initially other than needing feeding and changing, before they become a playmate.

ONCE BABY ARRIVES

Continue to involve your existing child in care for the new sibling. Build their confidence by giving them specific tasks. Apply the tips on sleep and naps for you all. One aspect that others in this position have wrestled with is guilt – if the birth, bonding and early days are much better this time, then mothers have said they have felt bad then for their first one 'missing out'. As I have said before, you cannot undo or relive the past. Be thankful and enjoy motherhood this next time round. You did not ask for the challenges previously, so why punish yourself if you are well the next time?

Perhaps the idea of the memory book could be useful, especially if Mum is not well. Most children love to be involved in creative activities, so perhaps other adults could help them create a scrapbook of the new baby to make them feel more involved. One mother shared that she has been told that her sister gave her her favourite teddy to have in hospital when she was born and she was only 3.5 years old – siblings clearly love to help and be involved!

Also remember that any mother who has another child may at times feel a little tired, snappy or impatient with their older children. It does not necessarily mean that you are mentally unwell. If it becomes regular you may need to seek help. As with all of the aspects of a subsequent pregnancy and birth – acknowledge and deal with areas of challenge rather than hiding from them.

WHAT TO DO IF YOU DO SUFFER FROM A PERINATAL MENTAL ILLNESS AGAIN

If you are unwell again, the impact on your existing child will depend on how ill you are, of course. The main thing is that they are cared for by others whom you and they trust. If this has been considered and arranged as part of your risk plan, then it will be easier for all concerned. Ease the worry on the adults so it is less for the child.

It may be a concern as to how to explain a mental health challenge to youngsters as it is not as tangible as a physical injury. Theresa Borchard[3] recommends seven things to say to a child, depending on their age:

1. Explain that you are sick.
2. That depression is invisible.
3. They are not to blame.
4. It's okay to cry.
5. Don't take it personally.
6. They are still loved.
7. It can be treated.

She has also written a picture book called *What Does 'Depressed' Mean? A Guidebook for Children with a Depressed Loved One*.[4]

ADDITIONAL SUPPORT

If the siblings need extra help, especially if they are older, it may be useful for them to contact organisations who offer counselling and listening facilities to help them adjust to the situation, e.g. www.relate.org.uk/relationship-help/ help-children-and-young-people/children-and-young-peoples-counselling, www.youngminds.org.uk/for_children_young_people/better_mental_ health/friends_family; www.childline.org.uk/

Healthcare professionals may find support and information for older children from organisations like Barnardos, who offer help to Young Carers www.barnardos.org.uk/reaching_families_in_need.pdf They also have a range of resources, reports and policies for assisting families affected by poor mental health. The 'Keeping the Family in Mind' pack is one example. www. barnardos.org.uk/resources/research_and_publications/keeping-the-family-in-mind-resource-pack-2nd-edition/publication-view.jsp?pid=PUB-1600 There are others available via their website too. www.barnardos.org.uk/ what_we_do/policy_research_unit/research_and_publications/mental_ health_policy_research.htm

Other charities may offer support for young carers too, such as providing trips outs and groups, e.g. www.family-action.org.uk/what-we-do/ children-families/young-carers-services/

Families may also be referred to charities such as www.home-start.org.uk/ who may be able to organise for a volunteer to help with the practical tasks. The local children's centre or Sure Start group may offer helpful services too. www.actionforchildren.org.uk/ may provide family support.

Find out what is available in your area for a local support group or centre at www.gov.uk/support-group-for-children-young-people-families Also enquire at your local community centre and places of worship that offer sessions for young families.

Remember too that if you are mentally unwell again and your older child has to manage that in addition to the introduction of a new sibling, ultimately it may build their character and understanding of others. If you, and the other significant others in their lives, treat mental health problems as a 'normal' illness that requires care, compassion and treatment, you are helping them to grow into empathetic people. I know that my son is far more aware of mental health as a teenager than I ever was. We cannot shield our children from illness and challenges of life – what we can do is show them ways and give them tools to manage them.

One comment from a couple who decided to have another baby after a previous perinatal mental illness advise:

> Don't be put off from considering more children if you've always wanted a bigger family. You could feel more guilt and disappointment in the long run if you let the illness stop you, and there's a chance you could become unwell again even if you

don't have another child. If you have unresolved issues about your illness seek counselling to talk these over and help you decide what's best for you regarding future children.

TOP TIPS FOR PARENTS

1. Remember that parents may still consider the needs of their existing children when contemplating another baby, even without any history of perinatal mental illness.
2. Consider how much, if any, consultation your existing children should have in the decision.
3. Make plans for if you become ill again, without the need to involve or concern the older sibling(s). You may remain well and they will have been worried unnecessarily. Deal with 'what' happens rather than 'if'.
4. Involve them in plans and bonding during pregnancy.
5. Involve them in age-appropriate tasks when the baby is born and be sensitive and alert to any 'usual' sibling rivalry.

TOP TIPS FOR HEALTHCARE PROFESSIONALS

1. Be familiar with the available resources and local support for older siblings.
2. Listen to any concerns the parents may have about their existing children and signpost appropriate help.

REFERENCES

1. Maternal depression and child development. *Paediatr Child Health*. 2004; **9**(8): 575–83. Available at: www.ncbi.nlm.nih.gov/pmc/articles/PMC2724169/
2. Beardslee W, Podorefski D. Resilient adolescents whose parents have serious affective and other psychiatric disorders: importance of self-understanding and relationships. *Am J Psychiatry*. 1988; **145**: 63–9.
3. Borchard T. 7 Things a Depressed Parent Can Say to a Child. *Psych Central*. 2013 Available at: http://psychcentral.com/blog/archives/2013/11/13/7-things-a-depressed-parent-can-say-to-a-child/ (accessed 1 December 2014).
4. Borchard TJ (author), Alley RW (Illustrator). *What Does 'Depressed' Mean? A guidebook for children with a depressed loved one*. St Meinrad, IN: Abbey Press; 2011.

FURTHER READING AND RESOURCES

- Kitbag for Families is a set of tools designed to help children become calm, relaxed, resilient and confident, helping to build positive relationships in school and in families. www.internationalfuturesforum.com/p/kitbag-for-families

- www.barnardos.org.uk/reaching_families_in_need.pdf
- www.familylives.org.uk/ and www.getconnected.org.uk/ offer specific advice aimed at young parents.
- Family Rights Group. www.frg.org.uk/images/Advice_Sheets/4-family-support-services. pdf?gclid=Cj0KEQiAwPCjBRDZp9LWno3p7rEBEiQAGj3KJsy-gPj2UvS-6S9Hzdqi 6in-0omYHGnZxAXbRaTVbh0aAnRO8P8HAQ
- Cooper-Abbs N. *The Need to Know Guide to Life with a Toddler and a Newborn: how to prepare for and cope with the day to day challenge of raising two young children.* (Central YMCA Mums' Health Guides Book 2, 2013) London: Central YMCA; 2012.
- Chase-Brand J. Effects of maternal postpartum depression on the infant and older siblings. In: Stone SD, Menken AE, editors. *Perinatal and Postpartum Mood Disorders: perspectives and treatment guide.* New York: Springer; 2008.
- www.babysleepsite.com/tag/new-baby-and-toddler/

Picture books

- Cole J. *I'm a Big Brother* and *I'm a Big Sister*. New York: William Morrow; 1997. A 'big sibling' classic!
- Falwell C. *We Have A Baby*. New York: Houghton Mifflin; 1999. This one is great to read as a family – it shows how the new baby will affect everyone in the entire family.
- Kubler A. *My New Baby*. Swindon: Child's Play (International); 2000. This is a 'pictures only' book – no words! This makes it a great choice for young toddlers.
- Berenstain S, Berenstain J. *The Berenstain Bears and Baby Makes Five*. New York: Random House; 2000. Excellent book for pre-schoolers and young elementary children.
- Faulkner J. *A Monster Ate My Mum!* 2013. Available at: www.lulu.com/shop/jen-faulkner/ a-monster-ate-my-mum/paperback/product-21305413.html

CHAPTER 18

The role of the partner

Coming together is a beginning; keeping together is progress; working together is success.

Henry Ford

Most people would probably agree that ideally we bring a child into this world with someone whom we love and are in a stable relationship with. Having a child is a symbol of that love and we hope to raise a family together. For some people poor mental health can impact upon this either antenatally or post-natally, adding additional pressures to deal with. Generally it is the mother who suffers from postnatal illness; yet it is also recognised that their partners may also be affected by a depressive illness in the first 12 months after a baby arrives. Either way the dyad has become a triad, so a 'new' balance, routine and a new 'normal' has to be created. When that new routine has become 'normal' and another child enters the family unit, then there is the risk again for either parent to have challenges. The demands of another new baby, sleep-lessness, financial pressures, adjustments to additional parenthood can all take their toll on the relationship of the new parents. Looking back, that was certainly the situation for us first time round. We both did what we felt was best, yet really we approached it from naivety and ignorance.

Historically we know that by the mid-nineteenth century puerperal insanity was firmly established in medical literature as an easily recognisable condition, triggered by the specific event of childbirth and its aftermath, and usually setting in soon after delivery. In 1831, Robert Gooch explained how:

> Nervous irritation is very common after delivery, more especially among fash-ionable ladies, and this may exist in any degree between mere peevishness and downright madness. Some women, though naturally amiable and good tempered, are so irritable after delivery that their husbands cannot enter their bed-rooms without getting a certain lecture; others are thoroughly mad.[1]

After experiencing this situation with one child, how and why do others go on to repeat it? Forty-one per cent of the people in my survey had gone on to have another baby. Here are some examples shared with me:

- I'm currently pregnant. I'm nervous and extremely scared that I'm going to end up with PND again! However my partner and family know exactly what to look out for this time! My partner's thoughts on everything that happened are that he is furious that the mental health team didn't keep a closer eye on me, however he always wanted more than one child, but two is the limit, ha ha!

- My hubby said my PP didn't put him off having another baby as it was a short-lived incident and rectified itself (or started to) once I had my blood transfusion. He therefore felt quite relaxed that it was unlikely to happen again. His view, not mine. He didn't want another baby anyway but PP would not have put him off if he had.

- After thinking hard for a long time about having another child, both my partner and I decided the time was right. Two and a half years it took for us to feel ready again. My husband has always dreamt of having 3 children. Sadly though, our son is almost 5 now and we still only have him. At first, my husband couldn't wait, albeit a little scared as we both were. Thankfully, he paid a lot of attention when I was ill the first time around and I'm almost certain he knows the signs to look out for if and when I suffer again. Having gone through a hard time with my illness, I can understand why he is scared. I left him many a time throughout the course of the illness yet he provided nothing but love and support. He suffered constant rejection from me and I can still see that I hurt him although he doesn't blame me. After 2 and a half years of infertility, he's starting to sway a little from the '3 kids dream'. He wonders whether it would be worth the heartache of me suffering again although he remains optimistic that I would get lucky next time around. He's also starting to wonder whether our son is enough and that we have come such a long way since our 'dark times' that to do it again might be the breaking for us. As I call him, fearfully optimistic. My husband has been my rock and I hope to one day give him the children he longs for and enjoy those first months/years with him. Together. As a family. But who knows. Maybe our son is our angel and he was and still is worth every tear we both shed in that year.

- I think my partner's main concern was finance. I don't feel he ever understood postnatal depression. I have postnatal depression second time around – he is a bit more understanding. I watched *One born every minute* and was so pleased to see I was not the only one against epidural and C-section. The decision was out of my hands and I felt so cheated and upset the same as the fact of not being able to breastfeed. I think ladies need to be prepared if they are not able to do either or both of these. If they can't and it's an issue then counselling should be on offer. I was lucky (well if you can call it that) that on the second pregnancy I had a natural birth and it cancelled out all the negativity I felt. The same with breastfeeding – I couldn't second time around but dealt with the disappointment. I wish I had more support from my partner but as they say, 'Men are from Mars'.

- At first, it was a definite 'no more babies'! But after a few years he agreed to discuss the very emotional and difficult subject. Our daughter was conceived through IVF so we had some frozen embryos in storage. We agreed to go and speak to our GP about the difficult decision that we had to make and he referred us to the psychiatrist I had been under at a Mother and Baby Unit. An appointment was arranged and we went to see her. She suggested that if I became pregnant again, I should stay on my PND medication throughout the pregnancy and that I would be admitted to the unit a few weeks before the baby was due. I would have delivered the baby at the same hospital and then be admitted back in to the Mother and Baby unit until they felt I was definitely stable enough to go home with my baby. We both felt that this was the best way to move forward and I felt confident in my GP and psychiatrist with their suggestions. We went for further IVF treatment but it was unsuccessful. We both felt that another baby in our family wasn't meant to be and my husband was quietly relieved that we didn't have to face the possibility of going through what had been the most horrendous period of our lives. My husband still struggles to talk about my PND and feels that the subject should be put in a box and archived! I understand how he must feel as he was helpless and so scared and it was a very dark period of our lives. However, the birth of our daughter has turned out to be the best thing that has ever happened and although those few years were traumatic and almost feel like a figment of my imagination, I feel that it was all worth it. I must emphasise though, that after many weeks in a variety of psychiatric units and under a variety of NHS specialists, I did eventually receive some excellent treatment. I do feel that if this hadn't been the case, I would not be here today.
- His first reaction was utter shock – it wasn't planned. It takes two but he wanted me to have an abortion and refused to speak to me. In fact it got so bad we split up till after his birth. He wouldn't come – I had one of neighbours attend. He just couldn't understand how I could go through it all and my baby was born exactly a year and two days after the last. He did come round in the end and four years later has a very strong bond with him. We actually had another child together 2 years afterwards and with both, I was fine.
- My partner's thoughts and feelings were 'never again!' It caused a lot of tension and unhappiness. Eventually he agreed to another baby, but with lots of conditions – I took a career break, we paid for a daily mother's help in the early months, we had a lot of family help, etc. Even then, he would have been happy to stick at one, and though he loves number two dearly he still feels that it would be less tiring and easier with one. He only agreed to a second because I was so desperately unhappy about not having another baby. If I'm honest, I wanted a chance to 'do it right this time', and although that is NOT a good reason to have a baby, it has worked out fine. Breastfeeding was much easier because at

least one of us knew what we were doing, she wasn't colicky, I had an emergency C-section but not a crash one, I just let her live in the sling and trusted she would sleep in her cot when she was ready.
- After my PND we waited a good 3 years. It was my desire for another child, however my husband made it clear our marriage would not survive another PND diagnosis which worried us both. I worked alongside amazing health visitor who monitored me and was amazing after the birth of my second child to ensure I had full support.

So what can be done to minimise the risks or perinatal mental illness, maximise recovery and strengthen the bond within the parental relationship?

WORK AS A TEAM

Work out your plan for a healthy experience this pregnancy and beyond. If health professionals are involved in treatment, both of you should be consulted and play your role. Depression is difficult to talk about. In short appointments, the sufferer may feel rushed, ashamed, embarrassed or uncooperative. Write down your thoughts and take them into the appointment. Even better, go as a couple so you have an advocate. If you felt there were gaps in services or care previously, discover and ask for them next time. Many of the mothers said that the support of their partner was invaluable, e.g.:

- Best part of having my second baby was that Richard was there and I had total faith in him standing up for me and my care.

Identify the triggers and areas of stress from the previous episode and know what helped then – set it up again this time.

Remember that, where possible, minimise the stresses of everyday life, including moving house; big career changes; decorating. One mother mentioned:

- We moved house 4 months after our daughter was born which put a huge strain on both of us. Looking back, I don't know how we did it. Try not to make any big decisions too quickly – pause, breathe, count to 10 and focus on the priority of your family unit – baby, partner and relationship.

If you are a healthcare professional, be alert to the involvement of the partner during this pregnancy. Be alert to the fact that they may need additional emotional support and/or counselling to help prepare them. If the mother or partner do become mentally unwell, always ask the question: 'Who is caring for the carer?' Look back at the resources I listed previously for this, e.g. www. reachingoutpmh.co.uk[2]

One couple advised:

- Caring for the carer – when I was sectioned, the hospital offered to take our daughter into the nursery ward for a night to give my husband time to sleep. Ask health carers if this option is available, and don't feel guilty about need to rest. Your baby will be well cared for and not miss you for one night.

A good diet and exercise can both aid mental wellbeing – work on these together. If one of you is working all day, think out and plan (the night before) what the next evening's meal will be as this will reduce the anxiety on the sufferer. Such decisions can appear huge if you are not well. Plan for walks, swimming, etc. as a family.

Be there – physically, practically and emotionally. As much as possible, take time off work to enable you both to adjust to the new family dynamics. As a couple you may decide that it works better for you if the partner takes a career break, rather than the mother. Perhaps this is the time to cut back on other usual clubs, meetings, etc. Remember that this is a short phase. What is your priority? The wellbeing of your family and yourself should come before your concern about 'what others might say'. The chances are that others would understand and, after all, it's not their business.

Forgiveness is giving up the hope that the past could have been any different.

Oprah Winfrey

Practically help each other as much as possible. If you have high standards of cleanliness and order, reassure one another that in the early days of a new baby, it does not matter! Praise each other for what you do that is okay, rather than nit-picking at what has been done 'wrongly' or not at all. There is more than one way to change a nappy – be gracious and appreciative with each other. A bitten tongue may be preferable to a head that is bitten off, creating tension and upset.

It may be that with your first child you had to 'work through' differences about bringing up a child based on your own respective family experience and upbringing. This may have been added to by pressure from in-laws about how child rearing and motherhood 'should' be done. Some sons can find it hard to adjust to what their mother did and what their partner does. Talk about this whilst you are pregnant and have the confidence and self-belief in making 'your' family ways and traditions that suit your lifestyle today.

HONESTY AND GREAT COMMUNICATION

Learn about the possible illness – its signs, symptoms and causes. In so doing, you should appreciate and understand that no one is to blame. It isn't a personal vendetta. How would you treat your partner if they had a physical ailment? This is the same … but generally invisible!

Sometimes it is hard to describe how you are feeling, especially when tired and time together is limited or strained. Why not write each other a letter (in your own time and space), exchange them and set enough time aside later to discuss them? Maybe you could both reflect on the previous pregnancy, birth and early days of parenthood, reviewing what you found most helpful and what could have been better. Next time you will not have to second guess.

Use the darkness of your past to propel you to a brighter future.

Donata Joseph

Be aware that we have different ways to communicate. I know mine is to tell anyone willing to listen! This is not always the case. These ladies commented:

- I think it is so incredibly hard for men to open up. I know my husband opted for the 'ostrich' approach in some ways to my illness, and threw himself back into work. But who did he turn to? He has no family and close friends lived away. Even if friends had been physically close, I doubt he would have confided in them as he never has before or since to my knowledge about any matters close to his heart or sensitive.
- Men and women approach things very differently – women need to talk but men can often mistake this as a woman's expectation that the man will have all the answers. Gentlemen we don't expect you to pull a rabbit out of the hat, just to listen!

Perhaps this is where healthcare professionals could make a difference. Think back to my earlier chapter about fathers, and how Mark Williams has encouraged the partners to speak out rather than use alcohol, for example, as a 'coping' method.

The use of language can make a big difference. Depression saps your confidence and minor comments of constructive criticism can be taken as massive attacks! Comments such as 'pull yourself together', 'snap out of it', 'all you ever wanted was a family – there is no pleasing you' are not helpful! If your partner had a broken leg, would you say such things? Remember that they are ill and haven't chosen to feel this way. They do need to take some personal responsibility for their own recovery though, and may need gentle persuasion to do some things for themselves.

With the stresses and strains on both parents, often anger and blame can be very real and can devastate the relationship. If one of you reacts to a situation in this way by reciprocating, the fire will be fuelled. Here are some practical thoughts for you to consider:
- Take time out (count to 10) before you reply.

- Suggest to your partner that you speak when you are both calmer.
- A warm, genuine and compassionate hug and an opportunity to cry might be what is needed.
- Remember that your partner is not expecting you to fix things – they want you to be there and be empathetic. At other times they may need a little space. And sometimes they haven't a clue what they want!
- Always keep a sense of humour through good and not so good times.

> The more things we can laugh about, the more alive we become: The more things we can laugh about together, the more connected we become.
>
> Frank Pittman

Depression, raging hormones and lack of sleep need an outlet. Find out together what helps the most ... and apply it. You may find it more helpful simply to use initiative and observation as to what wants doing. If a person is mentally low, being asked questions such as 'What do you need me to do?' can be too much – just do it!

If you feel that your relationship is an area of concern, then you may benefit from reading *Becoming Us: loving, learning and growing together – the essential relationship guide for parents* by Elly Taylor.[3]

PATIENCE

A depressive illness can be seen as a roller-coaster ride – some days or even hours are brighter than others, with few patterns and very erratic. You may plan something when you feel good yet when the event arises, you cannot face it. The partner needs to be patient and the sufferer needs to be kind to themselves and build in an alternative plan or compromise. Remain optimistic and hopeful that 'this will pass', even on days when it feels such a struggle. Consider each day as 'one day nearer to feeling better'. It is encouraging for the partner to point out and praise any small steps of progress, as often when you are depressed you are unable to recognise this for yourself. If you have trodden this path before, you can do so again, knowing that it will pass.

Consider that next time round with a baby you will be 'experienced' in all of the newborn care. Changing a nappy; finding ways to get them to settle, etc. will be second nature now. Enjoy that confidence!

As Dory says in the film *Finding Nemo*[4] – 'Just keep swimming!'

REMEMBER WHY YOU FIRST FELL IN LOVE

What were 'the little things' that you first appreciated when you got together? Did you leave small notes hidden in unexpected places? Send a text just to say 'thinking of you' in the middle of the day? Run a bath and put relaxing music on? Arrange a date night and a babysitter – even if you just stay in together. There may be a new baby in the house, but remember that as parents you need to look after yourselves so that you can look after them. Remove the guilt! Take inspiration from this website on making others feel special http://tinybuddha.com/blog/70-ways-make-others-feel-special/

> The best time to love with your whole heart is always now, in this moment, because no breath beyond the current is promised.
>
> Fawn Weaver

BONDING WITH THE NEW BABY

This is important for the partner too, especially if they are anxious about any potential challenges. There is much research around this issue, and it is generally believed that 'fathers who were observed interacting with their newborns went through the same sort of explanatory and synchronizing process as the mothers.'[5]

Michael Lamb,[6] a well-established researcher in the field of father–infant relationships, states that the relationship between a father and their child will have a great influence on the child's adjustment to society and development in later life. Fathers can be just as competent as caregivers and as a parent as mothers – especially if she is too ill initially.[7] Current studies indicate that on the whole the high intimacy level between an expectant mother, her baby and partner appears to encourage a more rewarding birth and parenting experience.

During pregnancy the partner can become involved by going to antenatal visits and scans, feeling the baby kick, massaging the bump and talking or singing to the baby. Perhaps with the previous pregnancy, this was overlooked or thought to be embarrassing. This time perhaps they will be more aware of the impact of the bump! When the baby arrives, handle him as much as possible. Help with feeding and all of the practical tasks. During pregnancy it may be an idea to become more aware of some of the needs of the other child/children, so that you can also help more when the new baby is here. If you are both confident as a team as to what needs doing, how and when, this can greatly improve the chances of mental wellbeing for you all.

There is an increasing range of resources being created for the partners and inspiration for healthcare professionals. These include:

1. Best Beginnings Phone app that supports fathers through pregnancy and early parenthood. www.chimat.org.uk/resource/view.aspx?RID=223279 &src=pimh
2. iHV parent tips: how can new fathers get involved? A resource, published by the Fatherhood Institute for the Institute of Health Visiting, offering

practical tips on how to get involved in day-to-day hands-on baby care. www.chimat.org.uk/resource/view.aspx?RID=220557&src=pimh

3. All babies count: the Dad Project presents advice on working with and supporting new and expectant fathers www.chimat.org.uk/resource/view. aspx?RID=211760&src=pimh

4. Milgrom, J, Ericksen, J, Leigh, B, Romeo, Y, Loughlin, E, McCarthy, R (2009). *Towards Parenthood: preparing for the changes and challenges of a new baby.* Camberwell: ACER Press. The Towards Parenthood programme was found to be an effective antenatal preparation for parenthood, and in the randomised trial, it resulted in reduced anxiety and depression for both low and high risk women. Originally developed in Australia, it has already been translated into Italian and will soon be available in Dutch. It is also being currently trialled in the UK with Paul Ramchandani as lead as part of a comprehensive midwife programme (National Institute for Health Research – NIHR). The self-help workbook is for both mothers and fathers, includes communication exercises and can be used with supportive telephone coaches.

5. Elly Taylor[3] mentions that 'in his pilot study for Bringing Baby Home classes, relationship researcher John Gottman found that just two 40 minute "preparation for parenthood" classes reduced PPD by 60% and also reduced relationship distress. This claim is in his book *And Baby Makes Three*, I don't think the research was released or a paper published.'[8]

There are more listed below.

Tips from others who have been there all include 'support':

- I was 100% determined everyone knew the signs and where to get support and I was not ashamed. If I were to pass on any advice, it would be to take the help that is being offered. Don't push it away and become a recluse. It's so much harder to deal with this alone. A problem shared is a problem halved and what not. Also, try to look at the positives of having a child. Don't dwell (very hard I know) on the dark days because, well, they aren't worth the bad memories and emotional scars and in no way does the illness define you as a mother nor should it determine your future path. Want another child? I say go for it. Just try to prepare yourself and look for the warning signs.

- I would say get a support package put in place whilst you're pregnant – make sure everyone agrees too.

- Timing is everything – as a couple, set some time aside on a regular basis e.g. weekly, to talk. Make sure that other things don't get in the way of this and ensure this time is taken in a quiet, calm environment. Don't rush it and try to squeeze it in to your routine when you are not in the right frame of mind. Make it a priority – it really matters!

- My advice would be to line up lots of support, for your partner as well as yourself. My more general new baby advice is to feed and cuddle/sling as much as the baby wants – it makes life so much easier than trying to get this tiny, confused, helpless little person to be 'independent'. And the sling gives you hands free to look after your older child so they don't feel too left out.

● My advice – be brutally honest and take all support on offer.

So what will you put into plan now for you and your partner?

If you are a healthcare professional, what will you investigate further and include in your support for parents?

TOP TIPS FOR PARENTS

1. Work as a team to minimise the risks or perinatal mental illness, maximise recovery and strengthen the bond within the parental relationship.
2. Be honest with one another and work out the best way to communicate.
3. Be patient – a perinatal mental health illness is not a personal attack.
4. Keep the romance alive.
5. Learn ways of bonding during pregnancy and once the baby arrives.
6. If your relationship needs support, ask for it and take it.

TOP TIPS FOR HEALTHCARE PROFESSIONALS

1. Be aware of the father/partner at every stage of a subsequent pregnancy. They can be such a strong support and may also need assistance themselves.
2. Take time to look at the growing bank of resources and information about the mental health of the partner.

REFERENCES

1. Marland H. *Maternity and Madness: puerperal insanity in the nineteenth century.* Warwick: Centre for the History of Medicine, University of Warwick; 2003. Available at: www.nursing.manchester.ac.uk/ukchnm/publications/seminarpapers/maternityand madness.pdf
2. www.reachingoutpmh.co.uk
3. Taylor E. *Becoming Us: loving, learning and growing together – the essential relationship guide for parents.* Sydney: ABC Books; 2011.
4. www.disney.co.uk/finding-nemo/
5. www.bondingandbirth.org/papers-and-articles-klaus.html
6. Lamb M. *The Role of the Father in Child Development.* Chichester: John Wiley & Sons; 2010.
7. www.midwivesonline.com/parents/parents1//105

8. Gottman JM. *And Baby Makes Three: the six-step plan for preserving marital intimacy and rekindling romance after baby arrives.* Reprint edition. Three Rivers, MI: Three Rivers Press; 2008.

FURTHER READING AND RESOURCES

- www.familylives.org.uk/ A useful website with an online chat facility for all aspects of parenting and a wealth of information.
- www.dailylife.com.au/life-and-love/parenting-and-families/the-eight-stages-of-early-parenthood-20150127-12z4we.html
- www.howtobeadad.com/2011/2765/another-baby Blog thoughts from a dad.
- www.havinganotherbaby.com/articles/dadsrole.html
- www.growingafamily.com/tips/preparing.htm
- www.yourtango.com/2013191628/ways-support-your-spouse-through-mental-illness#.VH8hzNKsXDU
- www.healthyplace.com/bipolar-disorder/bipolar-support/bipolar-spouse-support-survival-strategies/
- www.rethink.org/carers-family-friends/what-you-need-to-know
- Derbyshire Culture and Community Services. *Good Practice Resource: showing fathers how to play with their children.* Available at: www.healthyfe.org.uk/sites/default/files/shared/Derbyshire%20Culture%20and%20Community%20Services%20-%20good%20practice%20example.pdf
- Fatherhood Institute. *Bringing Fathers In: free resources for advocates, practitioners and researchers.* Available at: www.chimat.org.uk/resource/view.aspx?RID=220549&src=pimh A series of smart, punchy, evidence-based information sheets backed up with a series of online research summaries. These resources are intended for an international audience of health, education and social care professionals, policy makers, programme managers and designers, researchers and evaluators.
- Institute of Health Visiting. *Good Practice Points for Health Visitors: engaging with fathers.* Available at: www.chimat.org.uk/resource/view.aspx?RID=220555&src=pimh This resource, published by the Fatherhood Institute for the Institute of Health Visiting, is an evidence-based summary looking at why and how to engage with fathers.
- www.thecalmzone.net/ Charity concerned with suicide in young men.
- Fatherhood Institute. *Fathers and Parental Responsibility: a factsheet for practitioners.* Available at: www.chimat.org.uk/resource/view.aspx?RID=187686&src=pimh Explains parental responsibility, which is a key legal concept practitioners need to understand when working with fathers. It refers to the rights and responsibilities parents have to care and provide for their children and make important decisions about their upbringing.
- Tech times. *Young Dads are Prone to Post-partum Depression, Too: study.* Available at: www.chimat.org.uk/resource/view.aspx?RID=197703&src=pimh A new study suggests that men, young fathers in particular, are also vulnerable to developing depressive symptoms during the first few years of parenthood.
- Kerstis B, Berglund A, Engström G, *et al.* Depressive symptoms postpartum among parents are associated with marital separation: a Swedish cohort. *Scand J Public Health.* 2014; **42**(7): 660–8. Available at: www.ncbi.nlm.nih.gov/pubmed/25053465

- Iles J, Slade P, Spiby H. Posttraumatic stress symptoms and postpartum depression in couples after childbirth: the role of partner support and attachment. *J Anxiety Disord.* 2011; **25**(4): 520–30. Available at: www.ncbi.nlm.nih.gov/pubmed/21295438
- https://twitter.com/DadsMatterUK

CHAPTER 19

The single parent

I've been a single parent for a long time. It reminds me of being a waitress. As you walk back to the kitchen, requests come at you from all sides. You're doing the job of two – you have to be highly organised.

Cherie Lunghi

I know that there were many times when I was struggling with sleepless nights or stressful moments with a new baby, as part of a couple. I remember at the time wondering how people got through this stage on their own. Yet they do. Grace Sharrock published her experience as a single, young mother who suffered from puerperal psychosis in *Saving Grace: my journey and survival through postnatal depression.*[1] She has since gone on to have twins with a new partner with no relapse of her illness.

Most of us do not plan to bring children up without a partner, yet there are circumstances that happen which make this a reality. This can feel overwhelming and stressful. If you suddenly become a single parent, even without the additional risk of perinatal mental illness, you are probably more vulnerable to an emotional breakdown. The main advice is to seek support through this period of potential challenge. The end of any relationship can leave you feeling low and your self-esteem knocked. Your sleep and appetite may also be affected, all of which put you at higher chance of developing depression. Seek help from close family and friends and/or from healthcare professionals. Your GP may be able to refer you to support services such as counselling.

It may be that you are happy to be a single parent. If this is the case and you are at risk of having a perinatal mental health challenge, then it would make sense to consider the advice elsewhere in this book to ensure that you have all the necessary support in place. This is especially vital when it comes to the care of your child or children, as I am sure you will appreciate.

As with all the other areas of pregnancy and postnatal planning, there are some possible steps and sources of extra knowledge and information that you may find useful as a single parent or as a healthcare professional.

Of course, the majority of all the other aspects of this book will also apply. I have researched some of those that may be useful, relevant to why you have become a single parent:

1. UNEXPECTED PREGNANCY THAT THE FATHER DOES NOT WANT TO BE INVOLVED WITH, OR YOU DO NOT WANT THEM TO BE

This may be due to an abusive relationship and you feel that both you and your children are better away from the partner. Sadly pregnancy is a time when domestic violence increases. Here are some sources of help and information:

- www.nhs.uk/conditions/pregnancy-and-baby/pages/domestic-abuse-pregnant.aspx#close
- www.marchofdimes.org/pregnancy/abuse-during-pregnancy.aspx#
- www.refuge.org.uk/get-help-now/what-is-domestic-violence/domestic-violence-and-pregnancy/
- www.womensaid.org.uk/default.asp

2. THE BREAKDOWN OF RELATIONSHIP BETWEEN EXPECTANT PARENTS

There are many reasons why relationships change. There are services that will help you through this.

- www.relate.org.uk/relationship-help/help-separation-and-divorce
- www.fatherhoodinstitute.org/2008/fi-research-summary-separated-families/

3. YOUR CHOICE TO PLAN A PREGNANCY AS A SINGLE PERSON

You may need to consider aspects such as flexible employment – look at www.netmums.com/back-to-work/jobs/all-about-flexible-working Information about finances is at www.turn2us.org.uk/, with help to access benefits and grants.

4. ONE PARENT LEAVING WHEN A NEW BABY ARRIVES

- www.nhs.uk/Conditions/pregnancy-and-baby/pages/bringing-up-child-alone.aspx#close

5. THE LOSS OF YOUR PARTNER THROUGH ILLNESS OR ACCIDENT

The pain and shock of losing a loved one is awful at any time. When it is linked with the perinatal period, this has added implications. These organisations will all offer support.

- www.pregnancymagazine.com/mom/dealing-with-grief-during-pregnancy
- www.nhs.uk/conditions/pregnancy-and-baby/pages/coping-death-pregnant.aspx
- www.cruse.org.uk/
- www.merrywidow.me.uk/
- www.mummysstar.org/ In June 2013, Mummy's Star was born. It is the only UK charity with the aim of 'supporting pregnancy through cancer and beyond'. More specifically the charity focuses on supporting women/families:
  - › diagnosed or treated for cancer during pregnancy
  - › diagnosed or treated for cancer within a year of a birth
  - › who in the first year after pregnancy lose a spouse (female or male).
- http://singleparentdad.blogspot.co.uk/ Ian Newbold was widowed in 2005 with a baby to look after. He had his book *Parenting with Balls* published, then married again in 2014.[2] Ian and his wife Samantha were the proud parents of a beautiful seven-month-old baby boy, Max, when Samantha died suddenly from a heart attack. Overnight he became a sole parent. Ian gave up his job at an electrical firm to look after Max, who is now seven. Ian shares what he learned after being thrown into the parenting deep end – his story is told with humour and pathos and will be of help to any new father, single or not.
- www.uk-sands.org/ for anyone affected by the death of a baby.

Healthcare professionals may also find the tips and resources in the article 'Empty arms'[3] to be useful.

I have listed a range of other sources of support and knowledge for single parents at the end of the chapter. Generally they give advice on some of the main areas to consider. These are even more relevant if you are aware that your perinatal mental health may be challenged:

- Break the isolation by reaching out to others in a similar situation. Social media and telecommunication, e.g. Skype, are ways to connect with others even if you are unable to leave the house. Look into days out with the children, e.g. www.dayoutwiththekids.co.uk/
- Self-care. It is vital that you eat well, sleep when you can and find a way to exercise. It may be that other aspects of your life are relaxed for a while, e.g. housework. Forums can be a great way to find out how other single

parents do this creatively. Remember the importance of you – your children need you to be well, so take that responsibility!

- Be sociable. Find out what groups are in your area for parents with young families and go along. The more areas of support you find, the easier you can make it for yourself. Check community centres, places of worship, children's centres, etc. Remember that even other parents who are part of a couple can still feel isolated if their partner works away or long hours. For young single parents, have a look at http://ivebeenthere.org.au/
- Have an emergency plan. Consider the possible challenges of having one child ill and being unable to leave the other. Find out if there are emergency babysitting services near you. Ask family and friends if they would be willing to be called at such times. Be prepared and hopefully you will not need to put the plan into action.
- Be inventive for childcare. Investigate job sharing or consider a lodger who may also be okay to babysit (provided checks and trust are in place). Double up with another family to take it in turns to babysit, giving you both free times and playmates for your children.
- Be gracious and ask for help. Many people are only too happy to help out when a new baby appears. Sometimes they may not offer in case you are offended. Give them the opportunity to say no!
- Prepare your comments for being judged as a single parent. People can be very critical and unintentionally hurtful with their comments. They may assume that everything is difficult for you, when in reality it is not. If you have pre-thought what you can say in advance, you will be ready to be strong in such a situation.
- Remember that not all couples will be in domestic and family bliss! They may envy you the freedom and choices you have as a single parent. If you dwell on what you perceive you have not got or lost with a partner, then this can spoil the precious time you have with a new baby and older children.

You can still be an excellent parent as a single one!

TOP TIPS FOR SINGLE PARENT

1. Seek support through this period of potential challenge.
2. Ensure plans are in place for your existing child(ren) for if you become mentally unwell again.
3. Be organised; make plans for emergencies; ask for and be gracious in receiving help.
4. Have confidence in what you can achieve.

TOP TIPS FOR HEALTHCARE PROFESSIONALS

1. Know where to seek specific support for a particular situation, e.g. loss of a partner through bereavement.
2. Always be empathetic to the situation and avoid judgements and assumptions. A single parent may actually manage much better than some couples.

REFERENCES

1. Sharrock G. *Saving Grace: my journey and survival through postnatal depression.* Bloomington, IN: AuthorHouse; 2010.
2. Newbold I (2013). *Parenting with Balls.* London: New Holland Publishers; 2013.
3. McGuinness D, Coughlan B, Power S. Empty arms: supporting bereaved mothers during the immediate postnatal period. *Br J Midwifery.* 2014; **22**(4): 246–52. This article outlines the emotional support and physical care required by mothers who experience the loss of a baby, providing midwives with an understanding of grief theory and the grieving process to enable them to care for the bereaved mother.

RESOURCES

- www.netmums.com/parenting-support/single-parents
- www.onespace.org.uk/ OneSpace is the online community and information site for all single mums and dads who are raising children on their own.
- www.gingerbread.org.uk/ provide expert advice, practical support and campaign for single parents. They have fact sheets on many aspects of single parenthood.
- www.familylives.org.uk/advice/divorce-and-separation/thinking-about-divorce/advice-on-becoming-a-single-parent/
- www.lone-parents.org.uk/ have some links to great resources and also have some information geared to single fathers.
- www.daddymoms.com/

CHAPTER 20

The role of family and friends

Keep away from people who belittle your ambitions. Small people always do that, but the really great make you feel that you, too, can become great.

Mark Twain

The birth of a new baby is a gift for everyone involved. I have thoroughly enjoyed the arrival and subsequent joy of having my nieces and nephew in my life, along with the children of my friends. I now am stepping over the threshold into sharing the excitement as my friends become grandparents! On reflection I feel I should have shared the joy of my baby more when he was tiny. My feelings of inadequacies of being a good mother, and the (incorrect) belief that I needed to do it all, made me build a completely unnecessary wall against all those wonderful offers of help. Had I ever had another baby, I feel that I would have been much more willing to share the pleasures and the necessary chores.

Part of my reluctance to let go of my baby was that I did feel guilty that I felt I could not do everything. In my irrational mind I thought that if I appeared to manage the demands of early motherhood, then people would think I was coping well. I now realise that in allowing friends and family to have him at times would have been a win-win situation all round. For me as the mum it would have enabled me to have some time to myself. My son would have benefited with his social skills and ability to interact with others. The helper would have been delighted to have their own special time with baby and also felt good that they had been useful.

My dad judged this brilliantly. He was aware of how I was feeling and that if he came to my house and said he wanted to help, I would have probably snapped at him. Instead, he would simply appear and tell me that *he* needed time with his grandson and was just passing by. Firmly, yet kindly he would tell me that he wanted some time just with the baby to bond with him. He told me to go. It was my choice to rest, bathe, or whatever I wanted. He made me believe that it was *me* that was doing a favour, not him. A wonderful approach.

One new mother, Shirley, told me that not long after her daughter was born, she arranged for her mum to babysit whilst she went for a haircut. Everyone was happy about this arrangement until the following week at a 'Mums and Tots' group, other new mums made Shirley feel dreadful about this. They were incredulous about how she had been so selfish to be apart from her baby whilst she got pampered. I asked Shirley some questions:

'Did you leave your baby out in the street or with a passing stranger?'
'No.'
'Did you leave her under the loving care of her adoring grandma who will have been thrilled to have her?'
'Yes.'
'Did you feel better for having been pampered and a post-pregnancy new haircut?'
'Yes.'
'Were you and your husband pleased to see the results?'
'Yes.'
'Was baby well-cared for and safe?
'Yes.'
'So why are you feeling like a bad mother?'

Shirley realised that she had allowed the unfair judgements of others to upset her. She said that she now has the confidence to do what she feels is right and basically what others think is none of her business.

The approach by family and friends has emerged in my survey responses as an important one. I have used many examples here because most felt strongly their network helped or hindered with their challenges. I am hoping that you may recognise traits that were applicable too, so that you can identify what may be most helpful for you in the future. I asked other mothers how much support they had from family and friends during their first period of challenging motherhood. Replies varied from lots to none.

There were examples of some excellent support:

- On the whole very good. Got a lot of emotional support and some hands on stuff, looking after baby while I slept, etc.
- I didn't have a day to myself as my family and friends took it in turn to watch over/be there at some point every day for the first month.

Some had relatives to stay for a while or moved in with them:

- My mum was very supportive indeed. She initially came to stay with us for 2 weeks when baby was born. When I developed PND she came to stay for another 3 weeks.

Many ladies mentioned their mum (and mother-in-law), usually in positive ways. This should make us aware of those who no longer have their mum in their lives or are geographically miles away:

- My mum was brilliant. Since she had suffered with it before, she knew best how I could be feeling. She would talk sense into me and then leave me if I didn't want to talk. She would always support my decisions and that was exactly what I needed at the time.
- My mother-in-law brought us breakfast in bed every morning for the first few weeks (she lives very close) which was amazing, as we'd often only got a few hours sleep from about 3 a.m.

Others expressed sadness around their own mothers:

- Very little – my mum in particular did little to help me, which is something I really struggled with.
- I had some support from my parents. I couldn't have done without this practically but it was also very difficult. My mum was SO anxious and I became more anxious as a result.
- My sister was supportive but lives 150 miles away; my friends did not understand what was going on with me so they avoided me. My mum went to work abroad for a year when my baby was 12 weeks old.
- My mum came to stay for a couple of nights but that just created tension as she interferes and pushes my husband out.
- It would have been better if my mother had been more positive about my pregnancy. She put a downer upon it and thought I was going to have an abnormal pregnancy or a nervous breakdown.
- Keeping my mum and mother-in-law away would have helped me. In all honesty, they thought they were doing the right thing by visiting me all the time, but the psychosis was so virulent, I couldn't see this. They both talked a lot and said very damaging things to my recovery. Obviously they didn't mean to make it worse, but I wish I had of been protected from them by limiting their visits and maybe having them educated/counselled. E.g. mother-in-law complained that she didn't have enough time with her grandson and wanted to take him home – she thought I wouldn't notice as I was so sick ... This made me suspicious that she wanted to take him; that she thought I was a bad mother, and that she thought bonding with her was more important than with me. She insisted on taking over his care when she was visiting – again, I was so sick that I lost confidence in my own meagre abilities. Her insistence that it was her 'right' to feed him supported my complete lack of control over the few things I was able to do. My mum also hindered my recovery in just being there all the time, watching how I was doing things, talking quietly to other mums, and trying to force me to play scrabble/crosswords in an attempt to heal my brain. Obviously,

this was also innocent, but her persistence made me upset. I needed low stimulation.

Several expressed their loneliness:

- I had no family or friends close at the time and a husband who works a lot so I was quite lonely.
- I felt a bit abandoned by family. We would have to do a lot of the travelling to them to ask for a few minutes of having a hot cuppa while they had cuddles. My housework slipped and this didn't help my feelings.

Some felt support from family and friends was there yet due to their mental health issues, it was not always easy:

- Nobody knew how I was feeling so I did not ask for any, but my family were supportive generally. I had friends who wanted to help, but I wasn't in any position to take up their offer, as I panicked in company. My parents live over 200 miles away, so support from them was obviously intermittent.
- New friends I met through 'Sure Start' helped me loads, gave me a reason to leave the house. But I lost all contact with my original friends. I felt like a completely different person, and not one they wanted to know.
- They tried hard but no one knew what I needed and no one knew how to help.
- My mum and dad practically were a great support but didn't understand or know how to help me emotionally. Friends were very UN-understanding and thought I should just snap out of it.

A common misconception, which I shared, was that when breastfeeding new mums cannot leave their baby with anyone else.

- My parents and in-laws all tried to help as much as they could. But as I was breastfeeding it was difficult to hand over care.
- My friends and family were around but because of breastfeeding I couldn't get much relief and they just tended to 'be there'.

I also asked mothers what the support involved was. Practical support was evident for many:

- Always calling in and lightening the load for me. Just doing little jobs for me and taking my son to give me a break.

Some appreciated emotional and psychological support:

- My in-laws had my 15 month old whilst I was in hospital and also did my washing. My dad was there to talk to.

- One of my friends came round and watched the baby while I had a shower once a week and talked about non baby things.
- Family were fantastic, helped me a lot by just being there if I needed a cuddle.

Enabling the new mother to sleep and have some time to herself was important:

- They came over for a drink, took me out for lunch, took my eldest to the park so I could get an hour's rest.
- My mother used to provide me with time to sleep, and time away from the baby so that I could rest and be 'me' for some amount of time. I was restless when I was with my baby, and if someone else was looking after him – so some help wasn't helpful.

One of my friends, Sue, used to call me and even though she knew I would not answer the phone, she would chat via the answering machine (there were no mobile phones in those days). She would leave me snippets of her news and simply say she was around if I needed anything. Actions of friends that other mums appreciated included:

- Once I told friends, a couple told me of their problems after the birth of their children. I didn't realise that they had PND too.
- A close friend with a slightly older baby was amazing. I used to walk to her house with this screaming baby, and she welcomed me and held the baby for a bit.
- I appreciated those who asked how to help and did it, e.g. my husband asked people not to visit me unless I requested it, then only for half an hour at a time. They also provided meals to my husband.
- I have a friend who is a clinical psychologist, who helped me loads once I broke down. A few friends were really supportive and would come round for a coffee, when I felt like I couldn't get out.

Support with diagnosis and interaction with healthcare professionals was commented upon:

- Before diagnosis, my parents kept me going and eventually took me into their home for 2.5 months. My mam was my first port of call for any concerns I had about my daughter and was always there to help. She also came to doctor's appointments with me. When I became very poorly, my sister acted as advocate to try and get me some professional help.

The Royal College of Psychiatrists[1] have produced a leaflet on postnatal depression, with specific reference to ways of improving communication and partnerships between a woman, her carers and mental health professionals.

I asked mothers if there were any family members or friends who were a hindrance to them or if they felt pressured or criticised. The responses can be grouped in a number of ways:

1. LACK OF UNDERSTANDING AND INSENSITIVE LANGUAGE

- My mother told me to pull myself together and go to church and that I don't need medication.
- There was a feeling of I should snap out of it. That it was something that would just go away.
- My sister-in-law made comments if I was tired. She seemed to be jealous of the attention I received.
- Some of my closest friends at first tried to be understanding but got fed up and gave up with me.
- Yes, some couldn't understand. They said I had no reason to be depressed.
- Huge amount of pressure from one family member (who was probably trying to help) continually telling me 'you must say xxx or they will lock you up' or 'you mustn't say xxxx or they will lock you up'. In a time of massive confusion for me, being told what I should or must say was a huge pressure and made things even worse …

2. CRITICISM AND JUDGEMENTAL COMMENTS

- My mum thought that leaving my baby to cry herself to sleep, not having her in the sling all the time etc. were the right things to do. And, for my first baby, they were absolutely wrong, and made her so upset she couldn't feed or sleep.
- I was told I was molly-coddling my child. I picked him up because he was crying and needed a feed!
- Parents/parents-in-law – didn't understand. Bombarded me with calls, told me how disappointed they were!
- My dad banged on and on about stopping breastfeeding. My mother-in-law went a bit crazy as her daughter was going through infertility treatment and would take my baby away from me and criticise me.
- My partners' parents didn't approve of breastfeeding. Thought they knew best.

3. PERCEPTION OF PERSONAL FEELINGS

- A lot of my partner's family mentioned how I wouldn't cope and I felt pressured to prove them wrong.
- I felt too ashamed to admit I had PND to friends. When I did they looked at me in disgust as I had suicidal intentions to myself and daughter.

4. CHALLENGES OF THE FRIEND OR FAMILY MEMBER

- My mother was extremely anxious. This resulted in her criticising every decision I made. I remember her phoning my mobile every few minutes if she saw me take my son out for a walk, telling me that he was too warmly dressed, or not dressed warmly enough. She criticised the way I fed him, dressed him, bathed him, the fact that I couldn't stop him crying, literally everything. On more than one occasion I stood there completely helpless because I had tried to take him out and she would criticise every way I tried to do it, until I just didn't know what to do, and felt completely paralysed. Worst of all for me, one day in tears, I told her that I was not enjoying being a mother and that it all felt too hard. She told me that I was wrong and that I must be enjoying it as I had a lovely son.
- I should have stayed away from my parents. I would like to suggest that they should have had more faith in me, or at least approached my failures with support rather than damnation. But it became apparent that my mum had serious mental health problems in a way I had never seen before. I started to understand my own life and my own struggles in a new light.

These comments were made in hindsight:

- The support I would've liked is someone giving me a ring occasionally to see how I was, pop round to give me a few minutes. No-one seemed to notice I was struggling with my daughter and getting myself up in a morning.
- I think having close family staying with us immediately after the birth even for up to one month would have helped hugely. With hindsight, we should have employed a doula or similar. Nowadays as families live a distance apart the support network and experience is lost.
- They helped when I asked for it but I didn't ask enough.
- Parents stayed over and tried to help where they could, although to be honest I think they unwittingly made things worse …

I asked mothers too what they felt would have helped regarding support from family and friends. 'More' was a loud reply!

- More support, visits with offers of help after the first few weeks.
- I think meditation, counselling to calm me down and maybe having family around.
- I would have just loved some company, or just a voice at the end of the phone. Any support would have helped me.
- I wish my mum would have offered to help me, giving me a break, or cooking a meal. To this day I am still sad about how she left me alone to deal with the toughest time of my life. We'd always been close, but her actions affected our relationship to such an extent that I have recently emigrated overseas – I never

could have left her before, but her actions left me feeling that, although I love her, I don't depend on her for anything.
- I felt like I needed someone to just take the baby and look after him. Realistically though, even to have had a couple of hours' break would have helped. Also, I didn't feel able to say how I was feeling and health visitor didn't realise how mentally unwell I was.

The type of 'other' support that they felt may have been better included:

- In reality my parents were not in a good place to support me. With hindsight I should have declined their help (it caused months of panic afterwards) and taken up friends on their offers.
- If I had known there was something wrong I could have told them and they could have helped. I'd also moved to somewhere I felt extremely isolated though I had not realised this until I had given birth and was at home with the baby instead of at work. I'm convinced if I'd lived somewhere with an established community I would have coped much, much better.
- Someone to tell me it would be okay. Someone to make me go to bed and sleep for a few hours.
- If they had gone with the 'do whatever works now, if it's a problem later, we'll fix it later', way of doing things that my husband (very sensibly) was encouraging me to do.
- To support me in my choices. To not leave when I was breastfeeding.

Some were happy with what they had:

- Nothing as I was too ill. I had severe PND so I don't think even a team of staff could have made me feel any better! I just wanted my daughter to go and me get my life back.
- I was lucky that my family and the health visitors were so supportive. I can't fault them really.
- I don't know if my mum wasn't here constantly whether I would have asked for help sooner.

Some mothers wanted good advice and knowledge for themselves and those around them. This would then lead to better understanding:

- Knowing phone numbers for crisis teams, breastfeeding support, etc.
- People appear to understand PND in the first 6 months but then there's nothing. There is or was nothing for fathers at that time. They also need better education and support in order to support their partners.
- You cannot expect people to know what they don't know. You have to give people the knowledge if you want to enable them to be of help.

- By finding out more about my illness so they could understand.
- Ensuring they talk and discuss their thoughts and feelings when they feel they want to.
- By listening and understanding; no one asks for this to happen to them!

One plea was for peer support:

- Knowing other women who had gone through it, seeing/hearing others talk about it. A support group being available.
- If I had been able to meet other mothers going through the same experience; support from my local medical/health practice in relation to medical and mental health support. A support group and also help caring for my baby.

Relationships with family and friends can be affected by poor maternal mental health,[2] although some say they did not change in the long run. Some experienced sadness through changes:

- I grew further apart from them. Family members noticed but didn't ask or made any genuine offers of help, just very loose, general comments like: 'You know where we are.'
- I became distant from my best friend because she just didn't understand.
- I realised the only person I could wholeheartedly rely on was myself. At the time I felt let down by everyone.
- It strained friendships, my marriage and for everyone else around me
- I was very withdrawn, I lost a lot of friends, I didn't want to go out, I felt a failure, I felt a mess, I was an awful person, partly my fault my friends didn't stick around I guess.
- I feel like everyone knows my weakness and see me as fragile at times and I'm still embarrassed about parts of my illness.
- My relationship with the father failed due to my mental health problems.
- Difficult to talk about the whole episode to those who don't understand or don't want to understand.
- I leant too much on my mum and still do.
- My relationship suffered and I feel as though some with my friends as I didn't want to go out.
- I felt both really reliant on my parents and husband and yet quite emotionally distant from them. I felt a lot of anger towards them.
- My mum and mother-in-law still do not fully understand what I went through. This continues to hinder our relationships. To say 'you know if you get overtired you might get sick again' demonstrated ongoing poor insight into the psychosis I had. My mother-in-law often says she met someone who had a depression like mine ... I never had a depression, I had a psychosis – I was manic and later psychotic. There is a lot of information to read on the net and in books and for

two people so close to me, who I have spent many hours with trying to help them understand, this continues to irritate me. I will continue to work on our relationships, but I guess the crux of it is, it is almost impossible to understand mental illness unless you have first-hand experience.

There were others who reported positive changes:

- It has brought me closer, if anything, to my family and in-laws.
- My marriage is stronger and so are my relationships with siblings and friends. Crucially, I know myself better.
- On a positive note, my relationship with my mother improved as she played a big part in my recovery and her help with the baby when I was most ill was invaluable.
- I have moved away from some chaotic relationships and formed some genuine friendships over the last 14 years.
- I am now very open and honest with people and I think that, as a result, my friendships are deeper and more real.

Reading the accounts of other mothers and families makes me even more grateful for the help I had. I shall always graciously remember my friends and family who helped rebuild my life after the birth of my baby. I know that if I had gone on to having another child I could have relied on them again – with better knowledge and experience from us all.

IDEAS FOR THE MOTHER (TO BE) ON MAKING THE MOST OF YOUR FAMILY AND FRIENDS

I acknowledge that it will take assertiveness and courage to have what you may feel would be 'difficult conversations' about the possibility of having another baby and how you feel that your family and friends could best support you. Firstly I would suggest that you thank them for the role they played previously – you do not wish to alienate them by saying negative things or criticising what they did or did not do. Let them know that you have decided to have another child (or are accepting your unexpected pregnancy) and ask them to respect that fact and hope that you can count on their support. It may be worthwhile saying how much you all now love and enjoy your current child or children, and that is one reason why you want to add to the family. In fact, that might be a great way to start the conversation, e.g.:

Isn't it great that we all get so much pleasure now with little Annabel? I know it was a tough start, yet I feel it was worth it. That's why I have some exciting news for you ... I'm pregnant again.

Remember that they are likely to be concerned that you may become ill again. Share your knowledge and plans with them and ask how you feel they could help and how they may want to. Explain that harsh comments and judgements are not helpful – appropriate support will be. Perhaps you could let them get used to the news of your pregnancy first and approach the support aspect at a later date.

Generally family and friends want to help – be patient and gracious with them. They often do not know how to. Guide them if you can. If you ask for help about practical aspects, be prepared to change your expectations about standards. Accept that if ironing, cooking, cleaning and even dressing the baby aren't how you would do it, it is still okay. Be bold as a 'mother in distress'. Ask!

Be as candid and open as possible about how you are feeling and what you want or need. Often your brain may not know, so how can you expect others to? Being indecisive can be part of the illness. Explain this to others whilst you are pregnant and let them know that your responses may be inconsistent.

Let them know what really helped last time and what could have been useful in hindsight. If having the freezer full of your gran's homemade meals was an asset, prime her for next time. If your best friend calling every three hours was a nuisance, ask her to text in the future and explain that you appreciate her concern and you will ask if you need anything. One mum who has had a subsequent child after a previous postnatal mental illness recommends:

- Make a list of those who you know will be helpful for you to call and what exactly they can help you with, e.g. on my list was do call X because she is calm; do call Y because she will do your ironing, do not call Mum because she panics, do not call R because she cannot empathise … etc.

It may be that you consider lifestyle changes to be nearer family and friend support, for example by moving:

- As my husband worked long hours and was sometimes away overnight, we actually moved house because I didn't feel I had the support network around where we lived so we moved back to the area we had grown up in to be closer to family and a support network. Still years later I wish we did not have to take this decision as I loved our previous location and lifestyle, but it was necessary at the time. My husband's job frequently took him out of the house for 12 hours during the day which is a long time to be on your own. I felt I needed people around me as I was feeling very anxious and vulnerable. In essence, I therefore recommend just practically having people to hand for mums so they are not physically left alone.

Remember that next time round you are potentially forewarned and thus can be much more prepared. You also know that with effective support and treatment, you will get better. Trust yourself and have confidence in your views.

IDEAS TO SUPPORT THE MOTHER (TO BE) FOR FAMILY AND FRIENDS

> Sometimes our hearts get tangled and our souls a little off kilter. Friends and family can set us right and help guide us back to the light.
>
> Sera Christann

As a close family member or friend, I would imagine that you would want to be able to support the mother during her pregnancy and when the baby arrives. You might feel that you do not know the best way to do this. *Ask* what is really needed by the mother – and do it! If she isn't sure, then make suggestions about what you could do. Sometimes simply use your initiative for what obviously needs doing – and do it! Of course, if her partner is around, always consult them too. What we are focusing on here are ways to prevent or minimise the impact from poor mental health. All families with a new baby appreciate some form of extra assistance in the early days, depending on their needs. It might be that in the scenario that we are considering, it needs a bit more emphasis.

If you are aware that the mother, or father, is at risk of developing a mental illness again before or when the baby arrives, find out about their condition so that you can understand and show compassion. I know that I was very difficult to handle when I was mentally unwell. I would lash out verbally and sometimes physically at others. Remember these are not personal attacks – just a response to the illness. Find out for them what support is available locally or online. If there is a support group, gently encourage them to go, helping with a lift or childcare. Be interested in therapy and help/support in using coping strategies. You will find resources for these at other sections in this book. Praise them for making active steps towards their own recovery.

Recognise when to get help. Encourage them to seek and get professional support. Offer to go with them. You may need to be an advocate if any treatment does not suit her or further help is required. Sometimes you may have to be proactive in making choices about their treatment if they are too unwell. They may object, yet the whole family will probably thank you for it ultimately. Make sure she gets urgent professional treatment if she talks about wanting to end her life or harm herself or her child.

If the mental health issues arise again, remember that your loved one is unwell. Help them remember they are suffering from an illness, so that their possible feelings of guilt and shame can be eased. If you respond with shock or disappointment, then this will make them feel worse. Antenatal and post-natal mental health issues are temporary and can be overcome with effective support and treatment. How would you treat them if they were physically ill? Then do the same helpful things. It can be difficult to empathise if you haven't had a mental health problem yourself. Talking to someone else might help you to understand.[3] If you are prepared to be open and talk about it, recognising the problems are part of the way to overcoming them. Ignoring the elephant in the room and bottling it up are not helpful. Caring for someone who is suffering from depression can lead to frustration, unhappiness, impatience and anger in the carer. You are doing an important and needed role. You need to look after yourself so that you can then help them more effectively. Seek support and rest periods for yourself rather than add to the challenges of the mother by making her feel responsible for you and appearing to be a martyr.

Appreciate the power of listening and simply being there for them without the need to fix them. Be comfortable with silence at times, as Pythagoras said, 'Silence is better than unmeaning words.' Reassure, encourage and support them. Part of depression is often low self-esteem. When you recognise something of value – tell her. I once saw a mum wearing a t-shirt with the motto 'I'm dressed – what more do you want?' Brilliant! Look for the tiniest action or appearance to sincerely say something good about, even if she dismisses it. Use positive language. In the spiral of depression your brain tends to be aware of all the negatives around you, so you need encouragement to see the positives. Even if you feel like saying 'pull yourself together', 'it's time you chivvied yourself up', 'you have everything you wanted' – it will not help! The mum is likely to struggle with rational thinking at times, so listen to any of her concerns without dismissing them as 'silly'. The thoughts will feel very real to her. Be aware of being too gushing with positivity as this can have a detrimental effect sometimes and can sound patronising and annoying.

Be kind and loving and keep any judgements or criticism to yourself. Even though you may mean well by offering advice about what worked for you, she may interpret this as you being critical. Comment on what they have done rather than the list they have yet to achieve. She needs to know that she is loved and she will be supported through this temporary phase. I remember feeling that my condition was all my fault. Encourage her that she has people who are willing to guide her through. Mothers for Mothers[4] suggest:

> Sometimes, something as simple and obvious as a hug or a cuddle can help. We all like to be held and cuddled from time to time, not in a sexual way, but in a protective and caring way. The occasional cuddle will not suddenly make all your troubles go away, but it helps and feels good!

I am normally a very kinaesthetic person who loves to be hugged. When I was postnatally ill, I did not! Use your discretion and if a simple squeeze of the hand is all that is required, then leave it at that.

Look after baby (and/or siblings). Allow the mum some time for herself, simply to choose what she wants to do. If the baby is especially demanding this is vital. Be sensitive to saying how good they have been whilst with you – this can make a mum feel that she is the problem with the baby. At the same time, be mindful that they can trust you even if the baby doesn't settle. Mum must get rest.

Work as a team. The mother may not know what she wants so it can be down to those who are around her to give her support. Check with the partner (if they are involved) on help with practical tasks. Most people are very willing to have a meal prepared for them or washing and ironing done without fuss. Some mums may not want to be left alone – others will prefer solitude sometimes. Perhaps you will need to organise a rota until she is able to be more independent. Care from Home-Start, for example, may be available too. The importance of a good diet is well known. A team of support for meals can be made using www.foodtidings.com. Offer help with shopping, cooking and household chores. Be unobtrusive with help – just do it without expecting or needing a huge round of applause. Some days the mum will show her gratitude and may want to chat. Other times, a text or Post-it note is all that is required to say what you have done. If you get no response, remind yourself that she isn't being rude, she is unwell.

What treats can you organise? Any new mother often has limited time to look after her own personal routines. When you have additional mental health issues, this is often combined with the feeling that you are not worth the effort. Arrange for a mobile therapist to visit for a massage; look after the baby and children whilst they are being pampered. The internet is full of offers for such treats. What relaxation classes are held locally? Are there any that you could go to together? Arrange to take the mum and children out – just a walk around the block or for a coffee. It may be that she will opt out at the last minute as anxieties take hold. If this happens, reassure her that it is fine – you will do it again another time when she feels ready. Simply getting out of the house can help to lift depression.

Be patient. There is no timeline for mental illness. There are no rules to adhere to like after a surgical operation, when there are guides for when stitches come out, when to drive, etc. Recovery can be very spasmodic. Some days she will feel very low, and then there will be periods of wellness. I found that looking backwards at the progress I had made was more useful than being faced by a mountain of 'Can't dos'. Give help with tasks as they are needed. Some days, or even moments, she will actually want to do some tasks for herself. This will be great for her own confidence and recovery. If everything is done for her, that can add to her feelings of worthlessness. Seek to find the balance between support and overkill. Gradually the better feelings will increase. Keep on reminding her that that she is getting better. As Nick Vujicic says, 'remember that the light at the end of the tunnel might just be round the next bend'.[5]

Most challenges around mental illness do not come with a 'one-size-fits-all' approach. When I was very unwell I appreciated the cards I received, even if I could not manage seeing people who sent them. One mum told me though that:

- I begged my husband and mothers not to tell anyone. In hindsight, I don't mind that they did for their own support, but seriously, I received numerous cards from well-wishers – these were detrimental to my paranoid psychotic brain.

Helping a mother through another pregnancy and early months with a new child is a very personal and unique situation. It calls for sensitivity and flexibility. Pinky McKay[6] offers a variety of ideas and writes:

Be there: Don't disappear, don't give up on your friend and don't feel offended if she gets angry with you. Depression is a cruel illness and recovery will take months and longer – but with treatment and support, your friend will recover. And when she gets better, your friendship will be even stronger, because you have been there all along.

I asked my own mother about how she and my father would have felt if I had ever had another baby. She wrote:

We would have been delighted for Elaine to have had more children although we would have been very apprehensive to the news that she was pregnant again. Knowing children bring such love throughout our lives we would have been pleased and supported her without question.

However bearing in mind the severe illness she suffered the first time I, as her mum, would have fussed probably and over-reacted to her every physical and mental state for the nine months!

I would have been very conscious of her wellbeing throughout as the first time I wonder if I missed the tell-tale signs; she was so poorly leading up to her hospitalisation. Elaine would have made a wonderful mum to another child but it was sadly not to be. Nevertheless the outcome of her pioneering for care of new pregnant mums has been invaluable to many women. She is an inspiration to us all. The family are so proud of her.

IDEAS TO SUPPORT THE MOTHER (TO BE) FOR FAMILY AND FRIENDS FROM THE HEALTHCARE PROFESSIONAL PERSPECTIVE

It may be useful to ask who is in their circle of contact and then reassure the expectant family that support from family and friends can be extremely helpful. Research suggests that 'social support offered by family and friends has both positive and negative effects with which the postpartum mothers have to learn to cope.'[7]

You may be able to encourage the support to be the type that is needed by suggesting some of the ideas I have outlined for the respective parties, e.g. help the mother to use positive language to express what she feels she needs. Being judged by professionals and by family and friends has been found to be a key barrier to mothers expressing their needs and feelings.[8] The whole 'team' needs to be aware of appropriate responses to her emotional and practical needs to maximise her mental health.

One mum's plea for family and friends was that she wanted:

- SOMEONE to talk to ... SOMEONE who knew what to say and understood ... SOMEONE to just hug me!

Can you be that someone?

By identifying what and how family and friends can help a growing family, you will all be able to be proactive in asking for and receiving the correct support. Together you can help to maximise mental health for everyone concerned in the perinatal period.

TOP TIPS FOR PARENTS

1. Remember that a new addition to the family can bring joy to all involved – if managed well.
2. Have confidence to do what you feel is right and basically what others think is none of your business.
3. Rehearse the potentially challenging conversation that you may have if telling others of your plans.
4. Review with family and friends what you felt helped previously and ask for it again – modify where needed.
5. Share some of the ideas I have outlined to help them know how best they can support you.

TOP TIPS FOR HEALTHCARE PROFESSIONALS

1. Encourage the parents to identify their sources of support – if they are limited, explore alternatives.
2. If needed, help them to compose how they will tell others of their decision to have another baby and ways to ask for help.

REFERENCES

1. www.rcpsych.ac.uk/healthadvice/partnersincarecampaign/postnataldepression.aspx
2. Kelly L. *Effects of Maternal Mental Health on Child Behaviour and Development.* Glasgow: Scottish Centre for Social Research; 2010. Available at: www.parentingacrossscotland. org/policy--research/good-practice/health-and-poverty/maternal-mental-health.aspx
3. www.mind.org.uk/information-support/types-of-mental-health-problems/postnatal-depression/family-and-friends/#.Uv4xjM5FWMM
4. www.mothersformothers.co.uk/family-and-friends.html
5. www.lifewithoutlimbs.org/
6. www.pinkymckay.com/a-friend-in-need-helping-a-friend-with-postnatal-depression/
7. Ni PK, Koh SSL. The role of family and friends in providing social support towards enhancing the wellbeing of postpartum women: a comprehensive systematic review. *JBI Library of Systematic Reviews.* 2011; **9**(10): 313–70. Available at: www.joannabriggs library.org/jbilibrary/index.php/jbisrir/article/view/94
8. Dennis C-L, Chung-Lee L. Postpartum depression help-seeking barriers and maternal treatment preferences: a qualitative systematic review. *Birth.* 2006; **33**: 323–31.

FURTHER READING AND RESOURCES

- www.rcpsych.ac.uk/mentalhealthinfoforall/problems/postnatalmentalhealth/postnatal-depression.aspx
- http://apni.org/advice-for-carers/
- www.wikihow.com/Help-a-Friend-Going-Through-Postpartum-Depression
- http://lisajobaker.com/2012/02/100-ways-to-encourage-a-new-mom/
- Reid KM. The association between social support, stress exposure, and maternal postpartum depression: a stress process approach. *Electronic Theses, Treatises and Dissertations.* 2013; Paper 7570. Available at: http://diginole.lib.fsu.edu/cgi/viewcontent. cgi?article=7586&context=etd The primary aim of this dissertation project is to provide a more comprehensive understanding of the relationship between social support and maternal postpartum depression, drawing on a stress process framework.
- www.essentialbaby.com.au/life-style/nutrition-and-wellbeing/helping-a-friend-who-has-postnatal-depression-20131101-2woev.html

CHAPTER 21

Peer support

One of the greatest gifts a person can give another is support.

Unknown

Initially when I had my son I painted on a mask for the world and presented the expected image of a new mum who 'had it all'. A healthy baby, who was much wanted; a very comfortable home; supportive husband and family; a special needs teacher who should know all about children and a long summer break of maternity leave. What could I have to complain about? I met up on a regular basis with the mothers in my antenatal group who had all delivered within a four-week period. At our first reunion with our babies I listened to the other stories of their births. They all appeared to have been straightforward. I was the only one who had needed to be admitted to hospital during pregnancy. I was the only one whose plan had not happened. I remember feeling like I was an attention-seeking drama queen so played my story down. That was the start of my feelings of guilt and failure. We decided as a group to continue to meet outside of the health centre. Over the coming weeks I felt increasingly uncomfortable and useless as none of the other mothers appeared to be having the same challenges with feeding and sleep deprivation as I was. One of the ladies was pregnant again within months. I was dismayed as my husband and I still had not resumed any kind of sex life. Then my baby was admitted to hospital with a serious illness. I questioned my ability to do anything right in my new role as a mother.

I had also joined two other groups of new mothers. One was a mother and toddler group at the local church and also a nearby NCT[1] group. One lady, Sue, and her daughter Sophie went to both and we became good friends. We even met outside of the groups. I envied Sue as she had been able to take a five-year career break from her job. Even though we spent hours together and chatted about our new lifestyles, I still did not admit that I felt I was struggling with everything. When I walked into a group for mothers with postnatal depression, as suggested by my doctor, I was stunned to see Sue sitting there! She was equally amazed at seeing me. We both laughed as we confessed that we had thought the other one was doing brilliantly and daren't admit our true feelings. That opened the floodgates and gave us mutual permission to really be truthful to each other without fear of judgement or rejection. We became very close and a great support to each other. I wonder: if we had really been open in those early months, would we have needed as much professional help? Possibly not, yet it did teach me that sometimes our perception of others can be wrong and that how we choose to speak and behave can also be misleading. I never actually lied – I just hid the full truth.

A few years later, after my book was published and I took on a new supplementary career in selling cosmetics and jewellery for Virgin Vie, I would offer my presentations to mother and toddler groups, ladies groups as well as house parties. Part of the company sales dialogue was to introduce yourself and explain why you had joined the business. My cheesy line was that I had become a 'Virgin' because I had suffered postnatal depression, then would get my book out of my bag, before continuing to tell them the benefits of the products I was selling. I had been trained to apply make-up correctly and to appreciate that an attractive and well-turned out image was a big part of being successful. There I was looking 'the part' in contrast to the sorry image I painted of myself as a new mother. The wonderful outcome of this was that I could tell at a glance who either was or had suffered from postnatal depression, as soon as I said I had been ill. At the end of my presentation, more often than not, I would also hear the story of one or more of one of my customers' mental ill health associated with the birth of a child.

One evening a lady in her seventies told me that she had come along expecting to buy a lipstick – not get rid of 50 years of guilt that she had been a bad mother. She told me that she had kept her illness quiet for all those years because she felt ashamed. As I had been so open about it, I had given her the peace of mind she had never achieved. Another time, after talking about skincare to a group of new mums, three of them approached me and confessed that they were currently struggling. At that point none of them had mentioned it to their peers. We began a discussion and the realisation occurred that the two days of the week that they had a planned activity with this group or another one, they were okay. They found the other three days to be a challenge and very long. So they decided there and then to arrange to meet up with each other the other three days, or at least make contact just to check on how they were getting on. I heard from the group leader a few months later that all three of them were then doing well.

On another occasion I was asked to deliver a workshop on my experiences to a group of mums who were currently diagnosed with postnatal depression, accompanied by a health professional support worker. At the start of the day all of the mums came in with very poor body language. Eyes down, arms folded, very quiet. As I began to unfold my story, little by little heads lifted, arms unfolded and gradually comments increased about their own experiences. By lunchtime we had heard everyone's story develop using mine as a framework. The buzz in the room over lunch was brilliant, as I heard comments like 'So it's not just me?' and 'I can't believe you feel like this too.'

After lunch I asked the question, 'What's the worst thing about having postnatal depression?' The ladies identified some of their key concerns and we then discussed ways to deal with them. A big one was a feeling of isolation. At their suggestion they agreed that it would be good to swap mobile phone numbers and help each other. They asked for me to go back a few months later. I did so and was stunned to feel like I was in the room with completely different ladies. They looked and sounded brighter, more confident and definitely happier. I asked them what had made the difference. Firstly they agreed that having listened to my story, they did not want to become that ill. They had realised that they had a huge part to play in their own recovery and to become proactive in it by applying some of the ideas we had discussed. Secondly, they had formed their own peer support group. Simply by knowing that each of them were struggling they had an early morning 'check-in' by text. If any of them was feeling down, the others would give that mum what she needed, either by babysitting, help with practical tasks or just being there. On other mornings they reciprocated for each other. Thirdly, they shared their strengths. For example, one of them had just qualified as a beautician prior to becoming pregnant. She had lost her confidence through her postnatal illness. The other ladies volunteered for beauty treats for her to practise on, thus making them feel and look better and rebuilding her skill. This often turned into a social, fun event that others would bake for. The additional outcome was that they identified the strength and need for peer support and set up an official group in their area.

I am not suggesting that peer support is the answer to all poor mental health due to childbirth. For some ladies the need for health professional support and treatment is vital. Peer support can be a very strong positive influence for others and has been defined as:

offering and receiving help, based on shared understanding, respect and mutual empowerment between people in similar situations[2]

Often new mothers can feel distant from their pre-motherhood friends, who are still working and socialising as 'normal'. The gap widens often due to new routines and interests and can be even wider if a mental illness emerges. On the other hand, new life-long friendships are created out of new motherhood as the children become playmates too. One mum added:

- I found it very difficult to relate to other new mums from my antenatal group. Their birth experiences and problems seemed trivial and insignificant in comparison to the trauma of PP. This left me feeling very isolated.

If you are currently expecting or considering another baby and want to make it a better experience this time, it will be worth researching what is available in your area as opportunities to meet other new mothers. Also ask your health visitor and midwife if they know of any other community support groups. Some housing associations offer additional support; Sure Start children's centres are also a good place for support, practical help and friendships. Look at the noticeboard at your local community centre or place of worship, which also may have group or individual help for young families. If you go ahead with another pregnancy, find out about such avenues of help before the baby is born. A great source of local support groups can be found at Netmums.[3]

You may be lucky to live in an area that offers support to young families through the charity Home-Start.[4] If you decide to have another baby and are limited with support for practical aspects, then a visit on a regular basis by one of their volunteers may be added support. Have a look at the peer support system delivered by Family Action.[5]

The clinical research also recommends attending groups as they may help overcome social isolation and provide a break.[6] This would be another instance where I would encourage you to be assertive and get out there! I know that it is easier to stay inside wearing your dressing gown. You will have a sense of achievement simply by being able to get there. If you go when you are pregnant you can begin to make connections at that point. Even if the groups are not in your preferred area or you feel they will not suit you – just make an appearance. You may be pleasantly surprised. I am not expecting you to make firm friendships with everyone there. Just one or two may prove to be invaluable. You may find that your confidence improves as you share what you have found did work for you when you had your first or previous child. To a brand new mother, you will still be the voice of experience. Be aware of the words you use too – it's okay to share that you had problems last time and that you are going to do all you can to stay well this time. Avoid becoming the voice of doom!

Since my son was born, technology has increased beyond recognition. This has enabled new forms of social support. Telephone helplines are now far more common, especially through some charities, and have also been found to be beneficial. Dennis *et al.*[7] state that:

Telephone based peer support can be effective in preventing postnatal depression among women at high risk.

The internet has a wealth of information to help families with perinatal challenges. For example, Netmums[8] has practical tips for all concerned. I would recommend an air of caution as too much information can be harmful too. Limit your time in front of technology.

There is also an increasing number of forums available via social media, e.g. on Facebook. These can be invaluable, especially when you feel that the rest of the world is asleep and you don't want to disturb anyone.

NICE (2007) recommends receiving support from other women experiencing antenatal and postnatal depression and anxiety through dedicated internet chat rooms. One example is www.pni.org.uk. They can be very powerful in helping you realise that you are not alone and you can learn from the experience of others. They can be great support. One mother who felt very isolated in the Outer Hebrides found that Twitter helped break her isolation. She has now set up a regular session every week where many people join in to debate a particular issue at #PNDHour, between 8 and 9 p.m. every Wednesday.

I would offer a word of caution about chat rooms. Do be aware that the information can be in a very public domain. Be wise with how much detail you put on an open page. Some people can use them to make unkind or unhelpful comments and may make you feel worse. For example, I followed a debate on an open forum about the dilemma posed by the title of this book. A lady really did not know what to do. The many comments that followed in the main were helpful and based on the experience of others. Some, though, were cruel, harsh and very judgemental. The outcome was that the couple in question were left feeling even more confused.

Sometimes the people running such forums may also still be in recovery mode themselves and are not really strong enough to advise or support others. I believe very much in the role of peer support. Ensure that it is properly supervised and only 'go public' when you feel comfortable and safe to do so.

Online diaries can also be helpful, especially if you read how someone else is dealing with a similar situation. Research[9] recently stated that 'blogging may improve new mothers' wellbeing, as they feel more connected to the world outside their home through the internet'.

Postpartum Progress[10] is an American site that has been going over 10 years. There is a wealth of information there.

Other mothers and the research tell us that it does help to make connections with other people in the perinatal period. In the advice given regarding business networking that I feel is relevant here, surround yourself with people you 'know, like and trust'. If you are warm, open and friendly as you plan and possibly proceed with another pregnancy, you can build up your team of support. It may be that you are very well and you are then mutual support to them. There are some support groups that have sessions for both mothers and their partners. Also you may like to look at https://twitter.com/dads matteruk for male peer support.

Julie Smith, Family Action, National Perinatal Lead writes:

Research shows that anxiety and depression in and after pregnancy may cause problems for the child later in life, and recent research by the Maternal Mental

Health Alliance estimates that the cost of perinatal mental ill health to the economy is in the region of £8 billion. That is why Family Action, one of the country's leading family support charities, has developed highly successful befriender support services for women with low level diagnosed mental health issues or who are at risk of developing perinatal depression.

These services are early help, low intensity services that are coordinated by a professional project manager with an early years, health or social care background. Support comes from a team of volunteer befrienders who have experience of parenthood and sometimes have received help from the service themselves. The befrienders work with mums and families from before the baby is born to at least one year after offering emotional support, guidance on parenting and practical help and advice.

The service has been extensively evaluated on a number of occasions and is proven to be effective:

- Women vulnerable to perinatal depression who received support from the service were half as likely to escalate to depression serious enough to warrant antidepressants
- 88% of mums showed a reduced level of anxiety, and 59% showed reduced levels of depression
- There is a significant increase in mother–baby warmth and the overwhelming message from mums receiving support was that of relief and gratitude.

In 2014 a rigorous economic evaluation of the Family Action service showed that the benefit of receiving the service (when expressed in financial terms) exceeds the cost of delivering the service, and that is even before taking into account the long-term positive effects on both mum and child.

To find out more about Family Action's work visit www.family-action.org.uk/what-we-do/early-years/perinatal-support-services/

As a healthcare professional, encourage and support the mothers in your care to be with other people. Find what is available, and if there is nothing, perhaps that is the motivation to start something.

TOP TIPS FOR PARENTS

1. Be open with peers whom you trust as you may find that they are facing similar feelings and/or situations. This may give you mutual support.
2. Be open and willing to make new friends and contacts as you enter another phase of your life.
3. Use forums and public platforms with caution.
4. When you feel able to, you may choose to become a peer supporter for others.

TOP TIPS FOR HEALTHCARE PROFESSIONALS

1. Encourage and enable the parents in your care to make connections with others.
2. Explore ways of how you could introduce and develop peer support in your area.

REFERENCES

1. www.nct.org.uk/
2. Mead S, Hilton D, Curtis L. Peer support: a theoretical perspective. *Psychiatric Rehabilitation Journal.* 2001; **25**(2): 134–41.
3. www.netmums.com/local-to-you/local/index/support-groups/antenatal-postnatal-support
4. www.home-start.org.uk/
5. www.family-action.org.uk/what-we-do/early-years/perinatal-support-services/
6. MIND (2010) www.mind.org.uk/information-support/types-of-mental-health-problems/postnatal-depression/#.VWm5BdJVhHw
7. Dennis CL, *et al.* Effect of peer support on prevention of postnatal depression among high risk women. *BMJ.* 2009; **338**: a3064. Available at: www.bmj.com/content/338/bmj.a3064; Dennis CL. Postpartum depression peer support: Maternal perceptions from a randomized controlled trial. *Int J Nurs Stud.* 2010; **47**(5): 560–8. Available at: www.science direct.com/science/article/pii/S002074890900354X
8. www.netmums.com
9. McDaniel BT, Coyne SM, Holmes EK. New mothers and media use: associations between blogging, social networking, and maternal well-being. *Matern Child Health J.* 2012; **16**(7): 1509–17. Available at: http://link.springer.com/article/10.1007/s10995-011-0918-2
10. www.postpartumprogress.com/

FURTHER RESOURCES AND READING

● Implementing Recovery through Organisational Change. *Peer Support Workers: theory and practice.* Centre for Mental Health and Mental Health Network, 2013. Available at: www.centreformentalhealth.org.uk/peer-support-workers-theory-and-practice

CHAPTER 22

The working world whilst pregnant and beyond: next time round

I think if you love what you do, and the choice you've made in your life, somehow that drives you forward to enjoy it all – even the chaos, even the exhaustion of it, and even when it seems out of balance.

Angelina Jolie, actress and mother of six

In Western society today it is common for women to be in paid employment when they become pregnant. In the latest Maternity Allowance quarterly statistics: March to May 2014, 54,700 women claimed it.[1] I admit that I never wanted to be a 'working mother'. I would have happily left my teaching job to become a full-time mother. Mortgage payments and our desire for the luxuries in life meant that I had to work until my maternity leave and return to work at the end of it. That should have been straightforward.

My postnatal illness and the subsequent protracted absence, on an unknown timescale, caused challenges for the school where I taught. Perhaps if both my baby and I had been well, the maternity leave would have been adequate. It is much easier if you have a physical illness, as usually you are able to plan around expected recovery time for healing, such as from an operation, and people can often see tangible evidence that there is something which needs to heal which has not yet healed. There are guidelines to follow that everyone can use to plan accordingly. A mental illness is not so easy to accommodate. The local authority were good to me, adding occupational health support and finally a staggered return to work. I remember lurching from one sick note to another – each time hoping I would be considered to be fit to teach again yet also in a panic because I knew I was not ready.

Whilst pregnant I did too much at work, regardless of people telling me to slow down. I wanted to ensure that I left everything perfect for my class and supply teacher. I became ill with a urinary tract infection and had to go off before my intended date. This made me feel worse! When considering a second child I would ideally have planned to take a much more moderate approach during pregnancy and arranged for a maximum leave or even career break.

There is no moral right or wrong about working whilst pregnant or being a mother in paid employment. It is only in the last 50 years that mothers have increasingly had to juggle both roles. The Health and Safety Executive[2] advise on what is considered to be safe practice for both employee and employers. According to the 2014 Childcare and Early Years Survey,[3] more than a third of working mothers would like to give up their jobs completely and stay at home with their children.

Perhaps if I had been a mother without paid employment, I might have become bored eventually and felt that I had wasted my training and teaching experience. It is a personal decision that primarily may concern finances. Secondly, as you will read, some mothers actually feel better by going back to work. This is perhaps when it may suit a couple better for the partner to take a career break instead. This would depend on the type of work, whether the mother is happy with childcare arrangements and also the severity of the mental illness. At my worst there was no way I was fit to be a responsible teacher – I was not even responsible for myself. When I was well enough, over time it did help me find 'myself' again and gave me confidence that my 'loss of mind' had been temporary. On reflection it also made me a better teacher. My experiences of having to be involved with other professionals for my care taught me many lessons that I then used on my return to work, for example, really listening to people without showing impatience or distraction by clicking a pen! I also learned to be less judgemental and more patient.

If you are considering another child and you do have paid employment, what can you consider during the decision-making process to make it as good as possible and perhaps different from the previous time? Enquire at your workplace what services they may be able to offer. Of course this will vary depending on your size of employer, for example. Perhaps they are able to offer counselling, breastfeeding support and/or nursery facilities. Consider medication and how this may/may not affect your work or working whilst breastfeeding. Ask the difficult questions: how are you going to handle school holiday cover, nursery care, working hours? There has been a change in the law recently concerning flexible working: how can that help you? The whole basis behind these questions is to be informed to be able to take required actions to ease any possible stress and anxiety around your employment. This will reduce some aspects that may add to your chances of a repeat of perinatal mental illness.

Debate whether or not to discuss with your line manager about your previous mental illness associated with the perinatal period. Due to my illness and extended leave from teaching when I had my son, I am sure my employers would have been apprehensive had I ever announced I was pregnant again! I would have felt the need to have shared with them my intended plan for making it a better experience the second time around. Ideally I would have chosen not to have gone back at all. Remember that it is actually none of your employer's business whether or not you plan to have, or succeed in having, another child. It is your decision for what is best for your family, yet it may help to be sensitive to the employment situation. If you do approach any such conversation with your employer, do so from a purely work perspective. Cite, if necessary, areas that will be helpful to both you and your boss such as precedents, work policies, employment law and ways that you can manage your job. Give a thought to what the demands and needs will be if/when returning to work and managing an additional child. Be aware that it is ultimately up to the employer to manage the work scenario. This is applicable to either or both parents. As parents-to-be you can be co-operative and flexible, which will undoubtedly assist – there is no need to be guilty or apologetic.

These are some ways that may be useful for your employer to consider:

1. Identify with the employee ways in which their needs can be accommodated.
2. Encourage the employee to come to you with any concerns regarding her health.
3. Ensure the employee can identify areas where she can feed her baby without being disturbed.
4. Encourage the employee to download 'break time' software if relevant to her health needs.
5. Ensure confidentiality and respect is maintained in the workplace about the employees' health issues.

There is a great deal of help and resources for employers on mental health and the workplace at Time to Change[4] and Mind.[5]

If you are a healthcare professional helping families deciding whether to have another child after a previous perinatal mental health problem, share this information with them.

If you do become pregnant, then you are naturally very focused on time! Months, weeks and days are counted down to the due birth date. Another countdown tends to be around leaving work, regardless of whether you intend to return or not. What can you do to make this transition best for all involved?

Whilst you are still working when pregnant, be aware of your rights as an employee,[6] e.g. that you are entitled to take time off to attend classes if they have been recommended by a midwife or GP. In view of your previous problematic pregnancy/birth, this may be especially relevant. Also check on your allowed leave and maternity pay.[7]

While you do not have to inform your employer that you are pregnant, have given birth in the last six months or are breastfeeding, it is important (for you and your child's health and safety) to notify them in writing as early as possible. Until your employer receives written notification from you, they are not required to take any further action, such as altering working conditions or hours of work.[8]

Perhaps if you do share your news with your employer sooner rather than later, it may make the situation easier to manage for both parties. It could give you time to adjust, make plans and feel more confident about the new baby and in yourself. Also explore what paternity leave and support could be offered by the father's workplace.

The Citizens Advice Bureau[9] also produces some useful information. Maternity Action[10] is the UK's leading charity committed to ending inequality and improving the health and wellbeing of pregnant women, partners and young children – from conception through to the child's early years. There is advice here for fathers; same-sex partners; refugee and asylum seekers and employers.

Most of us would want to leave everything organised and efficient for people who will cover our role in our absence (if there is one). You may set your targets too high and attempt to be Superwoman completing all those tasks you have been meaning to do for ages – ask yourself if this is really necessary. I suggest that you make a list, with a timescale, of your tasks. Look at it again and divide it into three:

1. **Do:** What is essential and only you can do.
2. **Ditch:** What really is neither important nor urgent and can be done only if everything else is completed.
3. **Delegate:** What can you ask others to do, thereby giving other team members a new skill which will empower them and ease your worry that if you are not there, a certain task will not get done.

If you are leaving and not intending to return to your job, consider what the main tasks are that you need to complete in order to walk away and feel content that you have left everything as you would wish to find it. One mum advises:

- Make sure you don't leave start of maternity leave too late. You need time to put your feet up, rest and adjust to change before the baby is born. The temptation is to leave it as late as possible to have time with the baby after he/she is born.

If you are intending to return, consider what you want to return to and set up the conditions for this to happen, e.g. by passing on key knowledge to your covering person. This may require a certain amount of 'letting go' and lowering of your expectations when you do return, as you may go back to find that your requests and the way you do things have either not been done or not done to your standard. Prepare yourself for this and approach with an attitude of acceptance and appreciation for what has been achieved. Giving yourself permission to 'be okay with it' will actually be much kinder on yourself and for your colleagues. Why waste negative energy instead of simply getting on with the job? It is good practice for other areas of life – you will have changed over the months that you will have been off; the business will have too – roll with those changes to embrace them. Being resistant to change will add stress. One mum suggests:

- Returning to work can help you feel like you get back to the 'old' you, but make sure you take time for your recovery. Don't be too hasty

So what can you do if you are self-employed? Ideally you would allow yourself a good break to give time to adjust to the new birth and daily life with additional children. As I am now self-employed, I appreciate that this can be even harder than as an employee. You haven't a team that you can delegate to and if you do not work there is no pay. As part of your planning ensure, where possible, that you have the financial means in place to ease this period. Ask for help to allow you to at least keep up with emails and telephone calls rather than stopping completely. You would need to consider what would happen if you were to become ill again and what additional support would be needed to aid your recovery. Being at home may be better than in a workplace or vice versa.

I asked the mothers in my survey if they had returned to work after having another child. Some expressed emotions that are normal or common, yet may feel they would be perceived as shameful or secretive. Let's bring them into the light! Seventy-four per cent of the mothers said they had gone back to work. For some this actually aided their recovery as they found it helpful.

- Couldn't wait to get back to work to be me, Anna, it was the only thing that kept me going, and couldn't wait to go.
- I feel I manage well but have to make sure I look after myself in making sure I eat well and get plenty of sleep.
- Going to work was an escape; I didn't have to look after my baby and could pretend that my life hadn't changed since before the birth of my child.
- Glad, to get away from my son and get some of my life back.
- This made me feel more 'normal'.
- In fact I had planned not to return to work after the birth but in light of the depression I wanted to, so that my son could be away from me enough to develop more normally.
- Took time but was positive for me.
- I loved it – being back at work when my son was 10 months old was just what I needed to do, it helped me feel like my old self again.
- I was very worried about going back to work but I found it easier than I thought it would be.

- Initially I was really scared but work proved an excellent distraction.
- I felt better about it, but guilty for leaving her.

Some found that a new career helped:

- I started my first own business during second pregnancy. It helped to focus on something else – put energy into something, create something, succeed at something.
- I started my own photography business and it helped me massively! Just took my mind away from it all.
- Not to my original post as I was worried about facing people but I found a new job 18 months later.
- Found new job when baby was 14 months old (had been made redundant when pregnant).

Due to their illness some mothers changed or stopped their career as their confidence had been affected:

- I did not go back to the job I was in. In April 2010 I helped start a toddler group at my local children's centre which was terrifying at first, but managed to build up my confidence again and get to know other mums. I started work part time in a local pre-school doing admin. It took me some time to realise that I could actually do things and wasn't a complete failure and useless.
- I was anxious as the workplace was very stressful.
- Anxious. It was awful at first as I had a new manager who is a bit unsympathetic.
- I have recently started a job for just 5 hours a week but just doing basic admin, whereas before I was a nurse in a busy stressful environment.
- Almost 2 years after the birth. Worked part time for 18 months and then gave up work due to fear of being ill again due to having a high workload etc.
- Off and on but gave up work in 2004. I was unemployable because of my sickness record.

Look at options that may help such as part-time or job sharing, for example:

- Working part time has given me a good balance in life.
- Explore your employers' flexible working policy and talk to other mums ABOUT how they managed flexible working. I found one mum in my workplace really eager to share her experience and this really helped me when requesting flexible work routines.

If you have been forced to go back to paid work that has less responsibility, pay or demands than previously, remember that this may be a transitional phase. View it as another learning opportunity that will help you when you do seek other employment when your children are older and/or you feel better. Remember to give yourself credit for what you are doing as opposed to pulling yourself further down.

Being on medication does not necessarily mean that you are unable to work, although you may need to adapt, as in this example:

- I returned to work when baby turned 1. I was terrified I had 'mental' written on my forehead. I am an intensive care nurse and felt unprepared. Despite this, I had wonderful support and a very compassionate manager. I was unable to work in the mornings due to the sedating effect of the meds I was still on so only worked afternoons – 2 shifts a week. Despite my fears, work helped me gain control and structure in my life. I utilised extra care in my practice to avoid mistakes and relied heavily on protocol manuals to double check anything I wasn't sure of. I gradually told a number of my colleagues what I had been through and this further aided my recovery in the support and love that was shown to me.

If you are going to go back to work ensure that your plans are made for childcare arrangements in good time. If you feel confident and happy that your child/children are going to be well cared for it will help your confidence. My son loved his child minder. He was able to play with other children and it made him more confident for nursery and playgroup.

When you are returning to work remember that you need to give yourself permission to be kind to yourself. I know that the temptation will always be that your children come first – yet this is a time to put your needs as priority too. Although a new outfit and hair style may seem an extravagance, for example, it may help to give you a boost in confidence when you do return. Netmums[11] have some great tips, including the importance of regular breaks and remembering to value yourself.

If you are still breastfeeding, and did not do this previously, you will need to plan how to do this effectively.[12]

Going back to work after an additional child, if you choose to or have to, may be easier if you have organised as much as you can. A happy and fulfilled mother will greatly encourage her children to be the same. Having more than one child brings more challenges yet also more joys. It can take a few years for the effects of the perinatal period to lift completely, so remember to be as kind to yourself as possible and recognise all that you are doing.

TOP TIPS FOR BEING A PREGNANT AND WORKING MOTHER FOLLOWING A PERINATAL MENTAL ILLNESS

1. Accept that whatever decision is made concerning paid work is okay.
2. Be aware of all your maternity employee rights and guidelines.
3. Moderate your working tasks and apply DDD – do, ditch, delegate.
4. Engage in baby conversations only with those who are genuinely interested.
5. Rest as much as you can when maternity leave starts and leave work behind – acknowledge the change in life and its demands which is approaching.
6. If your workplace was affected by your previous perinatal period, reassure them that you will work with them to manage it effectively this time and have put plans in place to maximise your health.
7. Remember that some mothers find that going back to work helps their confidence and personal identity.
8. Make plans for your return to work including childcare and practical plans.

TOP TIPS FOR SUPPORTING A PREGNANT AND WORKING MOTHER FOR HEALTHCARE PROFESSIONALS

1. Ensure that you have done your role well in setting up the mother's care plan and liaise with occupational health if relevant.
2. Identify opportunities to minimise physical and mental demands.
3. Direct parents to the advice for maternity and employment rights and support.

REFERENCES

1. www.gov.uk/government/statistics/maternity-allowance-quarterly-statistics-march-to-may-2014
2. www.gov.uk/government/collections/statistics-childcare-and-early-years
3. www.gov.uk/maternity-pay-leave
4. www.time-to-change.org.uk/your-organisation/support-employers
5. www.mind.org.uk/for-business/mental-health-at-work/
6. www.gov.uk/working-when-pregnant-your-rights
7. www.adviceguide.org.uk/wales/work_w/work_time_off_work_e/maternity_leave.htm#h_other_parental_rights
8. www.hse.gov.uk/mothers/faqs.htm
9. www.adviceguide.org.uk/england/work_e/work_time_off_work_e/maternity_leave.htm
10. www.maternityaction.org.uk/wp/
11. www.netmums.com/back-to-work/jobs/working-mums/your-first-day-back-at-work
12. http://childdevelopmentinfo.com/child-development/preparing_for_birth/nursing-mother-working-mother-the-essential-guide-for-breastfeeding-and-staying-close-to-your-baby-after-you-return-to-work/

FURTHER READING AND RESOURCES

- www.aworkingmum.co.uk/ Extensive information for working mums including advice on: finances; childcare vouchers; tax credits; childcare fees; budgeting; creating routines.
- www.whattoexpect.com/first-year/week-12/back-to-work-transitions.aspx
- www.workingmums.co.uk/ Work from home and find part-time jobs, full-time jobs and flexible jobs here at Working Mums.
- www.mumandworking.co.uk/ The website for working parents seeking flexible employment, not just jobs for mums but work from home, family-friendly jobs and opportunities plus advice.

PART 4

The role of healthcare professionals and facilities

CHAPTER 23

The role of healthcare professionals: what parents have received, want and need

Body and soul cannot be separated for purposes of treatment, for they are one and indivisible. Sick minds must be healed as well as sick bodies.

C Jeff Miller

Usually the physical aspects of pregnancy are considered to be the main priority regarding health needs of the mother, baby and significant others. I would like to see a step towards much greater parity of esteem (equal approach to both mental and physical health), especially where couples are contemplating another pregnancy after a previously challenging one. The care I received in pregnancy was generally very good. I saw the same small group of midwives on a regular basis, and that continuity enabled one of them to immediately realise that something was amiss when I described how tearful and hot I was feeling. She ordered blood tests and was looking for a cause of my symptoms, during which time I deteriorated in great pain and needed to be hospitalised for a urinary tract infection. My treatment on the ward was very good apart from waiting for what seemed days without any guidance from the obstetrician as he was on holiday. Finally when I was moved to a different consultant, she was annoyed because my condition was a specialism of hers and she could not understand why no one had told her of my admittance of the ward. If so, I may have had the proper treatment faster and therefore cost the NHS less money by being an inpatient. Again poor communication to her happened again when no one told her of my problematic birth experience. She only found out at my six week check-up.

Throughout my period of failing mental health I was seen by my GP, my health visitor and at a support group. On paper it appeared that I was being well cared for. In reality I was not truthful about my feelings due to the shame and guilt I felt at being diagnosed with postnatal depression. I acknowledge now that I had a role to play in my own recovery. At the time I did not appreciate it. Additionally, other health professionals who have read my story say that I should have been referred to a specialist perinatal mental health professional much sooner, before I completely broke down. I also wonder: would it have changed things if the health professionals had spoken to each other more and to my family, along with me being more honest, if a more truthful picture had been painted, showing I needed additional care?

There were some wonderful examples of great care when I was in the psychiatric hospital, e.g. being allowed to sit with the team in the early hours when I was too distressed to sleep. Sadly there were also poor examples, such as when I was severely reprimanded for accidentally breaking a vase whilst wandering in a drug-induced state. That fear of being harshly spoken to led me to more self-harming because I was too scared to ask for help. I worried that I would be called 'trouble' again for 'complaining' about the effects of a new drug.

My community psychiatric nurse was wonderful in the counselling sessions that followed my stay in hospital. He helped me realise that I had been ill and not a failure. I changed my desire to have another baby from 'to do it properly next time' to 'enjoy it next time'. Had my ex-husband agreed for another child, I believe I would have been far more open and knowledgeable about what care I might need and requesting it.

I asked parents what main requests they would ask of health professionals who are in a position to give support to parents who face the dilemma of risking perinatal mental illness in order to have another child. These are their main ones:

- Listen to them! Postnatal illness is terrifying – it rips mothers from families and takes women to the depths of hell. They are not being neurotic or 'highly strung'. They are terrified and need specialist counselling.
- Don't belittle or dismiss their worries. Take any worries seriously. Respect their views.
- My experience would have been better if my psychiatrist made a plan. Instead he was totally against me bearing children, suggesting adoption. He was surprised by my pregnancy, which shows he was not listening to me.
- Be realistic (saying 'it might not happen again' doesn't help, because the reality is it is quite likely).
- Be available and flexible, for example, 'More regular visits from my health visitor to monitor how I was, as some days got really low and maybe I could have done with more support.'
- Be compassionate and empathetic as opposed to judgemental.
- Ensure parents are aware of all available help/treatment options and provide

information on resources, practical solutions, contact numbers, support groups. Offer advice that doesn't scare them.

- Make sure you are completely aware of the referral pathways in your area – what help is out there and for whom. I see some shocking misdirection of service users at times (for example – someone heavily pregnant and trying to kill themselves given a leaflet about counselling at their local health centre!)
- Be proactive rather than reactive leaving clients waiting for help.
- Support and monitor your clients with regular updates and check-ups, e.g. one mum said, 'Time is crucial, my GP gave me a check-up appointment every two weeks, and it was a lifeline.'
- ASK what the parents would like to happen.
- Effective signposting for all up front regardless of whether they know your history.
- To offer advice and similar stories of other mothers and success stories.
- Reassure them you would – and if necessary do – respond quickly if she does become unwell – a four week wait for an appointment is too long to be feeling so unwell.
- Be a friend to these women – don't consider them just another patient: 'Try to become a trusted friend to the woman instead of the healthcare professional who exists in her life because she is bonkers.'

There were also specific requests applicable to the different perinatal stages:
- Before conception:

  - To discuss that just because you have suffered previously doesn't mean you will again and you still have the right to extend your family.
  - Provide medical details and post birth debriefing, for traumatic births.
  - To discuss openly the risks and options and have a good assessment of risk.
  - To involve partner in the procedure of assessment, e.g. to gain an understanding of how much support he will give.
  - Offer support/pre-birth counselling.
  - Refer and take the risk of poor maternal mental health seriously.
  - Be aware of previous triggers.

- During pregnancy:

  - Work with the mother (and partner) to compile a birth and postnatal plan in detail in order to give every chance to avoid previous experiences, e.g. 'I feel that I was at an extremely high risk of PND due to the previous pregnancy ending in termination. I was practically told that it was for the best. I went against my huge instincts and suffered regret and loss. I had no help with this and I was haunted by it. A risk assessment during pregnancy would have picked this up.'

- Discuss all options before the birth, including what drugs are available for breastfeeding mums.
- Be well-informed about medication and understand that decisions around taking meds in pregnancy are extremely difficult.
- Reduce the stigma of taking – and prescribe if necessary – antidepressants during pregnancy. A lot of women, including myself, suffer unnecessarily because we are scared that medication might be harmful, for what is actually a negligible risk.
- To give women the opportunity for counselling during pregnancy.

- The birth:

  - Be there for the mother prior to birth.
  - Make labour/hospital experience less daunting being aware of emotions and history.

- Postnatally:

  - No breastfeeding bullying! Choice of feeding is far less important than a happy mother.
  - Any new mum in chronic pain and sleep deprived is at high risk, no matter how well she seems to be coping.
  - Never underestimate the power of loneliness and isolation and a lack of community to set examples.
  - Trust in the ability of the mother – don't treat the mum like she has done something wrong or is a danger to her children.
  - The depression risk questionnaire is great and have a support system in place to offer straight away.
  - Don't assume because a woman is intelligent and articulate that she knows what is best for her and is telling the truth about her situation.
  - More contact visits, better support spread *throughout first year* postnatally.
  - Offer drop in groups/classes, like antenatal classes for mums postnatally – 'More group meetings and more practical help. It would have been nice to be able to get a break from looking after my baby.'
  - Don't assume mums who have other children aren't coping just because the house is clean when you come to visit.

I also asked parents what they felt could have been better from the healthcare professionals that cared for them. The main aspect was early detection leading to correct referral and treatment.

- A GP who had a clue about PND and understood the systems in place to secure appropriate treatment. Early diagnosis would have made it far better and referral to the perinatal mental health team.

- Problem should have been picked up earlier – no need for full blown psychosis to develop. Should have never been separated from new baby – needed place in mother and baby unit.
- A week after the birth I knew there was something wrong with me and I asked for help but my illness was not diagnosed until 4 days later and I had to be sectioned which meant being taken away from my baby. I think if I had had professional help when I realised I was ill then maybe I would not have had to be sectioned.
- I should have been monitored closely after I told the health visitor at 10 days post birth that I didn't love the baby and felt daily dread and anxiety and couldn't sleep … instead I was left.
- Early interventions from mental health teams. I was extremely suicidal. I think the health visitor should have referred to the crisis team. Obviously a better relationship would have also made a massive difference.
- In retrospect, I needed a higher dose of antidepressants.
- Although flagged for an early visit from a support nurse (due to baby not gaining weight and mum nervous), this was cancelled twice in the first 2 weeks due to her being unwell. This was pivotal in missing the onset of my illness. I had a lot of insight at this time and wanted to discuss how I was feeling with her. When she cancelled the second time I am sure if the person who rang asked even one question they would have known something was very wrong, but it was simply cancelled and no questions were asked.
- I was visited after my daughter's illness weekly by the health visitor. She recognised I had PND and PTSD. I was terrified about going to the GP. In the end she contacted him without my permission. I ended up on a low dose antidepressant, but to be honest I was never completely honest about my thoughts and feelings to anyone. I was experiencing hallucinations on a regular basis as well as intrusive thoughts. I also became delusional. I don't think the GP assessed me properly. It was only when I asked to be referred to a shrink I got the help I needed. They should have done this a lot earlier and I shouldn't have needed to ask.

Perhaps one way to improve this situation would be by better training and awareness for healthcare professionals. There are improvements being made, e.g. perinatal mental health is now to be a key area in GP training.[1]

- More mental health specialist midwifery posts needed now. Midwives need better training. Women could have a convention to discuss various case experiences of antenatal and postnatal depression with health professionals, e.g. a weekend study conference to remove stigma and get message out there.

- Although all the health professionals I encountered were very kind and wanted to help, none of them seemed to know much about PND. It would have been more reassuring to have seen a specialist.
- Closer supervision by specialists would have made my experience better. I made the diagnosis myself, researched for hours on the internet about suitable support that was available for me. There was not much at all. In the form that nurses get you to fill out at the baby clinics, I scored high in all questions of how depressed I was feeling. The only feedback I was given is that I scored high.
- Information. It is not talked about. This needs addressing. I felt so ashamed, and completely incompetent as a mother.

Others would have preferred more support and a longer stay in hospital:

- Longer in hospital more help with breastfeeding support. My husband having longer than 2 weeks at home with me.
- Better support from midwives who were too busy to talk and really spend any time.
- A little more help from the health visitor – after coming home the second time, I was an anxious mess!
- Despite me having in my notes my history of mental health problems and the consultant in perinatal mental health recommending I start medication whilst pregnant and if not then immediately at birth – I was too scared to take medication as I was worried about the effects on the baby. I felt staff just didn't seem to deal with that aspect. I was crying in front of midwives and I think it was easier for them to just ignore it or put down to baby blues, but they didn't do anything to support me.
- I am convinced that I should have been advised that I needed a blood transfusion before I left hospital. I had the blood transfusion on day 6 post-delivery and within 24 hours was starting to return to normal. When I discharged myself the sister in charge asked me if I had considered a blood transfusion – I was in NO fit state to make this decision and needed advice/recommendation from the medical staff.
- Being treated like a human being in the hospital rather than a case and just another birth.
- If the nurse had come or at least discussed how we were doing over the phone. We had wonderful offers of support from friends and family – we just chose to have those first few weeks largely by ourselves.

I asked parents how much support they got from healthcare professionals whilst suffering with poor maternal mental health. Answers varied from lots, to moderate to 'F*** all'! These comments represent the overall perspective:

- Some professionals were excellent and others exacerbated my mental health problems.
- Good midwifery support. Varied health visitor support. Terrible support from GP, which was particularly damaging to my diagnosis and treatment.

Some mothers had excellent care and support for which they were grateful and appreciated:

- The HV did the PND test and sent me straight to the doctors, she also put me on a therapy group course held at a Children's Centre. She also realised that my son had eczema that needed treating, but I could not/did not see it. But at the time I could not face catching two buses to go to the eczema clinic, it scared me, so she arranged for the doctor in charge of the clinic to come to my house first.
- In hospital I got lots of support from the nurses and breastfeeding support workers who helped me to get my son to feed (we were on the reluctant feeder programme). Once at home, the health visitors were also very supportive and a breastfeeding support worker also visited me at home several times. If I phoned up needing help there was always someone to talk to or they would come round.

Others had a terrible experience, with long term effects. Often women felt the health professionals were simply too busy to help with their questions, basic care or concerns.

- The midwives in hospital were awful. They were rude and unhelpful. They weren't encouraging, I felt they had no concept of how much pain I was in physically and how hard it was to sit up, hold the baby, stand up, etc. The midwives who visited at home were much nicer, but discharged me after 10 days. I was then in hospital again the same night with a burst scar and an infection. The health visitor was very supportive and kind. My GP was very dismissive of my back pain, despite the fact I couldn't stand up unassisted. I was referred to psychiatric nurse who was very supportive and a great psychiatrist who signed me off work at the end of my maternity leave. My GP did not understand why I couldn't face the pressure of returning to a demanding teaching job and would only sign me off for 2 weeks so I handed in my notice despite this being my dream job.

I was also given examples of where mothers did not feel they were given the right support or asked the right questions. A common area of challenge concerned breastfeeding:

- Very little breastfeeding help which was where I was really struggling. I look back on photos of me after Olivia's birth and I look drugged to the eyeballs and totally out of it and so uncomfortable.

- I had good help from my health visitor but I don't feel she asked the right questions to see how I was coping.

There were other comments around mums feeling they were being judged or misunderstood:

- I begged for help from about day 3 but it still took 6 weeks before, on phoning the health clinic and threatening to throw myself down the stairs, that someone actually agreed 'postnatal depression'. In the meantime I'd even written letters to show the GP saying I didn't feel I was real anymore!! He said, 'Ah but you have a lovely healthy son and you are breastfeeding – you cannot be depressed!' WHAT!?!! I wanted to go to sleep and not wake up for 18 years.
- My health visitor wasn't much support. I was constantly ringing breastfeeding support workers and my health visitor but unfortunately felt quite isolated from them all and that I was just asking stupid new mum questions that they expected me to react better to.
- I got the initial month of support from the midwife, which then dropped to a healthcare professional through the doctor's surgery. Unfortunately this person was what I consider an 'earth mother', had 4 children of her own and couldn't understand why I wasn't over the moon with my situation.
- Health professionals can be quick to judge. I heard a nurse ask another if I was feeling sorry for myself or milking it. In fact I told them I was okay but they noticed I was anxious. More awareness needs to be in place. Professionals need to stop nagging about breastfeeding/nutrition/germs etc. All this made me paranoid and made me feel inadequate. Some make you think that there is a perfect parent out there when really no one is perfect.
- I had many trips to the GP. They were very unhelpful and one male GP asked me what I expected when I told him I couldn't sleep. He said I was a new mother – it was normal. Another GP told me it was not a problem that I couldn't sleep as he was an insomniac and sometimes only had one hour sleep every night and he was fine. I also contacted a community team and was told that he didn't feel I was depressed as I had make-up on.
- Doctors being more aware/using their initiative. I presented to the GP when I had slipped my disc, pleading for help as I could not lift my baby. She was dismissive of me. I believe I even used the word 'depressed' but she did not ask me any questions about this. I still feel extremely angry at this doctor in particular as she could have saved me years of sadness.

Sometimes mothers felt challenged by healthcare professionals telling them that things like housework do not matter, yet they do to that person:

- We are often told as new mums by well-meaning HCPs: 'Don't worry about the housework or the vacuuming!' But if you are the kind of person who spent a significant amount of time prior to the first baby ensuring your house was sparkling clean, this advice will not only sound alien to you but will undermine you as a person. Yes 'you won't have time for both but what can WE do about that?' As opposed to 'you won't have time for both so just ditch that part of your personality'. Mums who need a clean and tidy environment should have their needs taken seriously. It's not right to abandon everything she has previously striven for re: diet, good figure, housework, etc! She needs a realistic, sensitive approach.

Many mothers wanted to be introduced to other mothers, e.g.

- Having a local support group/unit that I could have attended to speak to other parents and medical staff would have helped, as I felt like an alien amongst friends who had children but weren't going through what I was, and they didn't understand why I was behaving the way I did. They were in the dark too.

Where a lady has needed to be hospitalised, there are concerns expressed where this was and if it could have been avoided. For some being admitted to a Mother and Baby Unit was the best course of action; one disagreed. Others felt the whole family would have been better if an MBU was closer to home.

- Not being apart from my son initially could have made my experience better as I had to wait for a space in the mother and baby unit for 3 days so he could only visit me and it made everything worse. Was awful as I had to stop breast-feeding but was still producing milk.
- In hindsight I should have been an inpatient and there was a mother and baby unit at the hospital my son was born in! I should have been in there and had proper full on support. I was too ill to be at home. My family really suffered but ultimately I did – I was told next time by the perinatal MH Consultant that I was incredibly brave to have got through it at home. I wish it had never been necessary.
- I was admitted to a normal psychiatric ward – it was a horrific time. The baby was not allowed there with me. I was there for a week as I was discussing suicidal thoughts. I was initially diagnosed with sleep deprivation and placed on Prozac. I felt like this was a huge error looking back as I had no support and would spend hours alone in the room trying to think of ways to hang myself.
- I think I would have recovered quicker at home with my baby beside me. I had a big issue with locked doors when I was ill as when baby in neonatal unit had to knock to be let in and in mother baby unit baby was locked in another room. This I think affected my bonding with baby.
- Going straight to the MBU rather than being in a general psychiatric ward.
- I wish now I was hospitalised but at the time I thought I was doing the right thing for my child. I relapsed when my son was 14 months old and was sectioned, diagnosed then for depression and anxiety. When my son was born I was diagnosed shortly after with puerperal psychosis.

- To have gone to a Mother and Baby unit would have been marvellous, it would have helped me so much I think.

My main message to parents in getting the best out of healthcare services is to be a good, clear communicator in expressing and asking for your needs to be met. I would also encourage you to seek a second opinion or ask to be moved to a different professional if you are unhappy. One mum recommends:

- I think in the modern world some of us have lost confidence in our ability to be parents and lack of faith in our own judgements. There is still a basic parenting instinct in all of us that we should trust – the message is go with your gut instinct and if you feel something is wrong, it probably will be!! Push for second opinion. An example is my own experience with community midwife. I had no rapport with her at all and know it wasn't me because two other midwives attended late in my pregnancy at a Bank Holiday and they were wonderful – just what you want – warm, kind, engaging, interested and reassuring. My own midwife (a team leader at that!!) flirted with my husband in my first consultation (I am not a jealous lady by the way!), came to my house stinking of smoke and showed little or no additional support to me in spite of PP. The only extra visit she made to me postnatally was to collect some notes that were at my house in error! In summary, in hindsight I should have requested changing to a different midwife but felt I couldn't ask to do so at the time for fear of 'making a fuss'. Just because somebody is qualified, they are not always right and trust/ have faith in your own instincts.

Where parents have felt supported through an additional pregnancy and post-natally, there are positive outcomes, such as these mother describes:

- My 1st birth was really traumatic. My second also ended with emergency C-section after a 3 day labour. The second was still a positive experience because I was in a good mental state and had excellent care antenatal and during labour. This time I was kept in for 4 days, until I had been through the baby blues and breastfeeding was truly established. They took care of all the nappy changes and passed my baby to me and put her back in the crib after feeds. I wasn't straining myself trying to lift and carry after surgery, so even with SPD and being on crutches/wheelchair, I felt ready to go home and wasn't in excessive pain.

Here are two final tips from those who have gone on to having another baby:

- Ensure all maternity staff are aware of your level of risk, and how important sleep is for you. Insist on a private room in the hospital if possible, so that you can sleep and get any additional extra support privately.

- Ensure you get specialist advice and support from a perinatal MH psychiatrist prior to, during and after the pregnancy. Work with them on an advanced care plan that aims to prevent relapse, which will probably include medication and ways of accessing extra support. Also include details of how you'd want your older children cared for if you became unwell again.

In the 2014 National Maternity Survey[2] they reported that:

since the birth of their baby almost all women (90%) had been asked about their own emotional and mental health by a health professional. Of those self-identifying with a mental health problem after the birth, 63% had received support and 49% had received treatment to date.

Clearly there are some positive situations and support happening – we need more.

TOP TIPS FOR PARENTS REGARDING HEALTHCARE PROFESSIONALS

1. Be open and candid about your past challenges so that you can give the people involved in your care the maximum opportunity to help this time.
2. Be informed of what you need and services you should have, e.g. look at www.joebingleymemorialfoundation.org.uk/category/useful-information/[3]
3. If you feel that you have a personality clash with a professional, ask to be moved to a different one.
4. Be aware that you are central to your care and treatment – know what you need and if you may need an advocate to help in making decisions.
5. You also have a responsibility in your care plans, prevention and recovery.

REFERENCES

1. www.ncb.org.uk/news/ncb-statement-on-health-education-england-mandate-measures-to-improve-gp-training-and-perinatal-mental-health
2. www.npeu.ox.ac.uk/maternity-surveys/news/808-new-national-maternity-survey-shows-women-are-seeking-pregnancy-care-earlier
3. Fact sheets on information www.joebingleymemorialfoundation.org.uk/category/useful-information/

FURTHER READING AND RESOURCES

- What mums need www.huffingtonpost.com/sarah-bregel/what-postpartum-moms-really-need_b_5343907.html?ncid=fcbklnkushpmg00000037
- Hanley J. *Listening Visits in Perinatal Mental Health: a guide for health professionals and support workers.* 1st ed. Abingdon: Routledge; 2015.

CHAPTER 24

The role of healthcare professionals: what can you, as an HCP, do?

A doctor who cannot take a good history and a patient who cannot give one are in danger of giving and receiving bad treatment.

Author unknown

I am eternally grateful for the services I received from the NHS professionals who cared for me and ultimately enabled me to make a full recovery from puerperal psychosis. When I vowed to speak and write further about maternal mental health as a former patient, I did so through a desire to make the journey of new parenthood easier for others. I also wanted to help the people treating them feel encouraged to do so with their present and future families in distress. I have found that this is common amongst those of us who have suffered poor mental health around a pregnancy. One of the mothers who responded to my survey illustrates this beautifully with this paragraph:

- Remember YOU have the power to make a massive difference to someone's life. Out there somewhere is a health visitor, a GP and a mental health nurse who at one time each saved my life for one more day. I will never forget them and the gifts they gave me with their compassion and care. You might feel like a drop in the ocean but you can be the drop that makes the difference to that person. The most important gift you can give anyone in that place is Hope.

This will be a message I shall continue to highlight. So often people working in a large organisation can feel demoralised and that their actions will make no difference. Take confidence and inspiration from being or becoming the 'drop' described above!

I have had some great care from some individuals, as have many of the people who responded to my survey. What is evident is the lack of consistency in care and services and amongst the different health professionals involved. The good practice outlined by the NICE guidelines,[1] does not appear to being followed in many cases, with very little networking around care being carried out. Considering we have a 'national' health service in the UK this is alarming. For example:

- Community Midwife – very good. GPs – first 3 useless, final one brilliant (that's how many I had to see to find one who would listen!). Health Visitor – first one AWFUL. Second one (after I sacked the first one!) – amazing. Life saving.

In the summer of 2014 the Maternal Mental Health Alliance[2] published a map of the UK showing the huge gaps that exist. The stories that I have heard would certainly back up this postcode lottery of care. This has to be one of the main drivers in the UK to ensure that we have a national system for specialist perinatal mental health. Imagine if you broke your leg only to be told that you needed a four-hour journey to find a specialist?

This has impacted upon the decision of one lady dramatically:

- I have been lucky to live in Australia during my second pregnancy, where I could pay privately for affordable access to a psychiatrist who is a specialist in perinatal mental health, and an obstetrician, who allowed me to have full control over my labour. If I was relying on the NHS, I would not have had another baby in the UK because the quality of care you receive is a matter of pot luck. I couldn't afford to take that risk again.

In November 2014 the Maternal Mental Health Alliance was able to commission an economic review on perinatal mental health by the London School of Economics and the Centre for Mental Health.[3] They highlighted the costs of undiagnosed or untreated perinatal mental health problems as including:

1. **avoidable suffering:** perinatal mental illness can cause intense, debilitating, isolating and often frightening suffering for women
2. **damage to families:** perinatal mental illness can have a long-term impact on a woman's self-esteem and relationships with partners and family members
3. **impact on children:** perinatal mental illness can have an adverse impact on the interaction between a mother and her baby, affecting the child's emotional, social and cognitive development
4. **death or serious injury:** in severe cases, perinatal mental illness can be life-threatening: suicide is one of the leading causes of death for women in the UK during the perinatal period
5. **economic costs:** the economic cost to society of not effectively treating perinatal mental illness far outweighs the cost of providing appropriate services.

From a review of the literature on perinatal depression, the estimates imply that only 3% of all cases of perinatal depression end up achieving full recovery (p. 22 of the report). The conclusion was 'If perinatal mental health problems were identified and treated quickly and effectively, all of these serious and often life-changing human and economic costs could be avoided.'[4]

As a healthcare professional, your first step could be to ensure that those who have the influence to channel funding into perinatal mental health are aware of the need and its impact. A useful tool to share with commissioners is the Guidance for Commissioners of Perinatal Mental Health Services by the Joint Commissioning Panel for Mental Health.[5] It has been written to assist specialised commissioners, as well as Clinical Commissioning Groups and Health and Wellbeing Boards. Send it to all the influential people – if you get no response, resend until you do! It will also be of use to provider organisations, service users, patients, carers, and the voluntary sector.

One of my teaching friends makes the point:

I always think that what the Government could get better is investment in prevention instead of having to fund additional services to 'pick up the pieces', e.g. instead of having a midwife with MH expertise they then need to fund psychiatric support services, hospital stays etc; instead of investing more into early numeracy and literacy they have to spend more in services like teaching in prisons!

Remember that as an individual within a healthcare profession, you can make a difference as an individual. Even if faced with tight budgets, if you have the will and determination to make a difference to people's lives, it can be done. Kathryn Gutteridge set up a postnatal support group in 1997 simply by finding a vacant room in Tamworth. It has since helped over 1000 women.

The NICE Guidelines stress the need for networks of professionals to work together – as perinatal mental health covers several, it takes just one person to arrange a meeting with a representative from each discipline. For example in Barking, Havering and Redbridge University Hospitals NHS Trust, Dr Farida Bano, Consultant Obstetrician and Gynaecologist, is also the perinatal mental health lead. She and her colleagues have set up a service for perinatal mental health with a joint obstetric and psychiatric clinic. This kind of system may even be possible without needing extra funding.

Another good example of a service is in Oxford Health NHS Foundation Trust. Gerry Byrne is clinical lead for the Family Assessment and Safeguarding Service (FASS) and the Infant Parent Perinatal Service (IPPS). Their award-winning service is described in their BMJ article.[6]

I believe that there is a growing interest within the government on perinatal mental health. They now award prizes via the All-Party Parliamentary Group on Maternity.[7] For example, the Perinatal Mental Service led by Nigel Perks from Lewisham and Greenwich NHS has just been recognised. They stress the need for 'identification through communication' and how professionals need to be aware of picking up the signals to access the mental state of a new parent. Also you may like to get involved with the First 1001 Critical Days,[8] a cross-party manifesto, looking at the importance of conception to age 2.

Again I encourage healthcare professionals to believe that they *can* make a difference. As Dalai Lama XIV said, 'If you think you are too small to make a difference, try sleeping with a mosquito.'

Let me remind you that from the ward to the board you have a role to play. I used to believe that I was not in a leadership role because I am self-employed. I now accept this quote by John Quincy Adams:

If your actions inspire others to dream more; learn more; do more and become more, you are a leader.

We all cast a shadow by our thoughts, words and deeds – what is the impact of yours and what can you do to improve perinatal mental health?

I have already mentioned the financial aspects above that tend to be one of the initial reasons people use to say they 'can't' do anything. The other challenge I am often given is time. You may find it helpful to look at some of the tips I included in the chapter about the mother who is in employment, e.g. 'the do, ditch and delegate' principle. Another approach I find useful is Parkinson's time law that states 'work expands to fill the time available for completion'. Think about how much you actually achieve in 15 minutes before you have to leave on a work day. How much longer does it take you to do the same chores when it is a day off? Set yourself scheduled times into a diary rather than making a list. You may find that you achieve more in a shorter time.

I know that often healthcare professionals tell me that the time they get with patients is too short. Let me share this story with you. My sister is 10 years younger than me. When she announced her engagement I was delighted that she asked me to go looking for a wedding dress with her. We arrived in the first shop – stunning premises, designer gowns everywhere you looked. The assistant appeared, dressed extremely elegantly. She looked at me, back at my sister and asked, 'When is your daughter getting married?' We left. We go into the second shop. This one had a commercial radio station playing loudly, with special offer stickers everywhere. The assistant appeared, wearing slippers and slurping her coffee. 'Yeah?' she asked. My sister politely answered: 'I'd like a wedding dress – one with sleeves.' 'Oh, we don't have any of those – they're old-fashioned.' We left.

We went into the third shop, this time with our mum. As we entered, a smiling assistant appeared, making eye contact with each of us. Her first question was 'Who is the bride?' Once that was established, she complimented Claire on her engagement ring, the time of year she was getting married and told us that one of her other customers had just had a wonderful time at the venue we were going to. Guess where we got the dress? How long did it take us to decide where we wanted to shop?

You too can have that same impact on the people in your care. If you have 60 seconds or 60 minutes for contact, my message is make it count! Especially where mental health is concerned. Let me remind you again about the marathon runner – he does not run 26 miles – he runs a mile 26 times by putting one foot in front of the other. What small step can you do today to make perinatal mental health services better for those in your care? What if you did one small thing each day or week? What could that lead to or prevent? For example, in the case of this mother:

- In hindsight, the signs were all there even when I was pregnant but I can put on a good front. I think healthcare professionals would have been able to see through the front if they'd spent even a few minutes with me.

I would also like to encourage you using the Six Cs of enduring values and behaviours that underpin Compassion in Practice by the NHS.[9] I believe that whatever your role is working with young families, these are vital.

1. CARE

In the previous chapter I gave you many examples of what happened with poor care; additional trauma during births, for example. With an additional child, aspects of care are crucial to avoid anxiety of the parents. If you make people feel special, I strongly suggest that they will feel that you are. What do people do for you that makes you feel special? How can you apply this to others? Even a smile can make a difference, and simply acknowledging someone is there. Use names and 'be present' with the people you are with. One mum told me how her health visitor always used to jangle her car keys in her pocket during a visit – it made her feel like she was in a rush so there was no point in saying how she was really feeling. Remember this quote:

Too often we underestimate the power of a touch, a smile, a kind word, a listening ear, an honest compliment, or the smallest act of caring, all of which have the potential to turn a life around.

Leo Buscaglia

Think about the use of sensory stimulation to make yourself and others feel good. A blast of your favourite song in the car before a meeting can improve your mindset before seeing someone, for example, so that you can be at your best for them.

2. COMPASSION

I have mentioned at many stages about giving reassurance, 'being there' and hope in situations, no matter what treatment may be used.

> Drugs are not always necessary. Belief in recovery always is.
>
> Norman Cousins

You may need to draw on additional skills where loss is an issue. Ensure that you know the best ways to respond by looking at the advice by organisations such as Sands[10] and Child Bereavement UK.[11] If you are aware that you may face situations where you feel that you will not know what to say, research it. Did you know that the best public speakers, who appear to be so quick-witted in reply to hecklers in the audience, have actually thought out the likely comments and have rehearsed replies? Preparation is the key. Sometime patients need you to be their advocate and view their situation from their perspective. This may be by being aware of when 'the system' may overwhelm them, as demonstrated by this mum:

> Beware the dangers of overwhelming mums with too many healthcare visitors – please monitor and liaise. I remember a real low ebb where the phone and doorbell were constantly ringing at home with friends, family, flower deliveries, etc. Then on top of that was a stream of other people, I don't remember who, but could have been doctors, midwives, CPN, health visitors, social worker etc. The CPN arrived and I had to take myself upstairs to lie down. It was just too much to deal with.

3. COMPETENCE

When you are competent you instil faith and confidence in those that are seeking assistance from you. It helps ease their fears and worries. You have the ability to reduce perinatal mental anxiety in this way. Share your knowledge. Consider the different aspects in the book. What do you need to learn more about? For example, have you already looked at the Marcé Society website resources page?[12] There is a Marcé Resource Pack that can be used by groups or as self-training guide to update your knowledge and practice should this be of interest to you.[13] Are there some new methods that you could use, e.g. text-messaging?[14] Could you become involved in the Quality Network for Perinatal Mental Health Services[15] and their forum?[16] What can you learn from past reports on maternal deaths?[17]

From your knowledge then consider what you can ACT on:

A – apply
C – change
T – teach

Always remember to keep patients informed about their condition, care and treatment. It really does make a difference.

4. COMMUNICATION

I would highly recommend that you re-read my chapter on communication (*see* Chapter 9) and decide what you will 'ACT' on in both your internal and external dialogue. Remember about the need to reframe and use positive words about what you want to happen, as opposed to avoiding, e.g. 'hold the cup tightly with two hands' as opposed to 'don't spill the drink'. 'Remember' rather than 'Don't forget'. Think about the words and phrases you use and what their impact may be on those who are vulnerable. A key element throughout is for healthcare professionals to 'be there' for new parents. As one summed up – 'I knew I was ill. No one listened.' Always appreciate the need for 'someone to talk to' even if you are unable to 'fix' it. I love this quote by Alison Stuebe:

> We need to listen to the individual mother in front of us without judgement. We need to ask her what her goals are for her relationship with her baby, and find out how we can help her accomplish them.

Always remember that it is about how you say things as well as what, as in this example, provided by one of the mothers in my survey:

- For health carers, it is absolutely imperative the way they speak, introduce themselves and conduct themselves generally. I remember returning to hospital day 6 post-partum with suspected PP and in need of blood transfusion. I wasn't really psychotic, just spaced out and very, very unwell. A terribly clumsy locum psychiatrist entered the side room where I was with my husband and I do not recall any introduction, names etc. All I recall is her launching into questions starting with 'have you had any thoughts on harming yourself or your baby'. I hadn't, didn't and was shocked and horrified. I believe this pushed me over the edge from being unwell into paranoia and a slide into psychosis. Care, reassurance, politeness, sensitivity and time to build rapport, could have stopped this happening. My husband is very easy going but had an argument with her. I could not deal with the questions so simply turned my back on her and sat silently on the edge of the bed – it had all become too much. She then addressed my husband and asked why I was ignoring her?????!!! (I needed him to be my advocate.) He explained to her that I didn't know who she was or why she was asking me these questions. She could have approached me so differently and had a much more positive outcome for all concerned. So much can be learnt from this – it's not the 'what', but the 'how'!

5. COURAGE

As a healthcare professional I ask you to listen to your instinctive inner voice at times if you feel something could be better with a patient. I often wonder how the healthcare professional who drove away from a mother who said 'Please take me with you' felt the following day, when that mother's body was scraped up from a railway line? Have the strength and determination to act on your instinct. When a patient responds to the question 'how are you?' with 'I'm fine' and you have that gut feeling that they are not, what is the worst that can happen if you look them in the eye and simply ask, 'Are you really?' Our society tends to be so rushed today that people are worried about answering that question honestly. One mum said 'fine' stands for 'I'm Fed-up, Insecure, Neurotic and Emotional!' Get beyond the 'Fine' and ask more questions.

I have been told that some healthcare professionals are reluctant to ask because either they do not know how to respond if they really admit their thoughts and feelings and/or they do not know where to refer. Find out!

I have also suggested to parents that if they are not comfortable with someone who is supposed to be caring for them, to ask to change to someone else. I also encourage you to do the same. If you have a 'clash' for no other reason than that not all human beings connect, ask if you can swap with someone else. It may be that your skills are much better suited to someone who is currently having a clash too! Your courage at being honest could be the difference in a life being saved or at least improved.

6. COMMITMENT

The 6 Cs are meaningless unless you apply them. Embrace them. Choose and decide what knowledge you need to acquire to make your good practice great. Silence the inner critic (remember 'Shut the duck up') and investigate and apply what you *can* do.

We are all aware of why perinatal mental health is so important. We know how we can make it better. We simply need to identify what it is as individuals, groups and health and care organisations we can do to make a difference.

What if we all played our part in making a future pregnancy, birth and early parenthood better for those who previously were mentally unwell?

TOP TIPS FOR HEALTHCARE PROFESSIONALS

1. Listen to the parents and take their concerns seriously.
2. Be proactive in getting swift and correct referral or treatment as necessary.
3. Provide appropriate support and time at each stage of their journey.
4. Have relevant training in perinatal health.
5. Work towards a consistent national specialist perinatal mental health service in the UK.
6. Be compassionate and empathetic as opposed to judgemental.
7. Remember that with correct support and treatment, a positive outcome can be possible for an additional pregnancy.
8. Apply the 6Cs of Care, Compassion, Competence, Communication, Courage and Commitment to your role.
9. Believe that as an individual you can be instrumental in building a perinatal team to support many.

REFERENCES

1. www.nice.org.uk/guidance/cg45
2. Maternal Mental Health Alliance www.maternalmentalhealthalliance.org.uk/
3. http://everyonesbusiness.org.uk/wp-content/uploads/2014/12/Embargoed-20th-Oct-Final-Economic-Report-costs-of-perinatal-mental-health-problems.pdf
4. http://everyonesbusiness.org.uk/?page_id=46
5. www.jcpmh.info/resource/guidance-perinatal-mental-health-services/
6. www.magonlinelibrary.com/doi/abs/10.12968/bjom.2011.19.11.729
7. www.appg-maternity.org.uk/
8. www.wavetrust.org/our-work/publications/reports/1001-critical-days-importance-conception-age-two-period
9. www.england.nhs.uk/nursingvision/
10. www.uk-sands.org/
11. www.childbereavementuk.org/
12. http://marcesociety.com/resources/member-books-articles/
13. http://marcesociety.com/resources/education/
14. Rhyne EP, Borawski, A. Text messaging as an adjunct treatment for urban mothers with postpartum depression. *J Pediatr Health Care*. 2014; **28**(6): e49. Available at: www.chimat.org.uk/resource/view.aspx?RID=220662&src=pimh This study evaluated the feasibility of receiving scheduled text messages from paediatric providers as an adjunct treatment for postpartum depression in urban mothers identified in a high-volume, academic, primary care clinic.
15. www.rcpsych.ac.uk/workinpsychiatry/qualityimprovement/qualityandaccreditation/perinatal/perinatalqualitynetwork.aspx
16. perinatal-CHAT@rcpsych.ac.uk where questions and/or sharing good practice PMH can be posted.
17. www.npeu.ox.ac.uk/mbrrace-uk/reports

FURTHER READING AND RESOURCES

- www.nice.org.uk/guidance/CG192 The relationships between staff and service users need to change radically to improve outcomes in mental health services, according to a report published on 30 November 2010 by the National School of Government and supported by Centre for Mental Health. *Recovery Begins with Hope* by Su Maddock and Sophy Hallam finds that implementing recovery in mental healthcare depends upon radically changing staff and service-user relationships and the status of patients in making decisions about the support they get. www.recoverydevon.co.uk/index.php/news-a-reviews/news/154-recoverybeginswithhope
- Time management tips www.gettingagrip.com/

CHAPTER 25

The treatment of perinatal depression

Dr Carol Henshaw

A wide range of interventions is available to treat depression during pregnancy or after delivery. Which is most appropriate will depend on the *severity* of the depression, whether the woman has any past psychiatric history or other health problems, availability of treatment locally and her personal preference.

EDUCATION

Mild depression can be managed with self-help strategies or computer-based interventions. This can involve education about postnatal depression. One study involved women with symptoms of depression four weeks after delivery being randomised to receive an information leaflet at six weeks postpartum or not. The women who received the leaflet had lower scores when reassessed at three months.[1] Over 90% of those who received the booklet said that it was useful to them and their families. Most had not known about postnatal depression before reading it and because of this information gained more practical help and support from their families.

A web-based educational resource for both women and professionals, MedEdPPD, has been developed which uses a variety of strategies to promote learning.[2] Several organisations provide information via literature, websites, or run telephone support lines. Some also offer befriending or practical help in the home. However, be careful as some websites have been found not to contain much useful information or their information does not accurately reflect the evidence base and state of the science relating to postnatal depression.[3]

There has been a trial of internet-based behavioural activation in over 900 women with depressive symptoms recruited via a UK parenting website

(Netmums). The intervention involved 11 sessions lasting up to 40 minutes each to be completed over a 15-week period. It appeared to be effective in reducing depressive symptoms. However, although there was a huge interest in participating, many women dropped out and some had difficulty accessing the online therapy, lacked privacy, had issues around speaking face to face and were concerned that their child might be taken away.[4]

SUPPORT

Many small studies report that support and family-focused interventions such as home visits and peer support are effective. A systematic review found no evidence that universal provision of postnatal support improves maternal mental health but some evidence to suggest that high-risk populations might benefit.[5] A small pilot study involving 42 mothers suggested that those who had telephone-based peer support had a bigger decrease in depressive symptoms compared with mothers having usual care.[6]

A modified form of Gruen Therapy (encompassing relaxation techniques, problem-solving strategies and cognitive behavioural therapy (CBT)) delivered by telephone over a 10-week period by nurse therapists was reported in a small pilot study to reduce depression scores.[7] Telephone support is especially useful for women in rural areas or who have difficulty accessing supports outside the home.

INTERVENTIONS FOR DEPRESSION IN PREGNANCY

Mindfulness interventions are popular but there is only one study of a mindfulness-based group intervention for pregnant women. It reduced symptoms of distress, depression and anxiety but the numbers in the study were small and there were a large number of drop-outs.[8] A recent meta-analysis of antenatal interventions to reduce maternal distress (mindfulness, relaxation, acupuncture and a self-help workbook) reported a small but significant reduction in symptoms.[9]

Teaching partners to provide massage twice weekly for 12 weeks reduced depression and anxiety symptoms in pregnant women compared with a more general support group. Scores on a relationship quality questionnaire were improved and partners reported a reduction in depressed mood, anxiety and anger across the course of the massage therapy period.[10]

HEALTH VISITOR INTERVENTIONS

Many health visitors (HVs) in the UK have been trained in non-directive counselling and provide 'listening visits' to depressed postpartum women in their homes. Each visit usually lasts around one hour and 4–8 sessions are provided. However, training and supervision vary around the country and not all HVs in all areas have been trained. They can also be trained in cognitive behavioural (CB) counselling skills. This intervention comprises childcare advice, reassurance, encouraging participation in enjoyable activities, accessing support from others and setting targets and has been shown to be as effective as antidepressant treatment for postnatal major depression,[11] but adding either therapy to drug treatment did not confer any additional benefit. A large trial of trained HVs delivering sessions based either on CB or person-centred approaches reported benefit over usual care at six and 12 months compared with usual care.[12] Neither approach was better than the other.

Not surprisingly, qualitative studies of women who had received treatment from their HV reveal that they felt positive about the intervention if they had a previously good relationship but were less positive and might decline the intervention if that relationship was poor, they could not relate to her or did not know her. Women perceived the intervention as supportive rather than therapeutic and attributed their recovery to other factors.

INTERPERSONAL THERAPY

Interpersonal psychotherapy (IPT) is a time-limited, manualised psychotherapy focusing on four main problem areas: grief, interpersonal disputes, role transitions and interpersonal deficits. It consists of three phases. The first covers assessment, psychoeducation, selection of a treatment focus and negotiation of a treatment agreement. The problems are then worked on in the intermediate phase and a discussion of the progress made and how the patient feels about termination is carried out at the end.

IPT has been adapted to deal with issues facing women with postnatal depression such as her relationship with the baby and partner and returning to work. It has also been adapted for use in pregnant depressed women with a focus on role transition in relation to pregnancy, interpersonal disputes related to pregnancy and motherhood, and complicated pregnancies.[13]

A meta-analysis was carried out in 2011 and included 27 studies treating perinatal depression. All the interventions were superior to usual care and IPT was superior to those including a CBT component.[14]

EXERCISE

There is some evidence that exercise (group-based programmes such as pram-walking, group exercise sessions or individualised home-based interventions) can reduce postpartum depressive symptoms. Physical exercise is beneficial for women during pregnancy and in the postpartum period does not increase risks for the foetus or infant and can also lead to lifestyle changes that may confer long-term health benefits.

GROUP INTERVENTIONS

Many interventions can be delivered in groups. Being part of a group can reduce the sense of isolation that many mothers with depression feel and enable them to share experiences and coping strategies. It can also be a cost-effective way of delivering an intervention as several women can be treated at the same time. However, some mothers will have specific issues that may be better dealt with on a one-to-one basis, have difficulty talking openly in a group, be making negative social comparisons with others and may require some individual work before they feel able to cope with a group.

Most group treatments consist of several components, e.g. education, social support and CBT, and may involve partners in some or all sessions. Several reviews of group interventions including CBT, IPT and relational therapies for pregnant and postpartum women all report that group therapies appear to be clinically effective.[15,16,17]

Milgrom et al.[18] have described setting up, running and evaluating a group intervention. Their book includes material for all their group sessions. The development and content of IPT groups for postnatal depression has been described by Reay et al.[19]

Social support is often the main focus or an important component of group treatment. Many health visitors have set up such groups, with some becoming self-help groups beyond the lifetime of the original group. Groups may be open or closed and consist of just mothers, or fathers may attend some or all of the sessions. Services may also offer groups (which are usually closed) targeted at mothers with specific problems, e.g. survivors of childhood sexual abuse, those who have been bereaved or adolescent mothers.

ANTIDEPRESSANTS

More severe depression, or depression that has not responded to psychosocial interventions, may require antidepressant treatment. It is important to remember that antidepressants will take 10–14 days to begin to work and that they are not addictive, so after recovery and a further six months of therapy, they can be reduced and discontinued.

There have been several small studies of the antidepressant treatment of postnatal depression and most report some benefit. A systematic review of trials of the most commonly used antidepressants, selective serotonin re-uptake inhibitors (SSRIs), concluded that SSRIs are an effective treatment. They may be more efficacious than psychological interventions at the conclusion of therapy but there was no difference in outcomes at the follow-up phase and no benefit of combining SSRIs with a psychological intervention.[20]

DISCONTINUING ANTIDEPRESSANTS DURING PREGNANCY

Many women who become pregnant while taking antidepressants stop them. They may fear an adverse impact on the foetus, or may be advised to stop by a health professional. Deciding whether to stop or start an antidepressant in pregnancy should include an individual risk-benefit assessment. This should take into account the risk of relapse or recurrence and the impact of the untreated depression on a foetus if medication is stopped, versus any potential risk to the foetus by taking the drug. It should be noted that between two and three babies in every 100 are born with a birth defect even when no drugs are taken and that smoking or drinking excess alcohol may pose higher risks. The USA website www.mothertobaby.org has useful factsheets that can be downloaded on most of the antidepressants in use today.

Women whose depression is severe enough to be managed in specialist psychiatric care are more likely to relapse during pregnancy if they stop taking their antidepressant.[21] However, if depression has been managed in a community setting (by a GP or health visitor for example), there appears to be no difference in the risk of becoming depressed, whether antidepressants are continued during pregnancy or stopped.[22] Women with a history of four or more previous episodes of depression are more likely to become depressed after discontinuing treatment. Stopping an antidepressant abruptly can lead to unpleasant discontinuation symptoms and it is always advisable to taper off slowly to avoid this. Care must be taken when treating women with family histories of bipolar disorder with antidepressants, as there are reports of this triggering psychosis, a mixed affective episode or hypomania.[23]

HORMONES

The assumption that postnatal depression must have a hormonal aetiology led to attempts to treat it with oestrogens, progesterone and synthetic progestogens.

Uncontrolled studies performed by Dalton between 1985 and 1995 claimed success with progesterone as a treatment and preventive intervention but the studies had serious methodological problems and there are still no controlled data to support this. Synthetic progestogens can increase the risk of depressive symptoms.

Although there are small studies supporting the use of oestradiol in the treatment of severe postnatal depression, most of the women in these studies had previous or concurrent antidepressant or psychological therapy so the improvement cannot be attributed solely to oestradiol. There are concerns about using high doses of oestradiol in recently delivered women due to the increased risk of deep vein thrombosis, difficulties with breastfeeding and endometrial hyperplasia. The optimum dose and route of administration have not been established.

Until more data are available, the use of oestradiol is best limited to use as adjunct therapy for severe depressive disorders in women with no additional risk factors for thromboembolic disease or hormone-dependent tumours.

OMEGA-3 FATTY ACIDS

There has been interest in exploring the role of omega-3 fatty acids in the treatment of perinatal depression, despite no evidence that fish consumption or omega-3 status after childbirth are associated with depression. A review of seven trials observed that while depressive symptoms were reduced, the difference was only significant in three studies. The most common side-effects experienced were foul breath, an unpleasant taste and gastrointestinal complaints. There were no serious adverse events.[24]

BRIGHT LIGHT THERAPY

Morning bright light therapy has been reported as improving depressive symptoms in pregnant women and can trigger hypomania. Two randomised trials have compared morning bright light with a red placebo dim light. One reported no difference[25] and in the other, bright light produced a significantly greater reduction in depressive symptoms than dim red light.[26]

SLEEP DEPRIVATION

Sleep deprivation may help pregnant and postpartum women who are depressed. One small study exposed nine women with major depressive disorder who were either pregnant or postpartum to late (LSD) and early (ESD) sleep deprivation. More women responded to LSD and more responded after a night of recovery sleep. However, pregnant women responded to ESD and not to LSD.[27] Clearly further research with controlled conditions is needed before this can be recommended.

COMPLEMENTARY THERAPIES (CT)

Pregnant and postpartum women often use herbal medicines and complementary therapies. Deligiannidis *et al.* (2014) carried out a review of CT. In addition to omega-3 FA, bright light therapy and exercise (see above), they reviewed the evidence for folate, S-adenosyl-methionine, St John's Wort, massage and acupuncture. They found no evidence to support the use of folate as a treatment for perinatal depression and only one study of S-adenosyl-methionine reporting it to be superior to placebo in reducing symptoms of anxiety and depression. St John's Wort has not been evaluated for safety and efficacy in a perinatal population but there is some evidence that massage is effective when combined with group psychotherapy. They concluded that 'it is premature to recommend acupuncture as a first line treatment for perinatal major depressive disorder'.[28]

REFERENCES

1. Heh S-S, Fu Y-Y. Effectiveness of informational support in reducing the severity of post-natal depression in Taiwan. *J Adv Nurs*. 2003; **42**: 30–36.
2. Wisner KL, Logsdon CL, Shanahan BR. Web-based education for postpartum depression; conceptual development and impact. *Arch Womens Ment Health*. 2008; **11**: 377–85.
3. Summers AL, Logsdon MC. Web sites for postpartum depression: convenient, frustrating, incomplete, and misleading. *MCN Am J Matern Child Nurs*. 2005; **30**: 88–94.
4. O'Mahen HA, Woodford J, McGinley J, *et al.* Internet-based behavioral activation – treatment for postnatal depression (Netmums): a randomized controlled trial. *J Affect Disord*. 2013; **150**: 814–22.
5. Shaw E, Levitt C, Wong S, *et al.* Systematic review of the literature on postpartum care: effectiveness of postpartum support to improve maternal quality of life, and physical health. *Birth*. 2006; **33**: 210–20.
6. Dennis CL, Kingston D. A systematic review of telephone support for women during pregnancy and the early postpartum period. *J Obst Gynecol Neonatal Nurs*. 2008; **37**: 301–14.
7. Ugarriza DN, Schmidt L. Telecare for women with postpartum depression. *J Psychosoc Nurs Ment Health Serv*. 2006; **44**: 37–45.
8. Dunn C, Hanich E, Roberts R. Mindful pregnancy and childbirth: effects of a mindfulness-based intervention on women's psychological distress and well-being in the perinatal period. *Arch Womens Ment Health*. 2012; **15**: 139–43.
9. Fontein-Kuipers YJ, Nieuwenhuijze MJ, Ausems M, *et al.* Antenatal interventions to reduce maternal distress: a systematic review and meta-analysis of randomised trials. *BJOG*. 2014; **121**: 389–97.
10. Field T, Figueiredo B, Hernandez-Riaf M, *et al.* Massage therapy reduces pain in pregnant women, alleviates prenatal depression in both parents and improves their relationships. *J Bodyw Mov Ther*. 2008; **12**: 146–50.
11. Appleby L, Warner R, Whitton A, *et al.* A controlled study of fluoxetine and cognitive-behavioural counselling in the treatment of postnatal depression. *BMJ*. 1997; **314**: 932–6.
12. Morrell J, Slade P, Warner R, *et al.* Clinical effectiveness of health visitor training in psychologically informed approaches for depression in postnatal women: pragmatic cluster randomised trial in primary care. *BMJ*. 2009; **338**: a3045.
13. Spinelli MG, Endicott J. Controlled clinical trial of interpersonal psychotherapy versus parenting education program for depressed pregnant women. *Am J Psychiatr*. 2003; **160**: 555–62.
14. Sockol LE, Epperson CN, Barber J. A meta-analysis of treatments for perinatal depression. *Clin Psychol Rev*. 2011; **31**: 839–49.
15. Scope A, Leaviss J, Kalthenthaler E, *et al.* Is group cognitive behaviour therapy for postnatal depression evidence-based practice? A systematic review. *BMC Psychiatry*. 2013; **13**: 321.

16. Goodman JH, Santangelo G. Group treatment for postpartum depression: a systematic review. *Arch Womens Ment Health*. 2011; **14**: 277–93.
17. Claridge AM. Efficacy of systemically oriented psychotherapies in the treatment of perinatal depression: a meta-analysis. *Arch Womens Ment Health*. 2014; **17**: 3–15.
18. Milgrom J, Martin PR, Negri LM. *Treating Postnatal Depression: a psychological approach for health care practitioners*. Chichester: Wiley; 1999.
19. Reay RE, Mulcahy R, Wilkinson RB, *et al*. The development and content of an interpersonal psychotherapy group for postnatal depression. *Int J Group Psychother*. 2012; **62**: 221–51.
20. de Crescenzo F, Perelli F, Armando M, *et al*. Selective serotonin reuptake inhibitors (SSRIs) for post-partum depression (PPD): a systematic review of randomized clinical trials. *J Affect Disord*. 2014; **152–4**: 39–44.
21. Marcus SM, Flynn HA Blow F, *et al*. A screening study of antidepressant treatment rates and mood symptoms in pregnancy. *Arch Womens Ment Health*. 2005; **8**: 25–7.
22. Yonkers KA, Gotman, N, Smith MV, *et al*. Does antidepressant use attenuate the risk of a major depressive episode in pregnancy? *Epidemiology*. 2011; **22**: 848–54.
23. Sharma V. A cautionary note on the use of antidepressants in postpartum depression. *Bipolar Disord*. 2006; **8**: 411–14.
24. Borja-Hart D, Marino J. Role of omega-3 fatty acids for prevention or treatment of perinatal depression. *Pharmacotherapy*. 2010; **30**: 210–16.
25. Corral M, Wardrop A, Zhang A, *et al*. Morning light therapy for postpartum depression. *Arch Womens Ment Health*. 2007; **10**: 221–4.
26. Wirz-Justice A, Bader A, Frisch U, *et al*. A randomized, double-blind, placebo-controlled study of light therapy for antepartum depression. *J Clin Psychiatry*. 2011; **72**: 986–93.
27. Parry BL, Curran ML, Stuenkel CA, *et al*. Can critically timed sleep deprivation be useful in pregnancy and postpartum depressions? *J Affect Disord*. 2000; **60**: 201–12.
28. Deligiannidis KM, Freeman MP. Complementary and alternative therapies for perinatal depression. *Best Practice & Research Clinical Obstetrics & Gynaecology*. 2014; **28**: 85–95.

CHAPTER 26

Community support and counselling

Dr Jo Spoors

Mental health difficulties before, during and in the first year after pregnancy are best served by specialist perinatal mental health teams. Ideally such teams would consist of a perinatal community team linked to a local MBU inpatient unit. Mental health professionals with nursing, medical, psychological, social care and childcare expertise would be represented, enabling the community team to respond adequately to the needs of mothers and their families during the perinatal period.

CURRENT PICTURE OF COMMUNITY SERVICES

Sadly the current picture of perinatal mental health does not match the ideal, with little or no services in large areas of the UK. Fewer than half of all mental health trusts in Great Britain provide a specialised perinatal mental health team. There are at least 19 specialised perinatal community mental health teams in England, 11 of which are integrated within a Mother and Baby Unit.[1,2] All have a minimum of a consultant perinatal psychiatrist and community psychiatric nurse. These teams provide a maternity liaison service, manage new onset conditions and high-risk patients in the community, provide pre-conception counselling and will arrange admissions to a MBU when necessary.[1] In some areas a minimal or partial service is available, run by single or small numbers of professionals. Unfortunately they can't provide a comprehensive service, particularly to those with serious mental illness, and often have to refer cases to MBUs at some distance from patients' homes.

The good news is that this shortfall has been acknowledged. Although mental health services are under a great deal of financial pressure, there is a wider recognition of both unmet need and the urgency of commissioning specialised standardised perinatal mental health teams. Guidance written by experts in perinatal mental health is now available for commissioning good quality perinatal community teams.[3]

WHY DO WE NEED COMMUNITY PERINATAL MENTAL HEALTH TEAMS?

Perinatal mental health problems are those which complicate pregnancy and the year following childbirth. Although a time of expectant happiness, women are more vulnerable to mental health problems at this time.[4,5,6,7] Perinatal mental health problems can present as emergencies and can deteriorate rapidly. The diagnosis and management of such conditions is key therefore to the successful outcome for the mother and child; this is best met by a perinatal mental health professional working within the community. Serious perinatal psychiatric illness may require admission to an MBU. Women who do not require admission to hospital or are ready to be discharged from an inpatient stay continue to require specialist knowledge and skills from a community team. Poorly managed perinatal mental health problems may have devastating consequences not only for the mother and child, but for the entire family unit.

Perinatal mental healthcare should start as early as possible and preconception counselling should be provided by a specialist with up-to-date expertise in perinatal mental health, be it regarding previous illness or medication concerns. During pregnancy and breastfeeding, mental health should be optimised, with the risks and benefits of any medication and the risks of perinatal mental illness fully understood by pregnant women so they can make an informed choice about their treatment. Psychological treatment, regular nursing support, childcare and social care expertise should be available within the timeframes of pregnancy and the postpartum year. Professionals also need an understanding of the emotional and physical changes associated with pregnancy, childbirth and breastfeeding and the different organisation of maternity services.[3] Any concerns regarding the mother and baby relationship should be raised as early as possible and interventions to optimise attachment and bonding should start during pregnancy if possible. This cannot be provided adequately by overstretched general adult psychiatric services.

WHAT A PERINATAL MENTAL HEALTH TEAM SHOULD LOOK LIKE

The Joint Commissioning Panel for Mental Health asked several perinatal mental health experts to provide guidance to commissioners of good quality perinatal mental health services. This may be used in the provision of a new service or the continued improvement of an existing service.

A perinatal community team will assess and manage women with serious mental illness or complex disorders in the community who cannot be appropriately managed by primary care.[1] It should have close working links with a designated MBU and be able to serve the needs of the population covered by the local mental health trust. The community team should be able to arrange admission to an MBU if necessary and be able to facilitate the discharge process and continued management in the community.

The community team should provide care from pre-conception counselling up to a year following childbirth and ideally represent a variety of healthcare professionals in order to provide effective prevention, detection and management of perinatal mental health problems.

A community team should be able to respond in a timely manner taking into account the timeframes of pregnancy and the potential for rapid deterioration of mental health (particularly in the period immediately following childbirth). It should have the capacity to assess women and their families in a variety of settings, including their homes, maternity wards or hospitals and outpatient clinics. Communication between services is vitally important to optimise outcomes and there should be effective sharing of information between maternity services, primary care, adult mental health services, perinatal services and the woman herself. This is of particular importance if the woman has long-standing serious mental health problems or a history of such. Perinatal community services can take responsibility for co-ordinating an integrated care plan. This must ensure that all professionals are aware of their responsibilities and the plan must be effectively communicated with all parties, including the woman and her family if appropriate.[5]

The National Institute for Health and Care Excellence (NICE) guidelines recommend that clinical networks should be established for perinatal mental health services, managed by a co-ordinating board of healthcare professionals, commissioners, managers, and service users and carers.[8] Therefore a good specialised community perinatal mental health team will be a member of the Royal College of Psychiatrists quality network. This ensures the continued practice of high-quality standardised care.

COUNSELLING

Talking therapies and counselling form an integral part of perinatal mental healthcare. Mental health professionals should recognise that women may be reluctant to share information due to fear of stigma, negative perceptions of them as a mother, or fear their baby might be taken into care.[5] It is important therefore to provide a safe environment and a consistent relationship in which women feel able to engage with services.

Pre-conception counselling (as discussed in Chapter 10) should be delivered by a professional with up-to-date expertise in perinatal mental health.

Mental health diagnoses should be considered separately, as should medication (rather than discussing classes or types of medication). The influence on each trimester of the pregnancy and the period following childbirth including breastfeeding should be considered and any figures should be given in a standardised format (i.e. risk of illness occurring as a number out of 100 or 1000). The mother and baby relationship should be considered at this early stage, expectations and concerns may be discussed and taken forward for future engagement.

Mild to moderate perinatal mental health problems may be treated via Improved Access to Psychological Therapy teams (IAPT). IAPT is an NHS programme operating across England offering interventions approved by NICE for treating people with depression and anxiety disorders.[9] Patients can self-refer or be referred by their general practitioner or health professional. IAPT offers a stepped care model ranging from facilitated self-help to cognitive behavioural therapy (CBT) delivered by specialist practitioners. The current system does not consider the complexities of pregnancy, childbirth and the postpartum year when treating these conditions. In order to meet the needs of a perinatal population using IAPT, the joint commissioning guidance has made several proposals; routinely collecting data on whether referrals are pregnant or in the postpartum year, that IAPT practitioners should receive additional training in perinatal mental health and that pregnant and postpartum women should be assessed and treated within three months.[3,10]

NICE recommends that psychological interventions should be provided within one month of the initial assessment (if deemed an appropriate treatment).[8] This would include the IAPT model as above but would also include high-intensity psychological treatment such as CBT and interpersonal therapy (IPT) delivered by a psychologist or health professional receiving regular supervision to deliver such therapy. Other therapeutic interventions can also be used: behavioural couples therapy (particularly for those with bipolar illness), family therapy and trauma-focused work. Trauma-focused work may be considered in light of a particularly traumatic birth, a stillbirth or miscarriage or neonatal death and should be offered in accordance with NICE guidelines.[8]

A CASE VIGNETTE

The following case example from the Southern Health Mother and Baby Community Team illustrates the importance of a specialised community service and the positive experience it can offer women.

Sarah suffered with postnatal depression following the birth of her first child. She approached her GP and was referred and treated by general adult psychiatric services as no specialised service existed in her area. She waited for many weeks for her assessment and recalls this time as particularly harrowing.

She is certain that without the tireless support of friends and family she would have been admitted to hospital.

Sarah's second pregnancy was unplanned; she found out she was pregnant shortly after recovering from her depressive illness. Due to her partner's job, the family moved to a different area of the country. Sarah stopped taking her antidepressant medication as soon as she discovered she was pregnant and did not inform her new GP that she had done so. She was worried about what they would think and didn't believe her first experience with mental health services was particularly helpful. Sarah's depression returned towards the end of her pregnancy and continued into the first few weeks following a somewhat traumatic childbirth experience. The midwife alerted the crisis team when Sarah stopped eating, refused to leave the house and became fixated on the idea that the children would be better off without her. The crisis team then referred Sarah to the Southern Health Mother and Baby Community Team.

Sarah was assessed by the team as an urgent referral and following discussion she decided to restart her antidepressant medication. A perinatal community psychiatric nurse (CPN) was assigned Sarah's case and initially saw her twice a week, then weekly. Without the support of her family and friends Sarah was exhausted and felt isolated in her new surroundings with two young children to look after. The perinatal CPN was able to do some focused therapeutic work with Sarah to reduce her anxiety about leaving the house and exploring the local area. The perinatal nursery nurse introduced her to some local mother and baby groups, playgroups and a group for mothers who suffered with postnatal depression. She also focused on rebuilding Sarah's confidence in her childcare abilities and was able to advise on issues such as sibling rivalry. Sarah made great progress under the care of the perinatal team and reflects that her only regret is that her experience following her first baby shaped her expectations following her second. Sarah and her partner are now looking forward to their third pregnancy.

IN SUMMARY

1. The current picture of perinatal mental health services is patchy and inequitable.[11]
2. Pregnancy and the postpartum year are particularly vulnerable times for mental health problems impacting maternal and infant mental and physical wellbeing.
3. Specialised perinatal mental health teams are best placed to prevent, detect and manage perinatal mental health difficulties.
4. The Joint Commissioning Panel for Mental Health published guidance to health commissioners in order to commission good quality perinatal mental health services.

REFERENCES

1. NHS Commissioning Board. *Specialised Commissioning Specifications: perinatal mental health services.* London: NHS Commissioning Board; 2012. Available at: www.england. nhs.uk/wp-content/uploads/2013/06/c06-spec-peri-mh.pdf
2. Royal College of Psychiatrists. *Quality Network for Perinatal Mental Health Services.* London: Royal College of Psychiatrists; 2012. Available at: www.rcpsych.ac.uk/workin psychiatry/qualityimprovement/qualityandaccreditation/perinatal/perinatalquality network.aspx
3. Joint Commissioning Panel for Mental Health. *Guidance for Commissioners of Perinatal Mental Health Services. Vol. 2: Practical Mental Health Commissioning.* London: Joint Commissioning Panel for Mental Health; 2012.
4. Kendel RE, Chalmers KC, Platz C. Epidemiology of puerperal psychoses. *Br J Psychiatry.* 1987; **150**: 662–73.
5. Cox J, Murray D, Chapman G. A controlled study of the onset, prevalence and duration of postnatal depression. *Br J Psychiatry.* 1993; **163**: 27–41.
6. Jones I, Craddock N. Bipolar disorder and childbirth – the importance of recognising risk. *Br J Psychiatry.* 2005; **186**: 453–4.
7. Davies A, McIvor RI, Kumar R. Impact of childbirth on schizophrenic mothers. *Schizophrenic Res.* 1995; **16**: 25–31.
8. NICE. *Antenatal and Postnatal Mental Health: clinical management and service guidance.* London: DoH; 2014.
9. Improving Access to Psychological Therapies (IAPT). Available at: www.iapt.nhs.uk
10. Improving Access to Psychological Therapies (IAPT). *Perinatal Positive Practice Guide.* London: DoH; 2014. Available at: www.iapt.nhs.uk/silo/files/perinatal-positive-practice-guide.pdf
11. Elkin A, Gilburt H, Slade M, et al. A national survey of psychiatric Mother and Baby Units in England. *Psychiatr Serv.* 2009; **60**(5): 629–33.

CHAPTER 27

Inpatient treatment on Mother and Baby Units

Dr Angelika Wieck

(Note from Elaine Hanzak – I am an advocate of MBUs as I was hospitalised without my baby son and consequently forced to stop breastfeeding instantly. I still feel this loss 19 years later and now realise that it could have made my illness much worse. At that time as a family, we did not know such a facility existed. I have become increasingly aware that many healthcare professionals are also unaware of them. Hence I felt that I wanted to include MBUs in this book as they could be very useful for parents contemplating another pregnancy if they have suffered a previous mental illness associated with pregnancy.)

THE ORIGINS OF MOTHER AND BABY UNITS

Childbirth is a potent trigger for severe mental illness and it has been estimated that in the first few postnatal months up to six women per 1000 require an admission to hospital for psychiatric treatment. The practice of admitting mothers jointly with their babies to a psychiatric ward has a relatively recent history, with the first case recorded in 1948.[1] This was at a time of growing awareness of the importance of the mother–child relationship.[2] Observations of children who were separated from their mothers through placements in institutions, prolonged hospital admissions, or evacuations during the Second World War had shown that they were profoundly affected in their behaviour and emotional development. It was also realised that mothers who were separated from their young children became less competent and confident as caregivers, developed intense feelings of guilt and suffered anxieties whether they would be able to mother their children again when reunited with them. Because of this, paediatric services had for some time encouraged mothers of young children requiring treatment in hospital to visit frequently or even stay with them overnight. When a woman requested to be admitted to the psychiatric Cassel Hospital with her toddler son, who had no one else to care for him in the community, Main agreed.[1] The experience of this and subsequent cases was so positive that it became a condition of admission at this hospital that mothers should bring their babies and young children with them. They were accommodated with other patients in the general psychiatry ward. All mothers had non-psychotic disorders and treatment mainly consisted of group therapy or psychotherapy informed by psychoanalysis. The average duration of admissions was as long as 6 months.

Another pioneering psychiatric service at Shenley Hospital, England, allowed joint admissions from 1956.[3] Since they observed that the quality of the parenting did not seem to depend on the mothers' psychiatric diagnosis they did not exclude any diagnoses. The philosophy of the ward was to let women have as much responsibility as possible for the care of their child, whilst being supported by staff, and to encourage them to contribute to the cleaning and cooking on the ward. Apart from a busy daily routine and somatic treatments, mothers were offered group and individual psychotherapy.

The first unit dedicated to only mother and baby admissions was set up in Banstead, England, in 1959.[4] It provided accommodation for eight women and their babies less than 12 months old and was staffed by psychiatric nurses and nursery nurses. When the outcomes for a small group of women with psychosis and their babies admitted to this new unit were compared with those for women who had been previously admitted without their babies to a general psychiatric ward but under the same consultant psychiatrist, the former appeared to do much better on discharge.[4] They had a shorter length of stay in hospital and were all able to take full care of their child on return home whereas only a proportion of women admitted to a general ward were able to do so. However, the study sample was small, with only 20 mothers and babies in each group, so that no definite conclusions could be drawn.

Several other dedicated units have since then been established in England, Wales and Scotland, but progress has been overall slow over the last six decades. The development has largely depended on local enthusiastic and dedicated champions, which were usually psychiatrists.[5] Some of these units were closed again when local support ceased. In France, the first MBU did not open until 1989, but within a few years 17 more units were set up.[6] There have also been local initiatives in several other countries, including the Netherlands, Belgium, Germany, Hungary, Sri Lanka, India and the United States.

RECENT DEVELOPMENTS IN MOTHER AND BABY INPATIENT SERVICES IN GREAT BRITAIN

In Great Britain, the perinatal psychiatrist Margaret Oates pioneered a model of an integrated perinatal mental health service delivered by a specialist team in Nottingham.[7] This led to the first recommendations by the Royal College of Psychiatrists on perinatal mental health services.[8] It recommended that all women requiring secondary psychiatric services following childbirth should be treated by a consultant psychiatrist with a special interest in their condition, supported by a multidisciplinary team. This treatment should take place wherever possible in the women's own locality. In the event of them requiring inpatient care, they should be admitted, together with their infant wherever possible, to a specialist facility.

In the last 15 years there have been major developments driven by national policy that was to a great extent influenced by the Royal College of Psychiatrists. In 2000 the Department of Health for England issued guidance how to ensure that all patients were protected from physical, psychological or sexual harm whilst being treated in mental health services.[9] A specific reference was made to MBUs: 'Mother and baby units should be self-contained and separate from the general psychiatric ward. Health visiting staff or, where appropriate, midwifery staff attend the mother and baby in hospital.' In some hospitals in England, facilities were available for occasional joint admissions onto general adult wards or a 1–2 bedded annexe. This practice poses a number of problems, including concerns over the safety and security of the child and the level of specialist skills of staff. The Department of Health was also concerned about women's dignity and privacy on general adult psychiatric wards and stated that mothers should not be 'routinely cared for in general acute inpatient wards with their babies; in the absence of a local mother and baby unit, PCTs [primary care trusts] act collaboratively to ensure that mothers within their locality have access to a high-quality mother and baby unit within reasonable travelling distance'.[10] The Scottish Government went further and enshrined in the Mental Health Act (2003) that Health Boards have 'to ensure the provision of mother and baby units to allow a mother being admitted to hospital for the treatment of post-natal depression (*meaning probably any postnatal mental illness severe enough to require inpatient treatment*) to care for her child in hospital.[11]

The second report of the Royal College of Psychiatrists[12] aimed to support regional health authorities and local clinicians to plan and develop perinatal mental health services in their area. The document set core standards and provided formulae for estimating resources needed derived from the epidemiology of perinatal psychiatric conditions. Another milestone in the recent history of perinatal mental health service development has been the endorsement of specialist services by the first Clinical Guideline on antenatal and postnatal mental health by the National Institute of Health and Care

Excellence:[13] 'Women who need inpatient care for a mental disorder within 12 months of childbirth should be admitted to a specialist mother and baby unit unless there are specific reasons for not doing so' and that these units should 'be closely integrated with community-based mental health services to ensure continuity of care and minimum length of stay'. These recommendations have not been altered in the recent guideline review.[14]

These national guidance and recommendations have been helpful to support the survival of existing MBUs, but an equal access for women to joint inpatient admission with their baby has not yet been achieved in Great Britain. The recent survey of service provision by the Maternal Mental Health Alliance[15] has identified 17 dedicated mother and baby units with four or more beds and cots which are centred in some areas of the country but leaving others uncovered.

It is estimated that 0.25 inpatient mother and baby beds per 1000 live births are required if Specialised Perinatal Community Psychiatric Teams are available or 0.5 per 1000 if no specialised teams are provided.[16] The current bed provision in England needs to increase by up to 50% to meet the overall national need.[14,16]

THE QUALITY NETWORK FOR PERINATAL MENTAL HEALTH SERVICES AND SERVICE STANDARDS

The College Centre for Quality Improvement of the Royal College of Psychiatrists has in recent years established several professional networks to improve the quality of mental health services. The aims are that participating clinical teams support and learn from each other but also that patient and carers as well as commissioners and regulatory authorities have the confidence that teams are providing a high-quality service.[17] Each quality network develops its own specific service standards. For inpatient MBUs these were developed through literature review, a workshop with a wide range of disciplines from MBUs and service users, and consultation with all other MBUs in England, Wales and Scotland.[18] The over 400 standards cover in detail access and admission to MBUs, environment and facilities, staffing, care and treatment, psychiatric care, care of infant, information and confidentiality, rights and consent, audit and policy, and discharge. Each participating unit is visited annually by a multidisciplinary peer review team which examines whether the facility is concordant with the standards by review of evidence, questionnaires and meetings with staff, patients and carers. When all of the essential and legally required standards and the majority of the desirable standards are fulfilled a unit receives accreditation status. MBUs have experienced receiving feedback from peers as very helpful in improving their service. It has also supported them locally in obtaining the necessary resources, where needed. Most MBUs in England have now been accredited.

There is also a health regulatory system that is aimed at improving quality. Health service commissioners can reward service providers financially for achieving set quality standards, the so-called CQUIN targets (CQUIN stands for Commissioning for Quality and Innovation). There is some overlap between the two systems and experts in perinatal mental health have contributed to the formulation of CQUIN targets for perinatal mental health.

FUNCTION AND FACILITIES OF CURRENT MOTHER AND BABY UNITS IN THE UK

NHS England has defined the main functions of MBUs as being to:

> provide appropriate facilities, treatments and interventions to meet the special needs of mothers and their infants including both physical and psychological care. They provide support, assistance and supervision to the mother so that the physical and emotional needs of the infant are met and promote the developing mother–infant relationship.[16]

MBUs are separate from other psychiatric wards, should not share facilities with them and have their own entrance. Each MBU has access to an outdoor area so that patients have the option to take their babies or visitors outside without having to leave the unit. There is a range of communal and play areas on the unit as well as laundry facilities, a milk kitchen area and private meeting space. In addition to equipment for physical care that is standard in other acute admission wards there should be equipment to monitor the infants' development and physical health as well as provide emergency resuscitation for infants. As elsewhere in mental health services, the patients' rights and need for respect and dignity are important and the premises on MBUs are laid out to reflect the special needs of pregnant or postnatal mothers for privacy, including single accommodation for every mother and child pair.

ADMISSIONS TO MOTHER AND BABY UNITS

Three groups of women may require admissions to MBUs. The first are mothers who develop an episode of psychosis or severe depression after childbirth and may have never been ill before or have made a complete recovery after a previous episode. These illnesses often present abruptly, escalate rapidly, fluctuate dramatically and represent high risks for the mother and her baby. They need to be considered as psychiatric emergencies. If a specialised perinatal community mental health team is available, home treatment may be appropriate from some of these women. Experience with the outcome of home treatment by generic community mental health teams is limited and has not been summarised to date. Because the incidence of new postnatal psychosis in any given catchment area is low, general community mental health staff are likely to be inexperienced with the course of illness and may not recognise the specific risks.

Once the need for a placement on an MBU is identified, this should be arranged as soon as possible. MBUs operate 7 days a week, 24 hours a day, so that there should be no unacceptable delay of admissions. In fact, units are expected to conduct regular audits of the time it takes from an initial referral to admission and of inappropriate stays on general adult wards. MBUs have the capacity to manage patients detained under the Mental Health Act as any other acute admission ward.

Women who have a pre-existing serious mental illness have quite different needs. They should have been identified in pregnancy and referred to a perinatal psychiatrist and perinatal mental health community team in the first or early second trimester. They require a comprehensive assessment and a care plan that is agreed with the patient and her family and tailored to their specific needs. Part of the plan should also be how a possible deterioration in mental state after the child is born is managed and an admission to an MBU may be considered. MBUs should be aware of the potential need for a bed in advance of the delivery and be familiar with the woman's specific circumstances. Admissions in these cases are likely to happen in a more planned fashion.

In pregnancy, new onsets of severe mental illness appear to be less common but can occur. Recurrences of pre-existing severe illnesses are probably at least as common as in non-pregnant women, especially since psychotropic medication is often discontinued when the woman or her prescriber learn of the pregnancy. Because of their specific vulnerability and need for specialised care pregnant women should also be offered treatment on an MBU. Some facilities will admit these women in the second and others only in the third trimester of pregnancy.

The service specifications set by NHS England[16] also stipulate certain exclusions from admission to MBUs. This concerns women who have severe personality disorder, learning disability or substance misuse unless they are also suffering from, or are suspected to suffer from, another serious mental illness, or there is a suspected/potential, serious or complex mental illness. Secondly, mothers should not be admitted for the sole purpose of parenting assessments unless they also are suffering from, or there is suspected, serious mental illness.

A national audit of 11 MBUs in the UK summarised features of 1217 admissions and found that the most common diagnosis was depression (43%), followed by schizophrenia (21%) and bipolar disorder (14%).[19]

STAFF ON MOTHER AND BABY UNITS

Pregnant women and recently delivered mothers with mental health problems have specific and complex needs. Management during this time requires mental health practitioners to be knowledgeable and experienced with the specific nature and course of perinatal mental illnesses. They also need to be able to recognise and make a balanced assessment of the specific risks to mother and child. They should have a working knowledge of normal and abnormal physical and emotional changes during pregnancy, delivery and the postnatal period. Prescribers should have up-to-date knowledge of and be able to evaluate the current evidence on the safety of medicine use in pregnancy and breastfeeding and how dose requirements and side-effects may change during this time. They need to have experience in how to communicate and discuss the risks and benefits of taking or discontinuing medication in a way that is helpful to patients and their carers. Practitioners should also have a working knowledge of the normal and abnormal development of children in the first year of life and have the skills to support women to meet the emotional, developmental and physical needs of their infants. Gaining this expertise requires working regularly with pregnant or postnatal mothers and can only be acquired on MBUs or perinatal community mental health teams. These are the reasons why consultants appointed to posts in perinatal mental health services usually have had at least one year of training in perinatal mental health. Ward staff also receive regular formal training in areas of perinatal practice that are defined by the national standards.

The multidisciplinary teams of MBUs consist of consultants specialised in perinatal psychiatry who are supported by ward-based doctors, registered mental health nurses and healthcare assistants. Other members of the team include nursery nurses, a clinical psychologist, an occupational therapist, and a ward clerk. Units should have access to health visitors, midwives and obstetricians. There are usually links with GPs for routine basic medical care of the children and arrangements with the local hospital for any required paediatric care.

ASSESSMENTS, THE PLANNING OF CARE AND REVIEWS

The quality perinatal mental health network[20] have set clear standards for the timescales, frequency and comprehensiveness of the initial and subsequent assessments of mother and baby by the multidisciplinary team. Some of these standards are more stringent than one would expect for general adult wards, mainly because of the higher risks of physical illness in women shortly after childbirth and the often greater acuity of psychotic states in postnatal mothers. Apart from the physical examination, the psychiatrists will take a history of the mental illness, enquire about the woman's background, examine her current mental state and make a psychiatric diagnosis. They will make an initial assessment of whether there are any other causes than childbirth that could have contributed to the illness and which may need to be addressed in order to achieve and maintain recovery. They will also determine what further investigations are necessary to understand the woman's background, social situation and presentation better. The multidisciplinary team will assess whether the woman is at risk of self-harm or suicide, sexual exploitation or domestic violence. Potential risks to her own baby or to other mothers and babies are also being assessed and whether the baby needs to sleep in the ward nursery until the mother is less disturbed. The team should also enquire about the woman's other children and their wellbeing.

The multidisciplinary team formulates care plans reflecting each woman's current and individual needs and those of the baby. The mother's and baby's care plans should be developed as much as possible in consultation with the patient and her partner or carer. If there are concerns about the woman's parenting ability in the long term, the unit will make a referral to children and families social services who will determine whether further assessment and action is necessary.

Assessments are updated continually and the multidisciplinary care plans are reviewed at least once a week by the team and the patient in a ward round. Partners or carers and professionals involved with the woman's or baby's care should be invited to attend as appropriate. Patients should also have help to ask to meet professionals outside the ward rounds and discuss any questions or concerns. If a child social worker is involved with the family, they will usually request ward staff are to comment on the mother's parenting ability whilst she is on the ward as well as medical opinions on the diagnosis of the mental illness and prognosis.

TREATMENTS ON MOTHER AND BABY UNITS

In some women with severe psychosis or depression, the most important initial concern may be to ensure the safety of the mother and baby and others on the ward. This may require close or 1:1 observations by ward staff of the mother on her own or when she is caring for her baby. Observations are regularly reviewed and reduced when the mother improves and the risk lessens.

Many women with severe mental illnesses during pregnancy and after childbirth require psychiatric medications to get better. Because of the strong evidence of beneficial effects for children, women are now encouraged to exclusively breastfeed for the first 4–6 months if they can.[21] Medication with most drugs used for the treatment of mental illnesses is compatible with breastfeeding because only very small amounts are transferred to the child. There are exceptions, however, and the reader is referred to Chapter 25, by Carol Henshaw. In pregnancy the exposure of children to medication is greater but there is some evidence that untreated mental illness may also affect the intrauterine development of the child (*see* Chapter 25).

MBUs also offer treatments by a clinical psychologist, which may take the form of cognitive behavioural therapy, mindfulness or other therapies. Some units also offer other types of psychotherapy such as art therapy (for further details *see* Chapter 25). Until recently some MBUs could not offer occupational therapy, which was the most common area of dissatisfaction in a survey of patients.[22] Now units usually offer access to a range of activities on the ward or the local community.

Whilst in hospital pregnant women should have the same access to midwifery and obstetric care as they would have in the community. Experience shows that the collaboration between MBUs and maternity services is usually very good.

During the mother's stay on the MBU it is essential that the fathers of the babies continue their relationship with the child. MBUs usually allow partners, but also other family members or close friends, to visit freely during the day unless this is detrimental to the woman's current mental health.

THE MOTHER–BABY RELATIONSHIP

The philosophy of MBUs is to encourage the woman to carry out as much of the care of the baby as she can herself. Initially the mother may be too unwell to engage with this and nursing staff may meet most of the infant's needs. The level of nursing involvement will be gradually reduced as the mother is improving. Women may also require advice from ward staff on the physical care of the baby and how to stimulate its development. Some women have lost their confidence as mothers when recovering from a severe illness and require encouragement and emotional support to resume childcare fully. Ongoing symptoms of the mental illness can affect the quality of parenting in some mothers. This has been particularly well researched for maternal depression where a mother's sensitivity to her infant's needs, her interactions with the baby, her safety practices and her overall quality of parenting have been found to be impaired.[23] These early problems can negatively affect the behavioural, emotional and physical development of the child and its relationship with others in the longer term. Women with schizophrenia are at an increased risk of losing custody of their children because of parenting difficulties. It is therefore very important that women with severe mental illness receive early and focused help to minimise these difficulties.

One way of working on the mother–infant relationship is by taking a short video clip of the mother playing with her baby. When the video is played back to the mother the therapist can give feedback and work with her on interpreting the baby's cues, responding sensitively to them and enhancing turn-taking behaviour. This method was originally developed for women with postnatal depression in the community but has also recently been evaluated in an MBU setting. In the study by Kenny *et al.*, mothers and babies who had this intervention on a MBU improved significantly.[24] On discharge their interaction was rated as no different from a group of healthy women and their babies in the community but better than in a group of mothers who were ill but had not been admitted. Video-feedback interaction guidance is offered on several MBUs in the UK. A number of other parenting interventions are being used in community settings but have not yet been tested on psychiatric MBUs. One promising approach is the positive parenting programme, for which a baby version has recently been developed (Baby Triple P). It is based on social learning, cognitive behavioural and developmental theory. In a recent pilot study on an MBU, feedback from patients and staff was positive and they felt that the method was suitable and beneficial.[25]

PREPARING FOR DISCHARGE

When a mother begins to improve it is important that she gradually resumes her normal activities and responsibilities. Initially she may leave the unit with her baby accompanied by her partner, family or nursing staff until she is able to comfortably and safely do this on her own. Ward staff will support and advise the woman and her partner if she experiences any difficulties or setbacks on leaves. A flat with independent kitchen facilities and a separate entrance are available on some MBUs so that she can test being more independent whilst support is available from the ward if needed. There is a possibility for the partner to spend time with the mother and child in the flat.

The MBU team should also discuss the mental illness with the mother, how likely it is to return if she has another child, what she can do to remain well, the safety of her medication in a future pregnancy and family planning.

The MBU works closely with community mental health professionals, who should attend any pre-discharge meetings. The aims are to get to know the woman and her family, and to facilitate smooth transition of care. It is also helpful for other professionals involved in the mother's and child's care after discharge, including the health visitor and child social worker, to attend these meetings.

OUTCOME OF ADMISSIONS TO MOTHER AND BABY UNITS

In two surveys of discharges from MBUs, mothers were very satisfied with their stay on the ward and the great majority of aspects of their care.[22,26] All women preferred to stay on the MBU than on a general adult psychiatry ward.[22] In-depth interviews with mothers[27] revealed that they valued the expertise, empathetic approach and advice on parenting that scheduled time with staff on the MBU provided them. The MBU was felt to be a safe and appropriate setting in which to bond with one's child. More relaxing and skill-enhancing structured activity and peer support were identified as areas for improvement.

In the large national audit of UK MBU discharges, senior clinicians rated the majority of women (78% of 1081 patients) as having good outcomes of their mental health, with 43% being symptom-free and 35% having considerably improved.[28] With regard to parenting problems, 80% or more were not judged to have significant problems in practical baby care, emotional responsiveness or being a risk to the baby. When there were problems with parenting, these were mostly identified in the group of women with schizophrenia. Nevertheless, in a more detailed analysis of statutory parenting outcome, 50% of women with schizophrenia were discharged home with their babies without any social services supervision.[29]

Although these results are encouraging and women treated on MBUs are clearly very positive about their experience, it is not known whether objective outcomes are better than they would have been if the mothers had been treated elsewhere. This is an important question since joint admissions to MBUs are costly and access to these facilities is not available to all women. At present a prospective study is being conducted in England which compares maternal, parenting and infant outcomes in postnatal women admitted to MBUs, and those treated in general adult psychiatry wards or by home treatment teams. It is hoped that this will shed light on this important question.

REFERENCES

1. Main TF. Mothers with children in a psychiatric hospital. *Lancet*. 1958; **2**(7051): 845–7.
2. Margison F, Brockington IF. Psychiatric mother and baby units. In: Brockington IF, Kumar R, editors. *Motherhood and Mental Illness*. London: Academic Press; 1988. pp. 223–8.
3. Glaser YIM. A unit for mothers and babies in a psychiatric hospital. *J Child Psychol Psychiat*. 1962; **3**(1): 53–60.
4. Baker AA, Morison M, Game JA, *et al*. Admitting schizophrenic mothers with their babies. *Lancet*. 1961; **2**(7196): 237–9.
5. Robertson KE. The diffusion of joint mother and baby psychiatric hospital admissions in the UK: an historical analysis [PHD thesis]. Stirling: The University of Stirling; 2012. Available at: http://hdl.handle.net/1893/11295
6. Cazas O, Glangeaud-Freudenthal NM. The history of Mother-Baby Units (MBUs) in France and Belgium and of the French version of the Marcé checklist. *Arch Womens Ment Health*. 2004; **7**(1): 53–8.
7. Oates M. The development of an integrated community-orientated service for severe postnatal mental illness. In: Brockington IF, Kumar R, editors. *Motherhood and Mental Illness*. London: Academic Press; 1988. pp. 133–58.
8. Royal College of Psychiatrists. *Working Party Report on Postnatal Mental Illness. Council Report CR28*. London: Royal College of Psychiatrists; 1992.

9. NHS Executive. *Safety, Privacy and Dignity in Mental Health Units*. London: NHS Executive; 2000. Available at: http://webarchive.nationalarchives.gov.uk/+/www.dh.gov.uk/assetRoot/04/01/46/53/04014653.pdf

10. Department of Health. *Mainstreaming Gender and Women's Mental Health*. London: DoH; 2003. Available at: http://webarchive.nationalarchives.gov.uk/20130107105354/www.dh.gov.uk/prod_consum_dh/groups/dh_digitalassets/@dh/@en/documents/digital asset/dh_4072069.pdf

11. Scottish Executive. *The New Mental Health Act. What's it all about? A short introduction*. Edinburgh: Scottish Executive; 2004. Available at: www.mwcscot.org.uk/media/71869/a_short_intro_to_the_mental_health_act.pdf

12. Oates, M. *(2001). Perinatal Maternal Mental Health Services: recommendations for provision of services for childbearing women*. London: Royal College of Psychiatrists; 2001. Available at: www.rcpsych.ac.uk/usefulresources/publications/collegereports/cr/cr88.aspx

13. NICE. *Antenatal and Postnatal Mental Health: clinical management and service guidance. Clinical guideline 045, guidance*. London: DoH; 2007. Available at: www.nice.org.uk/cg045

14. NICE. *Antenatal and Postnatal Mental Health: clinical management and service guidance: Full guideline. NICE clinical guideline 192*. London: DoI I; 2014. Available at: www.nice.org.uk/cg192

15. Maternal Mental Health Alliance. *Accredited Mother and Baby Units*. London: Maternal Mental Health Alliance; 2014. Available at: http://everyonesbusiness.org.uk/wp-content/uploads/2014/07/FINAL-Maps.pdf

16. NHS England. *NHS Standard Contract for Specialised Perinatal Mental Health Services*. London: NHS England; 2013.

17. Royal College of Psychiatrists. *College Centre for Quality Improvement*. London: Royal College of Psychiatrists; 2015. Available at: www.rcpsych.ac.uk/workinpsychiatry/quality improvement/abouttheccqi.aspx

18. Royal College of Psychiatrists. *Centre for Quality Improvement. Quality Network for Perinatal Mental Health Services. Standards for Mother and Baby Inpatient Units*. London: Royal College of Psychiatrists; 2008. Available at: www.rcpsych.ac.uk/perinatal-network

19. Salmon MP, Abel K, Webb R, *et al*. A national audit of joint mother and baby admissions to UK psychiatric hospitals: an overview of findings. *Arch Womens Ment Health*. 2004; **7**: 65–70.

20. Royal College of Psychiatrists. *Centre for Quality Improvement. Perinatal Quality Network for Perinatal Mental Health Services. Standards for Mother and Baby Inpatient Units*. 4th ed. London: Royal College of Psychiatrists; 2014. Available at: www.rcpsych.ac.uk/perinatal-network

21. World Health Organization. *Global Strategy for Infant and Young Child Feeding*. Geneva: World Health Organization; 2003. Available at: www.who.int/nutrition/publications/infantfeeding/9241562218/en/

22. Neil S, Sanderson H, Wieck A. A satisfaction survey of women admitted to a Psychiatric Mother and Baby Unit in the northwest of England. *Arch Womens Ment Health*. 2006; **9**: 109–12.

23. Field T. Postpartum depression effects on early interactions, parenting, and safety practices: a review. *Infant Behav Dev*. 2010; **33**: 1–6.

24. Kenny M, Conroy S, Pariante CM, *et al*. Mother-infant interaction in mother and baby unit patients: before and after treatment. *J Psychiatr Res*. 2013; **47**: 1192–8.

25. Butler H, Hare D, Walker S, *et al*. The acceptability and feasibility of the Baby Triple P Positive Parenting Programme on a mother and baby unit: Q-methodology with mothers with severe mental illness. *Arch Womens Ment Health*. 2014; **17**: 455–63.

26. Antonysamy A, Wieck A, Wittkowski A. Service satisfaction on discharge from a psychiatric mother and baby unit: a representative patient survey. *Arch Womens Ment Health*. 2009; **12**: 359–62.

27. Sapre B, Wieck A, Chew-Graham C. *Women's Perceptions and Experiences of Staying on a Mother and Baby Unit and Working with Children and Families Social Services* [poster abstract]. Annual Scientific Conference of the Perinatal Section of the Royal College of Psychiatrists, London, 25 November 2011.

28. Salmon M, Abel K, Cordingley L, *et al*. Clinical and parenting skills outcomes following joint mother-baby psychiatric admission. *Aust NZ J Psychiatry*. 2003; **37**: 556–62.

29. Abel KM, Webb RT, Salmon MP, *et al*. Prevalence and predictors of parenting outcomes in a cohort of mothers with schizophrenia admitted for joint mother and baby psychiatric care in England. *J Clin Psychiatry*. 2005; **66**: 781–9.

CHAPTER 28

Black and minority ethnic (BME) women and postpartum depression

Dr Dawn Edge and Dr Fatimah Jackson-Best

Like postnatal mental illness itself, contemplating another pregnancy following mental illness in the postnatal period is an issue that affects women from all ethnic backgrounds. In this chapter, using examples from the United Kingdom (UK) and the Caribbean in particular, we argue that socio-cultural factors impose additional levels of complexity and challenge into this decision-making process for women from Black and minority ethnic (BME) communities. To support this assertion, we focus on postnatal depression (also known as 'postpartum depression'), one of three main psychological conditions that affect women following childbirth. It is beyond the scope of this chapter to examine the factors that might influence decision making for all ethnic groups. Accordingly, to illustrate our argument, we explore these issues in relation to women of South Asian and Caribbean origin in the UK and their countries of origin. We adopt this approach as the available evidence suggests that global figures mask significant inter-ethnic and trans-cultural differences in prevalence, presentation and outcome of postnatal mental illness. This is significant as, due to globalisation, Western societies such as those in Europe and North America are increasingly multi-racial/multi-ethnic. Understanding the health needs of all citizens is a fundamental aspect of developing appropriate services and reducing ethnicity-based inequalities in access, experience and outcome.

POSTNATAL DEPRESSION

In terms of prevalence and seriousness, postnatal depression (which affects approximately 15% of women giving birth to live babies worldwide) falls between the 'baby blues' and puerperal psychosis, which affect around 75% and two women in every thousand respectively.[1] Due to its frequency, 'baby blues', commonly referred to as 'the blues', is generally regarded as a transient, relatively benign condition, although over several decades researchers have highlighted its strong association with and predictive ability in relation to postnatal depression.[2,3,4] Puerperal psychosis is regarded as a serious mental illness. Symptoms include hallucinations, delusions and high risk of suicide.[5,6] These features together with rapid onset render puerperal psychosis more amenable to detection and treatment than postnatal depression, which is often missed in primary care despite being regarded as a 'common mental illness' and the high level of postnatal contact between women and practitioners.[7]

However, despite not being regarded as serious mental illness (SMI), both clinical and anecdotal evidence suggests that, compared with psychotic episodes, the morbidity and long-term impact of postnatal depression are significantly greater for women, children and their families as postnatal depression can herald the onset of chronic, life-long mental ill health.[8,9] Children whose mothers experience postnatal depression are more likely to experience physical and psychological ill health and conduct disorders – especially among minority women.[10,11,12] Given these issues, surprisingly little is known about the long-term impact of postnatal mental illness on Black and minority ethnic women more generally or their decision making about whether or not to have subsequent pregnancies following depressive episodes. This may be at least partly because, although increasing, the evidence base for minority women's experience of postnatal depression remains relatively under-developed.

BLACK AND MINORITY ETHNIC (BME) WOMEN AND POSTNATAL DEPRESSION

The available evidence indicates that postnatal depression is a global phenomenon that affects women from all social classes, ethnic/racial backgrounds and cultures. Meta-analyses have shown that around 15% of women experience depression in the postnatal period.[13,14] However, closer scrutiny of these data indicates less homogeneity than immediately apparent. Whereas lower than expected rates were found among some ethnic groups such as Jewish Israeli women,[15] postnatal depression affected more than one quarter of Brazilian women,[16] South African women,[17] Jamaican women[18] and Arab Bedouin women in southern Israel.[19]

Explanations for higher rates of postnatal depression among Black and minority women of African and Asian descent in particular vary but include different psychosocial conceptualisations and expressions of psychological distress.[20,21] Whilst biological explanations for onset of postnatal depression exist, most research focuses on bio-psychosocial models.[22] In this context, BME women's greater exposure to social stressors such as isolation, and socio-economic deprivation, discrimination and racism increases their risk of developing postnatal depression and other mental illnesses.[23,24] Higher rates of pregnancy and larger families are additional risk factors, particularly in societies where there are a large number of single, women-headed households, as this is likely to reduce the availability of social support from a partner, which is known to protect against onset of postnatal depression.[25,26] However, even here there are differences between ethnic groups. Whilst lone parenthood has been implicated in the onset of postnatal depression for white and South Asian women, this is not the case for Black women.[27]

Despite greater risk of postnatal depression and long-term morbidity, BME women are less likely to receive appropriate care and treatment; even when residing in affluent societies.[28,29,30] This may be because whilst symptoms of postnatal depression may be common to all women, their impact and ways in which they are experienced and expressed will vary according to social and cultural contexts. For example, it has been reported that although depressed Black women experience problems with appetite and sleep, the ways in which they are affected differ from white women.[31] In other words, the very factors that make women diverse (ethnicity, culture, socio-economic status etc.) also impact their experiences of postnatal depression and influence their decisions about subsequent pregnancies.

Furthermore, in communities where depression is conceptualised as an inappropriate response to life's 'ups and downs', it is unlikely that women will seek help. If they do so, it is likely to be from non-medical sources.[21] Community-level stigma[32] coupled with social and cultural imperatives,[21,33] such as fulfilling role expectations and prioritising the needs of their families and members of the wider community over their own needs, also influence women's ability to acknowledge depressive feelings and seek or accept appropriate help and support.[23] Where women's identity and role performance are linked to child-rearing and bound with the need to cope with difficult feelings, help-seeking both within and outside their families is especially challenging.[30,31]

FACTORS INFLUENCING BME WOMEN'S DECISION MAKING ABOUT PREGNANCY FOLLOWING POSTNATAL DEPRESSION

Despite advances in gender equality and a shift towards male involvement in child-rearing, in most societies women remain the predominant caregivers and retain primary responsibility for child-rearing.[23] However, gender-based power imbalance and socio-cultural expectations that many women do not have ultimate control over their reproductive health.[34] In most societies where fertility is highly prized, especially when coupled with the perceived or actual pressure to produce male children and the unavailability or restrictions on the use of birth control, this can mean that some women have little control over the timing of a pregnancy subsequent to postpartum depression. This is important because emerging evidence suggests that depressed mothers may be at greater risk of recurrent and chronic depression.[35,36]

Although, in comparison to research into postnatal depression in white Western women, the evidence base amongst women from other countries and cultures is still growing, the existing evidence indicates that some BME women use culturally specific coping strategies to help them deal with postpartum depression. For example, research in the UK reported that women of Black Caribbean origin drew heavily on social and historical ideas about what it means to be both Black and a woman and their capacity to manage hardships.[21] In this context, women from this ethnic group rarely regarded depressive feelings following childbirth as warranting medical intervention.[37] However, when they overcame socio-cultural imperatives to minimise and 'deal with' persistent depressive feelings that hindered their ability to function to seek help and support,[21] they found that health service providers lacked the training and confidence required to identify and manage the needs of BME women.[38,39] Women's perspectives were endorsed by healthcare professionals who, by their own admission, lacked the cultural competence to understand and manage the needs of BME women from the range of ethnic groups that now comprise the UK population.[40]

These findings have been endorsed by research from the Caribbean. In Barbados, Black women who experienced postnatal depression also reported using culturally specific techniques to cope with the condition and highlighted barriers within the local healthcare system that prevented them receiving the care they needed.[41] Both examples illustrate that social, personal, cultural and structural factors can intersect to impact women's experiences with postpartum depression and their ability to access postnatal mental healthcare. This is significant because, in BME communities where there tends to be high levels of mental health stigma, women are less likely to be able to discuss their past experiences of postnatal depression in the context of feelings about becoming pregnant again.[32] Accordingly, we shall now briefly examine barriers to accessing support that may particularly affect BME women in decision making when contemplating pregnancy following postnatal depression. Specifically, we examine the potential impact of ethnic identity, cultural awareness of services and stigma.

ETHNICITY, CULTURAL AWARENESS AND DECISION MAKING

All women contemplating having another child after experiencing postnatal depression are faced with considering several factors. For example, women, their partners and families might be understandably fearful of recurrence of postnatal depression with subsequent pregnancies and want to 'protect' women from another bout of postnatal depression. However, women who have recovered might want to have another child to fulfil expectations of more 'natural' postnatal interactions with their babies and others without the challenges of depressive feelings. Furthermore, there might be great personal and social imperatives to have further children. To help with the decision-making process, women need access to accurate information about risk, likelihood of recurrent depressive illness and strategies to ameliorate risk, and to restore and maximise mental health and wellbeing.

Healthcare providers are the obvious sources of this kind of information. However, BME women have reported challenges navigating maternal mental health services in general and particular difficulties in interacting with health professionals.[42,43] Although this is partly due to structural factors such as lack of translation and interpreting services, other factors influence minority women's perception of the way they are treated as individuals and the quality of clinical care they receive.[44] For example, the ways that women think and talk about depressive feelings postnatally differ according to ethnicity and culture. Social and medical anthropologists have therefore challenged the view of universal categories of mental illness. From this relativist standpoint, they suggest that there are as many categories of mental illness as languages and culture in which they may be expressed.[45] Cultural expressions of clinical syndromes such as postnatal depression might therefore differ significantly between ethnic groups or symptoms may cluster in different ways across cultures. In addition, women might use culturally specific language terms to describe feelings which correspond to Western models of 'depression', even when there is no equivalent terminology in their original language.

Although from the English-speaking Caribbean, members of this ethnic group in the UK have reported difficulties during consultation with health professionals.[46,47] In common with women from other minority groups, there is evidence that they may be more likely than white British women to express psychological distress in terms of physical pain or to speak about hardships like financial difficulties or lack of social support rather than depressive feelings per se.[48] Health providers, who are unaware of the different ways in which women discuss mental health and illness or whose care strategies for dealing with psychological distress are modelled on provision for White women, might overlook or misunderstand the experiences and expressions of BME women during consultations. As a result, BME women may feel unacknowledged and unheard, which can negatively impact their health-seeking and engagement with service providers, thus hindering their ability to receive the care they need.[49]

It has been suggested that BME women's perceptions of inferior care and treatment is because, even in a multi-cultural context, health professionals' training prepares them primarily to deal with a standardised woman. By implication, this is a white woman.[41] Basing care provision on a 'one-size-fits-all' representation of women can lead to BME women feeling disconnected and disenfranchised from healthcare providers.[49] This might particularly affect Black Caribbean and other English-speaking minority women due to perceived similarities between them and the dominant culture. For, unlike minority ethnic women who experience language and/or religious-based barriers to accessing care, shared characteristics can lead to the needs of minority women being subsumed into the dominant culture, resulting in their particular needs being overlooked.[43] This is important because feeling invisible in healthcare settings makes it difficult for women to establish sufficient trust to disclose personal information, which is a prerequisite for effective psychological care. Whilst it is important for all women to be able to reflect on past experiences of postpartum depression with their healthcare providers, this may be crucial for BME women because of elevated risk of recurrence.[38,42] However, lack of trust can be an insurmountable barrier to such engagement, leaving women unable to access the support they need when contemplating another pregnancy following postnatal depression.

CONTENDING WITH CULTURE-BASED MENTAL HEALTH STIGMA

Mental health stigma is universal, affecting people from all ethnic and cultural backgrounds. However, women from minority ethnic groups contend with additional distinct and culture-based stigma about mental health and illness. For example, in a report commissioned by the UK's Department of Health, it was reported that some women were inhibited from seeking help with postnatal depression because this had serious implications for the perceptions of their families and the marriage prospects of affected women's siblings. Fear of stigma and social exclusion were therefore powerful barriers accessing mental healthcare.[49]

These findings have been endorsed by studies on mental health stigma from the Caribbean and minority women in the United States (US).[32,41] For example, in qualitative research undertaken in Jamaica, it was reported that participants held strong beliefs about the perceived dangerousness of mentally ill people in their communities. This characterisation generated fear and marginalisation of people diagnosed with any form of mental illness from the rest of society.[50] Similar findings have been reported from Barbados, where anyone labelled 'mad' faced social exclusion.[51] These findings gain salience when one considers that women require support from their families and social networks to fully recover from postnatal depression.[52] When women believe they will be rejected, they are unlikely to disclose the true extent of psychological distress, especially if the woman has internalised stigma about mental illness and is therefore fearful of being labelled 'mad'.

These findings illustrate that BME women's views of mental health and illness and their ability to access care and support are profoundly influenced by their cultural backgrounds. Social constraints to be perceived as normal can cause women to be reluctant to disclose psychological distress. It is therefore imperative that health professionals working with BME women who are considering another pregnancy after having postpartum depression understand the social and cultural contexts in which such decisions are made.

CONCLUSION

Current evidence suggests that women from Black and minority backgrounds who are faced with contemplating another pregnancy following postnatal depression may require additional support to make informed choices. However, women's experiences and perceptions of inferior care including lack of culturally appropriate services means that some women may not receive the support that they need. This is an important omission in delivering postnatal care as BME women are at greater risk of postnatal morbidity. Understanding different culture-derived conceptions of mental illness is fundamental for the provision, delivery and evaluation of effective mental healthcare in increasingly multi-racial/multi-ethnic societies.[53,54] In the context of economic constraints, increasing numbers of potential patients and a shrinking voluntary sector have traditionally provided care for BME women; these are important considerations for delivery of fair and equitable services. To ensure that the needs of women from different ethnic and cultural backgrounds are met, it is imperative that health professionals' training and service delivery are commissioned with a clear intention to meet the needs of all women. Failure to do so could reinforce the 'inverse case law' where the most vulnerable women are least likely to receive the care they need.

REFERENCES

1. Stuart S, O'Hara MW, *et al.* Mental disorders associated with childbearing: report of the biennial meeting of the Marce Society. *Psychopharmacol Bull.* 1998; **34**(3): 333.
2. Cutrona CE. Causal attributions and perinatal depression. *J Abnorm Psychol.* 1983; **92**(2): 161.
3. Parry BL, Kaplan HI, *et al.* Section 15.4: Postpartum Psychiatric Syndromes. In: Kaplan HI, Sadock BJ, editors. *Comprehensive Textbook of Psychiatry/VI.* 6th ed. Baltimore, MD: Williams & Wilkins; 1995. pp. 1059–66.

4. Henshaw C. Clinical and biological aspects of postpartum blues and depression. *Curr Opin Psychiatry*. 2000; **13**(6): 635.

5. Terp IM and Mortensen PB. Post-partum psychoses: clinical diagnoses and relative risk of admission after parturition. *Br J Psychiatry*. 1998; **172**: 521–6.

6. Blackmore ER, Jones I, *et al*. Obstetric variables associated with bipolar affective puer-peral psychosis. *Br J Psychiatry*. 2006; **188**(1): 32–6.

7. Gilbody SM, Whitty PM, *et al*. Improving the detection and management of depression in primary care. *Qual Saf Health Care*. 2003; **12**(2): 149–55.

8. Patel V, Rahman A, *et al*. Effect of maternal mental health on income growth in low income countries: new evidence from South Asia. *BMJ*. 2004; **328**: 820–23.

9. Patel V and Prince M. Maternal psychological morbidity and low birth weight in India. *Br J Psychiatry*. 2006; **188**(3): 284–5.

10. Baker-Henningham H, Powell C, *et al*. Mothers of undernourished Jamaican children have poorer psychosocial functioning and this is associated with stimulation provided in the home. *Eur J Clin Nutr*. 2003; **57**: 786–92.

11. Adshead G and Bluglass K. Attachment representations in mothers with abnormal ill-ness behaviour by proxy. *Br J Psychiatry*. 2005; **187**(4): 328–33.

12. Chen YH, Tsai SY, *et al*. Increased mortality risk among offspring of mothers with post-natal depression: a nationwide population-based study in Taiwan. *Psychol Med*. 2011; **41**(11): 2287–96.

13. O'Hara M and Swain A. Rates and risk of postpartum depression – a meta-analysis. *Int Rev Psychiatry*. 1996; **8**: 37–54.

14. Bolton HL, Hughes PM, *et al*. Incidence and demographic correlates of depressive symp-toms during pregnancy in an inner London population. *J Psychosom Obstet Gynecol*. 1998; **19**: 202.

15. Fisch RZ, Tadmor OP, *et al*. Postnatal depression: a prospective study of its prevalence, incidence and psychosocial determinants in an Israeli sample. *J Obstet Gynaecol Res*. 1997; **23**(6): 547.

16. Da-Silva VA, Moraes-Santos AR, *et al*. Prenatal and postnatal depression among low income Brazilian women. *Braz J Med Biol Res*. 1998; **31**(6): 799–804.

17. Lawrie TA, Hofmeyer GJ, *et al*. Validation of the Edinburgh Postnatal Depression Scale on a cohort of South African women. *S Afr Med J*. 1998; **88**: 1340–4.

18. Pottinger AM, Trotman-Edwards H, *et al*. Detecting depression during pregnancy and associated lifestyle practices and concerns among women in a hospital-based obstetric clinic in Jamaica. *Gen Hosp Psychiatry*. 2009; **31**(3): 254–61.

19. Glasser S, Tanous M, *et al*. Perinatal depressive symptoms among Arab women in north-ern Israel. *Matern Child Health J*. 2012; **16**(6): 1197–205.

20. Bhugra D. Cultural identities and cultural congruency: a new model for evaluating men-tal distress in immigrants. *Acta Psychiatr Scand*. 2005; **111**(2): 84–93.

21. Edge D and Rogers A. 'Dealing with it': Black Caribbean women's response to adversity and psychological distress associated with pregnancy, childbirth, and early motherhood. *Soc Sci Med*. 2005; **61**(1): 15–25.

22. Haw C. Psychological perspectives on women's vulnerability to mental illness. In: Kohen D, editor. *Women and Mental Health*. London: Routledge; 2001. pp. 65–105.

23. Bhugra D, Wojcik W, *et al*. Cultural bereavement: culture shock and culture conflict

– adjustment and reaction. In: Bhugra D, Gupta S, editors. *Migration and Mental Health.* Cambridge: Cambridge University Press; 2011. pp. 139–48.

24. James C, Este D, *et al. Race and well-being.* Halifax & Winnipeg, Fernwood Publishing; 2010.

25. Marks M, Wieck A, *et al.* How does marriage protect women with histories of affective disorder from post-partum relapse? *Br J Med Psychol.* 1996; **69**: 329.

26. Crosby RA, DiClemente RJ, *et al.* Correlates of adolescent females' worry about undesired pregnancy – the importance of partner desire for pregnancy. *J Pediatr Adolesc Gynecol.* 2001; **14**: 123–7.

27. Lloyd K. Ethnicity, social inequality, and mental illness. *BMJ.* 1998; **316**: 1763–70.

28. Chaudhry N, Waheed W, *et al.* Development and pilot testing of a social intervention for depressed women of Pakistani family origin in the UK. *J Ment Health.* 2009; **18**(6): 504–9.

29. Edge D. Ethnicity and mental health encounters in primary care: help-seeking and help-giving for perinatal depression among Black Caribbean women in the UK. *Ethn Health.* 2010; **15**(1): 93–111.

30. Edge D and Mackian S. Ethnicity and mental health encounters in primary care: help-seeking and help-giving for perinatal depression among Black Caribbean women in the UK. *Ethn Health.* 2010; **15**(1): 93–111.

31. Beauboeuf-Lafontant T. Listening past the lies that make us sick: a voice-centered analysis of strength and depression among black women. *Qual Sociol.* 2008; **31**(4): 391–406.

32. Nadeem E, Lange JM, *et al.* Does stigma keep poor young immigrant and U.S.-born black and latina women from seeking mental health care? *Psychiatr Serv.* 2007; **58**(12): 1547–54.

33. Brown JS, Casey SJ, *et al.* How black African and white British women perceive depression and help-seeking: a pilot vignette study. *Int J Soc Psychiatry.* 2011; **57**(4): 362–74.

34. Holmshaw J and Hillier S. Gender and culture: a sociological perspective to mental health problems in women. In: Kohen D, editor. *Women and Mental Health.* London: Routledge; 2000. pp. 39–64.

35. Gater R, Tomenson B, *et al.* Persistent depressive disorders and social stress in people of Pakistani origin and white Europeans in UK. *Soc Psychiatry and Psychiatr Epidemiol.* 2009; **44**(3): 198–207.

36. Gater R, Waheed W, *et al.* Social intervention for British Pakistani women with depression: randomised controlled trial. *Br J Psychiatry.* 2010; **197**(3): 227–33.

37. Edge D. Ethnicity, psychosocial risk, and perinatal depression: a comparative study among inner-city women in the United Kingdom. *J Psychosom Res.* 2007; **63**(3): 291–5.

38. Edge D. 'Falling through the net': health professionals' views of perinatal mental healthcare for Black and minority ethnic women. (Conference Abstract). *J Reprod Infant Psychol.* 2009; **27**(3).

39. Edge D. Falling through the net – Black and minority ethnic women and perinatal mental healthcare: health professionals' views. *Gen Hosp Psychiatry.* 2010; **32**(1): 17–25.

40. Edge D. Perinatal mental health care for black and minority ethnic (BME) women: a scoping review of provision in England. *Ethn Inequal Health Soc Care.* 2010; **3**(3): 24–32.

41. Jackson-Best F. *Maternal depression in Barbados: exploring how Black women experience, understand, manage and cope with the 'baby blues' and postpartum depression* [PhD thesis]. Toronto: University of Toronto; 2015.

42. Collins E, Shakya YB, *et al.* Services for women: access, equity and quality. In: Guruge S, Collins E, editors. *Working with Immigrant Women: issues and strategies for mental health professionals.* Toronto, MH; 2008.

43. Edge D. 'We don't see Black women here': an exploration of the absence of Black Caribbean women from clinical and epidemiological data on perinatal depression in the UK. *Midwifery.* 2008; **24**: 379–89.

44. Edge D. 'It's leaflet, leaflet, leaflet then "see you later"' – Black Caribbean women's perceptions of perinatal mental healthcare in the UK. *Br J Gen Pract.* 2011; **61**(585): 256–62.

45. Fenton S and Sadiq-Sangster A. Culture, relativism and the expression of mental distress: South Asian women in Britain. *Sociol Health Illn.* 1996; **18**: 66.

46. Lloyd K. Depression and anxiety among Afro-Caribbean general practice attenders in Britain. *Int J Soc Psychiatry.* 1993; **39**(1): 1–9.

47. Lloyd K and Fuller E. *Use of Services – Ethnic Minority Psychiatric Illness Rates (EMPIRIC).* London: The Stationery Office; 2002.

48. Baker D, Mead N, *et al.* Inequalities in morbidity and consulting behaviour for socially vulnerable groups. *Br J Gen Pract.* 2002; **52**(475): 124–30.

49. Edge D. *Perinatal Mental Health of Black and Minority Ethnic Women: a review of current provision in England, Scotland and Wales.* London: Department of Health; 2011.

50. Arthur CM, Hickling FW, *et al.* 'Mad, sick, head nuh good': mental illness stigma in Jamaican communities. *Transcultural Psychiatry.* 2010; **47**: 252–75.

51. Potter RB and Phillips J. 'Mad dogs and transnational migrants?' Bajan-Brit second-generation migrants and accusations of madness. *Ann Assoc Am Geogr.* 2006; **96**(3): 586–600.

52. Campbell C and McLean C. Ethnic identities, social capital and health inequalities: factors shaping African-Caribbean participation in local community networks in the UK. *Soc Sci Med.* 2002; **55**(4): 643.

53. Bhui K, Fenton S, *et al. Ethnic Differences in the Context and Experience of Psychiatric Illness: a qualitative study.* London, The Stationery Office; 2002.

54. Fernando S. Inequalities and the politics of 'race' in mental health. In: Fernando S, Keating F, editors. *Mental Health in a Multi-ethnic Society – a multidisciplinary handbook.* London, Routledge; 2009, pp. 42–57.

ADDITIONAL COMMENTS

These comments are by Dr Jane Hanley, a perinatal mental health expert at Swansea University, immediate past president of the International Marcé Society, a charity dedicated to research and the awareness of perinatal mental health around the globe, and Principal Trainer for the Institute of Health Visiting.

As the UK becomes increasingly culturally diverse, it is important to recognise the differing health needs of the population. A small minority of mothers originate from outside of the UK, the greatest numbers of which are from the Indian subcontinent, and they represent nearly one half of the ethnic minority population. One quarter of these mothers are of Afro-Caribbean and African descent. The number of economic migrants and asylum seekers staying in the UK is growing annually (ONS 2011)*. Studies have indicated that perinatal mental illness is three times more prevalent in the lower and middle income countries than in resource-rich countries, and yet only one quarter of these mothers are able to access the care they need. The status of the migrant is known to be one of the risk factors for postnatal depressive symptoms.

The debilitating effects of poor perinatal mental health have been subject to extensive research whilst the negative consequences for the infants' cognitive, emotional and physical health have been well documented. The National Health Service within the UK has the capacity to offer mothers Care Pathways to meet some of their perinatal mental health needs, yet often resistance is encountered by the mother and sometimes by the healthcare worker, listing the lack of cultural norms, time, translation resources and signposting as some of the barriers to care.

Cultural norms

Some traditional cultures regard pregnancy as a rite of passage. Fertility is a blessing, and being a mother, as the provider of life, is a highly valued position within the community. Myths and legends suggest that she is also both feared and revered. The three phases of the rites of passage, postulated by Van Gennep (1909)†, serve to assure the physical, emotional and spiritual wellbeing of the parents and child. Initially there is a separation followed by the birth and the christening or naming ceremony and finally the reintroduction of the mother back into the community. Initiation processes may be performed by tribal elders, who ensure the continuity of moral instruction and social responsibility.

With so many differing ethnic minorities it is difficult to have a sound cultural awareness of each one. However, it is feasible for the healthcare worker to gain an understanding of an individual's needs and some insight into their principal attitudes towards pregnancy, childbirth and child-rearing practices, acknowledging the expectations of breastfeeding and who might provide the most support. Local knowledge is also important: knowing the location of the places of worship or the specialist grocer.

With the wealth of web-based knowledge it is not difficult to access this information, but discussing the impact of these and the rites of passage with

---

* www.ons.gov.uk/ons/dcp171776_346219.pdf
† Van Gennep, Arnold (1909). Les rites de passage (in French). Paris: Émile Nourry. Lay summary – Review by Frederick Starr. *Am J Soc.* 1910; **15**(5): 707–9.

an English-speaking compatriot may facilitate further exploration just as effectively.

The health worker may be anxious about their preconceived ideas and beliefs about the mother, which may be formed by previous experiences, stereotyping or prejudice. There may be a reluctance to verbally communicate as it may be felt to be embarrassing, difficult or even futile. It is important to examine these ideas to gain a greater understanding of the reasons for this and if possible to discuss these in more depth.

As would be expected in the UK, a few spoken words of English are always welcomed, likewise a few words in the mother's language would be equally appreciated. Some suggested phrases are: 'How are you?', 'I am fine thank you', 'You look sad', 'Who can you speak with?' and 'Who can I contact for you?'

This awareness can ensure that healthcare workers are responsive to cultural voids and the impact this may have on mother's mental health. The necessary background knowledge, a few seminal words, good non-verbal communication and an attitude that suggests real care can make a significant difference.

ADDITIONAL SUPPORT AND INFORMATION FOR MULTICULTURAL/BME FAMILIES AND PERINATAL MENTAL HEALTH

Added by Elaine A Hanzak

- Queensland Health Strategic Plan for Multicultural Health. *Cultural Dimensions of Pregnancy, Birth and Post-Natal Care*. Available at: www.health.qld.gov.au/multicultural/support_tools/14MCSR-pregnancy.pdf This has some excellent information on the differences and problems involved, e.g. over cultural aspects.
- West London Mental Health. *Cultural Competency Toolkit: a resource pack for clinicians who care for people from ethnic minority backgrounds*. Available at: http://wlmht.nhs.uk/docs/general/CCTK.pdf
- Cox J, Holden J, Henshaw C. *Perinatal Mental Health: the Edinburgh Postnatal Depression Scale (EPDS) manual*. 2nd ed. London: RCP Publications; 2014. The second edition of the EPDS manual is now published by RCPsych publications and has 50+ translations. Available at: www.rcpsych.ac.uk/usefulresources/publications/books/rcpp/9781909726130.aspx
- How other cultures prevent postpartum depression www.uppitysciencechick.com/how_other_cultures.pdf
- www.postpartumprogress.com/the-racial-ethnic-disparities-of-identifying-treating-postpartum-depression

Perinatal mood and anxiety disorders resources in other languages

- www.postpartum.net/Resources/Resources-in-other-Languages.aspx
- Translated Information – Postnatal Depression www.beyondblue.org.au/resources/for-me/multicultural-people

Factsheets on postpartum depression in a variety of languages

- www.heretohelp.bc.ca/other-languages
- Ponterotto JG. *Handbook of Multicultural Counselling*. Chichester: SAGE; 2009.
- MECOPP – supporting minority ethnic carers www.mecopp.org.uk/links-national_useful_links.php?section_id=219
- CPHVA 'How Are You Feeling?' Booklets and posters CPHVA, London www.cairnsbookshop.co.uk/categories/unitecphva/tab/general?topic=&pg=3
- You may find some cultural guides via UKTI – although these are based for business, there are some indicators around customs, e.g. www.china.doingbusinessguide.co.uk/

Research

- Minas H, Klimidis S, Kokanovic R. Depression in multicultural Australia: policies, research and services. *Aust NZ Health Policy*. 2007; **4**:16. Available at: www.anzhealthpolicy.com/content/4/1/16
- Cantle F. Tackling perinatal mental health among black and minority ethnic mothers. *Ethnicity and Inequalities in Health and Social Care*. 2010; **3**(2): 38–43. Available at: www.emeraldinsight.com/doi/abs/10.5042/eihsc.2010.0345
- Downe SM, Butler E, Hinder S. Screening tools for depressed mood after childbirth in UK-based South Asian women: a systematic review. *J Adv Nurs*. 2007; **57**(6): 565–83.

Example of good practice

Hammla Service based at Leeds Teaching Hospital – Haamla is a unique service that provides essential support for pregnant women, and their families, from minority ethnic communities, including asylum seekers and refugees, throughout their pregnancy and postnatal period. It aims to improve access within maternity services, empower and inform women of the choices available during their pregnancy and birth, thereby improving their health and wellbeing. www.leedsth.nhs.uk/a-z-of-services/leeds-perinatal-centre/what-we-do/haamla-service/ There are links and further information on their website.

PART 5

Self-help and complementary techniques for good mental health in the perinatal period

CHAPTER 29

General health and wellbeing

Nourishing yourself in a way that helps you blossom in the direction you want to go is attainable, and you are worth the effort.

Deborah Day

I remember thinking that I was totally prepared for the birth of my son and becoming a mother. Without all of the complications, perhaps I would have been. In reality I knew very little! So considering a 'take two' situation I would have explored some of the additional ways that perhaps could have helped to increase both my physical and mental health. I am not suggesting that these ideas would replace any measures offered by healthcare professionals. In cases of moderate/severe illness, such as psychosis, of course their involvement and treatment is required (*see* Chapter 25). My ideas here are for parents with mild to moderate difficulties and those in recovery from the more serious conditions, to be used alongside other methods that we have already considered. Even if you were aware of them with your previous pregnancy, I hope this serves as a useful resource of ideas which may be worth considering. There may also be new resources since your previous pregnancy. Build these aspects into your plan, as appropriate, so that it can help you to feel more empowered and keep well. There may be techniques here that you can use between appointments with healthcare professionals or whilst you wait for a referral. Debby Gould in Chapter 12 suggests that a birth library is created rather than a plan – I offer this range of ideas in a similar way. You may also use them at others times in your life and some may even become part of your daily routines. If you are reading this book as a health professional, you may find some useful ideas here for your own mental wellbeing and techniques to manage stress.

I feel that generally we have become far more aware of mental health in recent years through campaigns in the media, e.g. Time to Change.[1] In 2013, a number of established organisations including Tommy's, Boots and the Royal College of Midwives produced a report[2] on perinatal mental health.

One of the outcomes was the creation of a simple wellbeing plan. This is easy to download[3] and could be a great place to start for you.

FIVE WAYS TO WELLBEING

These are a set of evidence-based actions[4] which promote people's wellbeing. They are: Connect, Be Active, Take Notice, Keep Learning and Give. These activities are simple things individuals can do in their everyday lives. The NHS recommend them and give ideas on how you can apply them.[5] In the situation of having another child after a previously problematic experience, let's look at some specific ways these may be used.

Connect

We have covered this in the chapters dealing with peers, friends and family. I stress again the strength of connecting, by any means. Here is a reminder about this from Bob Beaudine, who wrote *The Power of Who:*[6]

> Life's fickle, just when U get comfortable with the rhythm of your life, BAM! It changes. But listen closely! All it takes is, one thought, one idea, one friend and your world can change to the better in a moments flash. Have U noticed, that some messages U are given are so timely, make so much sense, it's as if they were written just for U. Right then! They were! Receive the encouragement! Your best is still ahead.

Have you noticed how this seems to happen, e.g. when browsing social media? If you have a positive thought – share it, as you never know who else you may inspire. Remember to make that one small action to connect. I shall give more ideas in the next chapter on arts and creativity. It is also about surrounding yourself with strong, positive people. They are generally healthier than those without a social network. Make and build relationships when you are well so that you will have people to support you – and vice versa. That sounds like I am saying you should only make friends with the idea of them helping you! The best relationships are those with mutual pleasure and support. As the late Steve Jobs wrote:

> Your time is limited, so don't waste it living someone else's life. Don't be trapped by dogma – which is living with the results of other people's thinking. Don't let the noise of others' opinions drown out your own inner voice. And most importantly, have the courage to follow your heart and intuition. They somehow already know what you truly want to become. Everything else is secondary.

Be Active

No one is expecting you to become an Olympic athlete in your days with a new family. I know that I find that exercise tends to be the first thing I cut out when I feel pressured, when it should be one of the last!

> Evidence suggests that postpartum women, some of whom were depressed, report benefit from participation in exercise programmes.[7]

Kathleen Kendall-Tackett[8] stresses that exercise is great for breastfeeding mothers, and when done in groups it has the added advantage of social connection. Find out what structured perinatal classes are available in your area, e.g. www.makeamove.org.uk. In Australia they have a very successful group called Bay City Strollers.[9] Look at the NHS site for some great tips.[10] You can download Deborah Beard's guide on postnatal exercise for Kindle for free.[11] Yoga and Pilates are popular perinatal activities. Swimming and dancing are also great.

Remember here that we are also talking about the basics of movement. Remove that image of the well-toned, lycra-clad, size 8 model now! I must admit that I wish some of the images of new parents were more realistic, with bags under the eyes as opposed to gym bags. Just get moving! My late partner Clive used to say 'Motion creates Emotion'. I understand that some days you may feel that simply getting out of bed is too much. On those days I suggest you take the first step of uncovering yourself. Then sit up. Then stand up. Go to the toilet. Then take it from there. You are up! That is the hardest bit. Focus on one foot in front of the other. If you have a toddler and a new baby, let the energy of the older child encourage you. They will be thrilled if you all join in dancing to a children's television programme. All of the usual, common sense advice could be listed here, e.g. walk instead of using the car when you can; get outside as a family. It really does help to get moving. It is even better when you get outside for 'green therapy'. When I was a teenager I remember having a poster on my wall of a lush waterfall with the caption 'Find a place that makes you happy and go there'. Where is your place?

I also feel that the opposite of being active is vital for new and expectant parents, i.e. relaxation. These activities can be done by one or both of you. Anxiety can often lead to depression, with some symptoms of tense muscles and the inability to slow your breathing down to a restful level.

> Your breathing is your greatest friend. Return to it in all your troubles and you will find comfort and guidance.
>
> Unknown

By learning how to relax muscles and breathe more slowly, these methods may help to manage and reduce anxious thoughts and behaviours. There are two main forms of relaxation training. One type teaches the person to relax voluntarily by tensing then relaxing various muscle groups. Another involves visualising relaxing scenes or places. You can do this with a professional, e.g. hypnotherapist, or done as self-help. You can easily find MP3 and video clips on the internet by searching for 'guided progressive muscle relaxation'.

One technique I was taught whilst a patient in the psychiatric hospital was to take slow, deep breaths to get oxygen flowing around my body better. When you are anxious your breathing becomes shallow. The idea is to sit or lie comfortably and visualise a single candle in front of you. In your mind's eye, light the wick. Inhale deeply and slowly then hold your breath for a few moments. As you exhale, the idea is to 'flicker' the flame with your breath – not so fast that it goes out or so slowly that it stays still. Repeat several times. I still use this simple method today in situations where I find myself feeling anxious.

Some people find that meditation and prayer can help them. Research shows that meditation may help you feel calm and enhance the effects of therapy. The Headspace app[12] is proving useful for some to help guide them on this.

I also agree that the power of visualisation is a wonderful way to relax. Close your eyes, remember a time when you were really on top of the world, you felt incredibly well, where things felt easy, you felt 'Wow I really love this. This is what life is about. I want to feel like this forever.' What are you doing? What are you feeling? What can you see? What can you hear? What can you smell? Describe the landscape. Guided visualisation, either by self-help or with a professional, can lower blood pressure as well as the level of stress hormones in the blood. After quietening body and mind, you may feel full of energy and exceedingly relaxed. Once refreshed you are more likely to be able to manage your day.

This links into the next topic.

Take Notice

The NHS describes this as 'Paying more attention to the present moment – to your own thoughts and feelings, and to the world around you – can improve your mental wellbeing.'[13] This can also be described as 'mindfulness' and is being used increasingly to help perinatal mental health challenges:

> This refers to being completely in touch with and aware of the present moment, as well as taking a non-evaluative and non-judgmental approach to your inner experience. For example, a mindful approach to one's inner experience is simply viewing 'thoughts as thoughts' as opposed to evaluating certain thoughts as positive or negative.
>
> Matthew Tull, PhD

Gina Hassan[14] writes about the benefits of mindfulness in parenting:

> What I wish I had known at this vulnerable time – and which sadly seems all too obvious in retrospect – is that more important than whether I was providing this kind of stimulation or that, or whether I purchased the car seat with the absolute highest safety rating or not, was my ability to be present with my children, and that giving them my presence was more important than any other decision I might make as a parent.
>
> What does it mean to give one's presence? In short, it means to find moments, and more moments, to leave one's thinking/analysing/judging brain behind and to just be with one's baby, staring into their eyes, smelling their scent, trusting one's intuition, and being available to respond in a spontaneous and loving manner to the cues they inevitably provide us with.

I would agree with her. I feel that this approach would have been helpful for me in the perinatal period. I needed my mind to be quietened down and to stop racing. Instead of always thinking about what I should be doing next, I realise that we all would have benefited by me simply being in the 'now'. I apply this approach in all aspects of my life now and I feel I am a calmer and happier person as a result. For example, when my son is home from college I enjoy him being around and savouring those moments – I do not let my mind go into the 'he'll be gone soon' mode and spoil the present. If I close my eyes I can still remember how he felt as a tiny baby – his smell, sounds, touch. The shape of the back of his head, the feel of his hair. That memory makes me smile now. Take those moments and firmly lock them in your memory bank. I also found this approach useful in the latter stages of compiling this book. As the deadline grew closer to needing to finish my manuscript, I was aware that I was becoming over-focused and as a result more stressed and less productive. In the last few weeks I decided to focus during the weekdays and give myself the weekend completely away from writing. I told my loved ones that I promised not to even mention 'the book' on Saturday and Sunday. Even if it 'popped' into my head, I put it back in the proverbial box. I focused on fun and relaxation, simply being with loved ones. They deserved my full attention and my brain needed a break. I would then feel so much more prepared and ready to write again on the following Monday.

With another baby, take the responsibility and belief in your own instinct and knowledge of you and them to give you the confidence to appreciate and know what you both need at a specific moment. Free yourself of the perceived heavy burden of all the 'shoulds' that come at you from every direction. Trust in and be confident in yourself.

> We all have the tendency to believe self-doubt and self-criticism, but listening to this voice never gets us closer to our goals. Instead, try on the point of view of a

mentor or good friend who believes in you, wants the best for you, and will encourage you when you feel discouraged.

Kelly McGonigal

We now have the evidence and practice that mindfulness does help in the perinatal period. There is a great deal of work being done on this, especially in the Oxford area. They run courses and training on this, along with providing resources.[15,16] Take a look at the article written by Sian Warriner.[17] There is a growing presence online too, with information such as www.bemindful online.com/, http://bemindful.co.uk/ and www.mindful.org/mindful-magazine/mindful-pregnancy

A new app has been designed specifically for the perinatal period using these approaches, called 'Mind the Bump'.[18]

You may find it helpful to notice and record the things that make you and your loved ones feel good during a day. That way, when you need a lift of your spirits, you will have a bank of 'feel good' ideas to apply. Remember that I have recommended a number of times about the value of music? I am not alone:

- I remember one of the first positive times when I started to appreciate my daughter, through all the gloom and horror of PP, was when she was about 3 months old. I was terrified of being on my own with her and my husband was working away. She had just started to smile and Lily Allen's hit 'Smile' was top of the charts and came on the radio. It's still a special song to me as I remember my mood changing and I looked at my beautiful girl smiling at me and started to dance to the song with her in my arms. Music is brilliant at helping us all feel more positive and lifting our spirits.

Keep Learning

My one word of caution in all of this is moderation. Please understand that I am listing all these suggestions for you to cherry-pick those that may be the most helpful to you. If you research them all your childbearing window could be over!

- **Books:** You are already doing that by reading this book. You could spend months reading about every aspect of mental health. The choices are overwhelming. I would suggest that when you have identified your biggest concern or trigger concerning your possible perinatal mental health challenge, focus on that to grow your knowledge of how best to help yourself. It is possible to get recommended books on prescription for different conditions.[19]
- **Internet-based:** This knowledge base is growing all the time. Explore the NHS site[20] for many general ideas for wellbeing. There are some audio guides under the 'Moodzone', to help you with a range of relevant issues, e.g. sleep, anxiety. Although they are not specifically linked to perinatal,

they are useful. There is also a postcode link to what services can be found in your area. The Mental Health Foundation also offer a range of podcasts that you may find beneficial.[21] Living Life to the Full[22] is an online course that teaches key knowledge in how to tackle and respond to issues/demands which we all meet in our everyday lives.

- **Documentation:** if you like to keep lists or write down your thoughts, goals, etc. you may find a printable workbook useful. There is one I have found for women living with depression during pregnancy, delivery and beyond.[23] It is also possible to find ready-made templates to record different aspects of your managing techniques.[24]

- **E-therapies:** if you have mild to moderate mental health issues, these may be effective in helping you to change your patterns of thinking and behaviour.[25] These online or computer-aided psychological therapy structured sessions are easy to access, can fit around your lifestyle and are ideal if you are in an isolated area or where there are long waiting lists for face-to-face appointments. In the UK, Netmums and researchers at the University of Exeter are currently running a study on a 12-week CBT course with telephone support.[26] Keep an eye out for when this is live. The Australian Government 'mindhealthconnect' website has a library of online programmes.[27]

- **Mobile phone apps:** There are now an increasing number available for use in the perinatal period. Many are aimed at first pregnancies when you are more focused on details such as the size of your growing bump! Some mothers have recommended them for subsequent pregnancies[28] as they have enjoyed both the technology advancements since their previous time and it has eased some anxieties. One that has been devised and researched[29] with mental and physical health in mind is called 'Baby Buddy'.[30] There is a Positive Pregnancy one by Andrew Johnson to aid relaxation and ease anxiety.[31] As the technology is growing all the time, I would recommend that if this is something that you feel may be helpful to you, look out for the latest ones recommended by others. Do beware of technology overuse!

- **Hobbies and interests:** What? With at least two children? Yes – I am putting this forward as a suggestion. As a parent you still have to find time for 'you'. This is even more important as we seek ways to keep you in good mental health. This can be as simple as doing a crossword puzzle or pottering in the garden. Plan how you can build these sessions in for yourself. Remember that you have to look after you so that you can look after others. Treat yourself with kindness and respect. Prioritise what is important and if that means loosening your attitude on wanting perfection, then so be it.

Accept yourself. Love yourself as you are. Your finest work, your best movements, your joy, peace, and healing come when you love yourself. You give a great gift to the world when you do that. You give others permission to do the same: to love themselves. Revel in self-love. Roll in it. Bask in it as you would sunshine.

Melodie Beattie

Give

There is a verse in scripture that says, 'There is more happiness in giving than in receiving.' By purposefully helping others, we add value and meaning to our lives. The message here is not about donating your salary to a charity or giving away all your possessions. The best gift we can give is one of time and ourselves.

> A wise physician said, 'The best medicine for humans is love.' Someone asked, 'If it doesn't work?' He smiled and answered, 'Increase the dose.'
>
> Author unknown

You can 'give' your time to yourself, your partner, children and other loved ones. What better way to spend an hour or so than with your child or children and your grandparents, if you are still able to? A lovely way to be 'mindful' with them all.

In the last 10 years since my first book was published, I have seen a growing network for former sufferers of perinatal mental illness that have begun to share their experiences and offer peer support to others. This may be a way that you feel that you can help and you may learn some new tips to help you if you do go on to have another baby. I stress that this should only be done when you feel strong and recovered. It will not help another sufferer to hear your tears.

Remember that by giving of your time and helping others you will feel a sense of purpose and fulfilment. For those who seek help, it is a sign of strength. When you are able to, give that time and support to others, without expecting anything in return. At another stage, if you do need help, remember to ask so that someone else can have the opportunity to feel useful.

OTHER ASPECTS OF IMPROVING YOUR PHYSICAL AND MENTAL HEALTH

Smoking cessation

There is a wealth of research and information that supports that smoking is bad for an unborn baby and for any smoker. We looked at this in the pregnancy chapter. If you are still smoking or have started again, please take steps to find an alternative way to relax or a different way to find the pleasure you get from smoking.[32] Other useful websites looking at smoking cessation in pregnancy are www.patient.co.uk/health/nicotine-replacement-therapy, www.ukctas.ac.uk/ and www.ncsct.co.uk/

Good diet

In reality, few new parents bask in the delights of creating stunning, organic meals from their kitchen-diner with bi-fold doors, to delight their appreciative offspring! Toddlers and children of all ages can be demanding about their likes and dislikes, and adding a new baby into the mix takes away more culinary time. You can guarantee that just as you may feel inclined to get something tasty rustled up, your attention will be distracted again. It is easy to fill up on 'rubbish'. In the first place avoid buying alcohol, refined sugar products etc. and ensure there is plenty of fresh fruit and vegetables in stock. Get into online shopping whilst you are pregnant so that you know this can be one task that is easier for you. Vitamin B is especially good for you and can be found in meat, eggs, fish, milk and whole grains. Omega 3 fatty acids are also recommended.[33] There is a very comprehensive fact sheet for 'healthy eating for people with depression, anxiety and related disorders'.[34]

Weight gain after pregnancy can affect some women and add to their lowered self-esteem. If this is a challenge for you, it may be worth looking at some newer ways to consider helping yourself. This may include the use of a hypnotherapy app for your mobile phone, e.g. Easyloss.[35] One mum reports that:

- I've suffered with PND since I had my daughter 2 years ago and have found that when I listen to the app I don't feel as bad. I am so much more relaxed. I'm enjoying everything more and not just food. Before I started I rarely left the house apart from taking my daughter to nursery or going to work and now I have been out shopping, to the park and even walked up to my sister's house 2 miles away. Losing weight is a plus but I am finally starting to get my life back.

Hypnotherapy

Sue Peckham of the Hampshire Hypnotherapy Centre writes:

So many people think of hypnotherapy as something a guy in a suit, standing on stage does to make an audience laugh as he gets subjects to cluck like chickens or jump around like racehorses. The truth is that hypnotherapy can really make a great difference to your mental health after your baby is born as well as during pregnancy and labour.

Using a series of simple mental relaxation exercises a good, professional hypnotherapist will help you to truly relax your mind and as a result your body too. My clients tell me it is the most the relaxed they have ever felt. Once in a really relaxed state your hypnotherapist will use powerful suggestions for your well-being and improved mental health that will help you to feel calmer, more relaxed and in control. You will be guided through exercises to help you to manage your thinking in different way and as a result your self-confidence grows and your self-esteem improves. These changes will have a dramatic, positive effect on how you cope with your feelings and thoughts and life in general becomes more manageable.

So whether you are looking to overcome the symptoms of postpartum depression, have a more relaxed pregnancy and birth or to lose weight after the birth of your baby, hypnotherapy is something that would be a great additional tool in your mental health tool box.

Massage and aromatherapy

Massage can help in the perinatal period, as massage stimulates nerve endings that in turn release feel-good chemicals into the body. Even if this has no effect on you, simply by taking time for yourself will ultimately help you feel calmer. Baby massage can also help to reduce stress levels in the mother and may help with bonding. Look out for local classes. If finance is an issue, teach yourself the techniques using books or the internet. Local colleges often offer massage and beauty therapy at reduced rates to enable their supervised students to have clients to practise on. Some women have found reflexology to be calming.

> Do something every day that is loving toward your body and gives you the opportunity to enjoy the sensations of your body.
>
> Golda Poretsky

A pilot study indicates positive findings with minimal risk for the use of aromatherapy as a complementary therapy in both anxiety and depression situations with the postpartum woman.[36] Essential oils such as lavender and camomile (which also helps insomnia) may help achieve a state of calm. Rosemary and bergamot are said to have an uplifting effect on moods. Oils can be used in a variety of ways including massage, bathing and inhaling. Create an uplifting oil aroma to waft around the house during the day and then relax into a hot lavender bath in the evening to unwind. A qualified aromatherapist should be able to come up with a blend of oils specifically tailored to your situation.

Herbal remedies and homeopathy

Plant extracts (herbal or homeopathic remedies) are available in tablet form from chemists and health food shops without prescription. Some of these are widely regarded as being effective supplements in the treatment of mild to moderate depression. It is wise to check with a pharmacist or GP that a complementary remedy won't interfere with any other medication you are taking. Breastfeeding mothers should definitely check with a reliable source as to any effects a supplement may have on their milk.

Look at the British Homeopathic Association[37] for more details and also at natural remedies.[38] For research look at Weir (2002).[39]

Other approaches

One system I have discovered that combines many of these techniques is called 'The Mommy Plan'.[40] It is based on a number of natural healing approaches, including diet and massage.

You can find more natural ideas in a downloadable document, 'Complementary Therapies for Postpartum Support', compiled and edited by Catherine Burns, RSMT[41] and also at other useful sites for natural approaches.[42]

Please refer to Chapter 25 for Dr Henshaw's comments about acupuncture and bright light therapy.

One approach that is beginning to emerge is Emotional Freedom Technique (EFT), sometimes referred to as 'tapping'. The team at the Brocklington Mother and Baby Unit in Staffordshire have been finding it a useful addition to the normal range of techniques following research by the university there, as mentioned in Chapter 11.[43]

Two more key areas that I feel are vital are laughter and goal setting. Even within the darkest days of depression, you need to find ways to make you smile. A good belly laugh is a brilliant medicine! Watch funny movies as a family. Research shows that laughter can boost your immune system, ease pain, relax your body and reduce stress.[44] Find simple joy and gratitude in your life and where you are right now. Sometimes faking a smile can actually lead to you feeling better, because if you smile at someone, the chances are they will smile back. Be careful who you choose though!

Some people find that setting realistic goals may help them. This can be a basic as 'get up', 'shower', 'get dressed' or bigger ones. Clive used to run marathons, and when asked how he ran 26 miles he would deny it – he'd say that he simply ran one mile 26 times. Each mile was a matter of putting one foot in front of the other. Take baby steps to achieve your goals and build in rewards along the way, e.g. a date night with your partner. Celebrating and acknowledging success will lead to more. Psychologist RY Langham[45] recommends:

> Get organized and avoid procrastination. Keep your home neat and clean; get help keeping your home and possessions (e.g. car) clean, if necessary. Get rid of clutter. If it has been there for more than a year, it probably isn't necessary. Get on top of your bills because finances can also influence your mental health. Sometimes professional services such as a coach or life coach can be of help in this area.

For healthcare professionals I have come across a range of information sources, in addition to all of the above that you may find useful. In Canada, I have found an organisation called Best Start. They have some information to download. One of the most relevant is a manual called *Creating Circles of Support for Pregnant Women and New Parents*.[46] They also have developed a ready-to-use workshop to meet the needs of service providers who are working with parents experiencing mental health challenges. There is no cost to the workshop and it can be downloaded from the Best Start Resource Centre website.[47]

In January 2014 the journal *Clinical Obstetrics and Gynaecology* published the whole edition on perinatal mental health. There is a research paper within it that reviews some of the complementary and alternative medicine therapies: www.bestpracticeobgyn.com/article/S1521-6934(13)00109-0/fulltext

Also refer to www.sign.ac.uk/guidelines/fulltext/60/section3.html

In Australia they have devised a range of materials for use in training for perinatal mental health. Take a look at their Think GP database.[48]

I was asked for a presentation to share some of my top tips for wellbeing. I planned them around my surname. I feel that this is a suitable place to share them again here to serve as a reminder.

THE HANZAK PRINCIPLES OF WELLBEING

Hope and honesty

If you feel that life is rather tough, always keep sight of the hope that it will be better soon. Being honest with yourself (and others) about how you feel and asking for help and accepting it will make a positive difference. Life is made of highs and lows. Identify your triggers and plan for ways to deal with them.

> Hope doesn't come from calculating whether the good news is winning out over the bad. It's simply a choice to take action.
>
> Anna Lappe

Attitude

Mental health is as important as physical health and when it suffers accept it in the same way as an illness, and accept that you need support to recover. By ignoring your feelings and hiding away in isolation with guilt and worry of stigma, it will make life worse for all. If you aren't 'fine', say so!

Needs

Remember that everyone has unique needs with the arrival of a new baby and you all need practical and emotional support to help you enjoy it.

Nurture: make yourself and others feel special around you, e.g. hand massage.

Education: learn about your new and changing roles in life as parents.

Exercise: together and separately.

Diet: ensure you have a good range of easy but nutritious food.

Sleep: remember that rest is far more important than an immaculate house!

Zest

Having a new baby can bring enormous pleasure, and that can help you through the times when you are tired. Create your own feel-good list so that you can turn to that when things get hard:

- What do you love to see, hear, smell, touch and taste? You can choose one thing off the list or if it's possible do all five things at once and see how you feel.

Altogether

Having a baby is a very special time which can be made easier if a 'team' approach is used. Share your new baby with trusted friends and relatives, who will be only too happy to get to know the new baby, leaving the parents with time for themselves and each other. There is more than one way to change a nappy, so be gracious and appreciative of help.

Kindness

Mental health and wellbeing starts with the simplest of all virtues – simple acts of kindness help everyone. A smile, a hug, just passing a bib can all make a positive difference. As a new mum (again), remember to be kind to yourself and treat yourself as you would your best friend.

If your mental health does suffer, remember that perinatal mental illnesses are treatable, you have support and a 'sisterhood' and you will get better if you take proactive steps.

REFERENCES

1. www.time-to-change.org.uk/
2. http://cdn.netmums.com/assets/files/2013/Boots_Perinatal_Mental_Health_9.10.13_WEB_2.pdf
3. www.tommys.org/file/Wellbeingplan.pdf
4. www.neweconomics.org/projects/entry/five-ways-to-well-being
5. www.nhs.uk/Conditions/stress-anxiety-depression/Pages/improve-mental-wellbeing.aspx
6. www.powerofwho.com/
7. Daley AJ, et al. The role of exercise in treating postpartum depression: a review of the literature. *J Midwifery Womens Health.* 2007; **52**(1): 56–62. Available at: www.ncbi.nlm.nih.gov/pubmed/17207752
8. www.uppitysciencechick.com/exercise.pdf
9. http://baycitystrollers.com.au/
10. www.nhs.uk/Conditions/pregnancy-and-baby/pages/keeping-fit-and-healthy.aspx

11. www.amazon.co.uk/New-Baby-You-Postnatal-Happiness/dp/1481912232/
12. www.headspace.com/headspace-meditation-app
13. www.nhs.uk/Conditions/stress-anxiety-depression/Pages/mindfulness.aspx
14. http://psychcentral.com/blog/archives/2012/12/29/the-benefits-of-mindfulness-in-early-parenting/
15. http://oxfordmindfulness.org/wp-content/uploads/Hughes-et-al-Mindfulness-Childbirth-Final-published-article.pdf
16. http://oxfordmindfulness.org/about/faqs/mental-health-resources/
17. Warriner S, Williams M, Bardacke N, *et al.* A mindfulness approach to antenatal preparation. *BJM.* 2012; **20**(3): 194–8.
18. www.mindthebump.org.au/
19. www.overcoming.co.uk/single.htm?ipg=6320
20. www.nhs.uk/conditions/stress-anxiety-depression/pages/self-help-therapies.aspx
21. www.mentalhealth.org.uk/help-information/podcasts/
22. www.llttf.com/
23. www.beststart.org/resources/ppmd/DepressionWorkbookFinal_15APR30.pdf
24. www.getselfhelp.co.uk/freedownloads2.htm
25. Griffiths KM, Mackinnon AJ, Crisp DA, *et al.* The effectiveness of an online support group for members of the community with depression: a randomized controlled trial. *PLoS ONE.* 2013; **7**(12): e53244. O'Mahen H. Internet Therapy may help postnatal depression. *Psychol Sci.* 2013.
26. www.exeter.ac.uk/news/research/title_174561_en.html
27. www.mindhealthconnect.org.au/online-self-help-programs
28. http://appcrawlr.com/ios-apps/best-apps-second-pregnancy
29. www.kcl.ac.uk/ioppn/news/records/2014/November/phone-app-to-strengthen-parents-engagement-with-health-services.aspx
30. www.bestbeginnings.org.uk/phone-apps
31. https://itunes.apple.com/us/app/positive-pregnancy-andrew/id349477846?mt=8&ign-mpt=uo%3D4
32. www.nhs.uk/conditions/pregnancy-and-baby/pages/smoking-pregnant.aspx#close
33. www.uppitysciencechick.com/can_fats_make_you_happy.pdf
34. www.bspg.com.au/dam/bsg/product?client=BEYONDBLUE&prodid=BL/0353&type=file
35. http://easyloss.co.uk/virtual-gastric-band/ and https://itunes.apple.com/gb/app/virtual-gastric-band-hypnosis/id504835984?mt=8
36. Conrad P, Adams C. The effects of clinical aromatherapy for anxiety and depression in the high risk postpartum woman – a pilot study. *Complement Ther Clin Pract.* 2012; **18**(3): 164–8.
37. www.britishhomeopathic.org/bha-charity/how-we-can-help/conditions-a-z/postnatal-depression-2/
38. www.help-me-natural-health.com/post_natal_depression.html
39. www.ncbi.nlm.nih.gov/pubmed/22789792
40. http://postpregnancywellness.com/
41. www.namihelps.org/assets/Word-Docs/PPDComplementaryTreatments-Handout.doc
42. www.womens-health-advice.com/postpartum-depression/natural-treatment.html
43. www.staffs.ac.uk/news/alternative-tapping-technique-good-for-mental-health.jsp

44. http://healthpsych.psy.vanderbilt.edu/laughter.htm
45. www.winmentalhealth.com/self_help_psychology_16_keys.php
46. www.beststart.org/resources/ppmd/circles_of_support_manual_2013.pdf
47. www.beststart.org/resources/ppmd/supporting_parents_modules.html
48. http://thinkgp.com.au/beyondblue

FURTHER RESOURCES AND READING

- www.mentalhealth.org.uk/help-information/mental-health-a-z/M/mindfulness/ A limited amount of research into mindfulness during pregnancy has shown encouraging results on the positive impact of mindfulness, finding 'significantly' reduced anxiety (Vieten C, Astin J. 'Effects of a mindfulness-based intervention during pregnancy on prenatal stress and mood: results of a pilot study'. *Arch Womens Ment Health.* 2008; **11**(1): 67–74.).

- Antenatal mindfulness intervention to reduce depression, anxiety and stress: a pilot randomised controlled trial of the MindBabyBody programme in an Australian tertiary maternity hospital. This pilot study was designed to explore the feasibility of a randomised controlled trial of a mindfulness intervention to reduce antenatal depression, anxiety and stress. www.chimat.org.uk/resource/view.aspx?RID=221621&src=pimh

- Hypnotherapy Directory (www.hypnotherapy-directory.org.uk) was launched to connect individuals with qualified professionals in the UK. They offer information about what hypnotherapy is, how it can help, upcoming events, articles written by professionals and the latest hypnotherapy news.

- Holmes J. *Chill Pill Hypnosis: weight loss, relaxation and mindfulness stress reduction.* Available at: https://itunes.apple.com/gb/app/chill-pill-hypnosis-weight/id918930867?mt=8

- http://pinnacletherapy.co.uk/issues-and-therapies/stress-management-therapy-in-london/

CHAPTER 30

Arts and creativity for easing perinatal mental distress

Creativity is allowing yourself to make mistakes. Art is knowing which ones to keep.

Scott Adams

MY HOBBIES THAT HELP ME THROUGH TIMES OF CRISIS

Art and I have always been a distance apart from each other! My proudest art picture was a swirly picture of pink and purple crayon lines whilst at infant school. I did play the cello for a number of years – painfully for anyone listening. The only time I sing (badly) is in the audience at a concert or by myself in the privacy of my car. Yet I do have two skills that could be considered as arts and they are creative. I write and I knit (not simultaneously). Almost subconsciously I used both of these to help me when my mental health was challenged. Now they are part of my tool kit when I am aware of having some healing to do, at any level. What are yours and what can you encourage others to do?

As a little girl I loved to come downstairs in the morning and find a number of knitted dolls clothes that my mum had lovingly made for me the night before. Her mother and auntie had taught her the skills years earlier and in time she passed them onto me. As a pregnant lady I loved to spend my evenings with my knitting needles creating a large selection of white items for my unborn child. It helped me to relax and as I love to be busy I got pleasure and pride from my achievements whilst 'just sitting'. To this day I have the same hobby and can justify autumnal Saturday evenings watching reality television talent shows if I have a knitted garment to show for it! As my postnatal depression spiralled down I could no longer knit – I found that I could not concentrate and also began to negatively feel that there was little point making anything for my son because he would grow out of it. He would not like it. I would make mistakes in the pattern. Sitting down evaded me. For a while my creativity vanished.

When I began to respond to treatment in the psychiatric ward, knitting was one of the things that helped my recovery. It was twofold, because I taught another young mum how to do it. She was being treated for her alcoholism and told me one day that she would love to make her little girl some dolls clothes when she saw me knitting. I asked my mum to bring us more wool, needles and patterns and we spent hours on the ward creating dolls clothes. I felt better for having helped another patient and in doing so I began to learn to sit and be creative again.

The second creative way I have naturally used when I am emotional is writing. As a child I used to write letters to myself if I was upset. I would commit the words to paper, have a cry, rip it up and then feel much better! During my recovery from puerperal psychosis my psychiatric nurse used to encourage me to keep a journal so we could begin to track my ups and downs and identify triggers or patterns and, most importantly, ways that I found to lift my mood and manage my life better. That still helps today. I realised when writing my first book that the process of putting down all of my thoughts, feelings and descriptions of my life at that time really helped. I found that it 'got rid' of many negative thoughts and it was a good way to keep happy ones. When I first wrote it, I knew that even if it went no further than me, it was worthwhile. The fact that it has helped many is a wonderful bonus. When my partner died, I knowingly used writing my blog[1] as a method of getting through each day – or even an hour.

THE HISTORICAL AND ACADEMIC BACKGROUND TO USING ARTS AND CREATIVITY

Not long after my book was published in 2005 I attended an event where Dr Hilary Marland from Warwick University gave a fascinating presentation about treatments of puerperal psychosis in the Victorian era. Knitting and writing were mentioned back then as suggested activities, amongst others. In the 1870s the Scottish alienist Thomas Clouston described recovery from 'puerperal mania', and therefore redemption, thus:[2]

> In a month she will be knitting a stocking, and will know her friends when they come to see her. Within three months she is well – a joyous mother, in her right mind, clasping her child, the whole of the disturbed mental period seeming like a dream to her, that is very soon altogether forgotten in her new duties and delights … few things are more pleasant than to see the restoration of the mother back to all that makes her life worth having.

Dr Marland has written a book, *Dangerous Motherhood: insanity and child-birth in Victorian Britain.*[3] This makes fascinating reading.

In August 1832 Sara Coleridge, daughter of the poet Samuel Taylor Coleridge, gave birth to her second child, and shortly afterwards wrote in her diary of her pains, bowel complaints, 'wretched spirits', 'nervous terror' and 'hysteria'. She went on to write many poems. According to Marland, in the nineteenth century:

> treatment consisted primarily of isolation from the family and new born, rest and quiet, building up the women with nutritious diet and tonics, light purgatives, and encouraging patients to occupy themselves. Heroic remedies were on the whole derided. For poor women, the asylum may have functioned as a refuge, a place where they could rest, receive proper food and a break from the hardships of their lives – and asylum superintendents often framed their care in these terms – and for all women, the gentle therapeutic regime may have allowed them a period of respite, a break from household duties and mothering. In a few cases, like that of Sara Coleridge, it offered the chance to follow more meaningful and creative pursuits; in her case literary work. Gooch, whose methods of treatment were taken up by many doctors, stressed the need to 'procure sleep at night' and 'to manage the mind of the patient, soothing it during irritation, encouraging it during depression, never to attempt the removal of her delusions by argument. I would rather allow a patient to think her legs were made of straw, and her body of glass, than dispute either proposition'. At one level this sounds terribly patronising, but it also outlines a regime of patience, carefulness and non-interference.

So what is the basis for using arts and creativity as an aid to good mental health? For me it was the advantages of sitting still, feeling I was producing something useful and I guess it also made me relax physically. It helped me manage my mind and soothe my irritation, as Marland described above. Although I refer to the mother in this chapter, it can also apply to the father and to the family unit.

An article written by Danielle Leigh[4] about ways in which art and creative therapy can help ladies suffering from postnatal depression reassures that this approach is about expressing your feelings through a therapeutic process – it is not about filling an art gallery. She states that it is a way to express hidden feelings and emotions that may be too overwhelming to deal with. 'Art therapy helps to put them in perspective, and to press the "deflate" button simply by bringing them into conscious awareness.' It offers an escape and relaxation from the daily chores, and if done in a group setting can help create new friendships.

Specific research around the use of creative arts with maternal mental health has been reported by C. Perry. *et al.* in 'Time for Me: the arts as therapy in postnatal depression':[5]

Time for Me describes a creative arts group for mothers with children under two years of age, who were experiencing mild to moderate postnatal depression or anxiety. Work in various areas of mental healthcare suggests that creative arts can be used to complement conventional therapy and that complementary therapies may be a valuable adjunct to conventional interventions for women with postnatal depression and anxiety.

USING HOBBIES AND THE CREATIVE ARTS TO AID RECOVERY

There are examples of good practice in some parts of the UK. For example, in Radstock, Somerset there is a group called My Time, My Space, which they describe as 'supportive creative workshops for women with PND'.[6] They say that:

> we have discovered that when women work together with an artist, take part in creative and artistic activities … women are able to creatively express themselves, make new friends, gain peer support, promote their well-being, and have fun.

Other examples of such groups are in Bath[7] and Halton.[8] The range of creative activities is vast. Using arts and creative skills can be done in a more formal group, either specifically focused on mental health or, if you are well enough, join classes or groups run locally for the public. These activities can also be done individually. Find out what is available locally. If there is nothing, consider making something happen. In Morley, Leeds, I was asked by a member of a church if they could do anything to help mothers in their area. We held an evening at the church and invited relevant people to attend. Out of that a regular art group was created for local mothers to help their mental health. The neighbouring Children's Centre offered crèche facilities; a trained group facilitator ran the art group with the mothers; the church was used as a venue and members of the congregation volunteered their time and practical support. No further monies were needed. What can you make happen in your area as either a healthcare professional or parent?

In Australia, new mother Hiromi Tango, along with the emotional turmoil of her early days of motherhood, also witnessed the environmental catastrophe in the form of massive dust storms that engulfed Brisbane and Sydney in September 2009.[9] As a thick blanket of dust turned the sky orange, Tango ventured out into the unbreathable air wrapped in a tangle of colourful fabrics, threads and material, which she documented in her 'Insanity Magnet' series of photographs and video. Five years later, those images of Tango in an apocalyptic landscape form the basis of *Dust Storm* at the Australian Centre for Photography. Hiromi says:

> Art has helped me to recover from certain times when I was having difficulties and has helped me cope with memories and emotions. I really enjoy art but maybe

more than that, if you have art in your life, it is easier to get through any difficult time.

Sometimes creativity during poor maternal mental health can launch a new career. Angie Stevens began to draw and blog when she had three small children. She told the *Guardian* newspaper:

> Drawing was how she rediscovered who she was after years of mothering – spending every second looking after others. 'You lose your identity. It's such a cliché to say that, but you need to find out who you are. You go for years not sleeping because you love them but you wonder how you fit into this. You look in the mirror and don't recognise yourself any more. What I've discovered through doing this is that I'm still me.'[10]

Angie still writes a very successful blog and has published a book with her cartoon drawings of family life, *Doodlemum: a year of family life*, published by Two Roads.[11]

Many women have written blogs about their mental health challenges as an expectant or new mother. In America, Katherine Stone began to write her blog just over 10 years ago to offer support and information around maternal mental health. It is now an award-winning site at www.postpartumprogress. com/ You can find some other top blogs listed at The Circle of Moms website.[12]

Another mum, Rachel,[13] was featured by Time to Change for her blog http://mummykindness.com/ Rachel writes:

> There will always be someone better at something than me. And you, too. There will be more inspiring writers, better dancers and funnier raconteurs. There will certainly be better singers. But, do you know what? I think we should sing anyway. Dance anyway. Write anyway. **Just … do it anyway.**
>
> Because someone, somewhere needs to hear your song, to feel your music. They need you to make them smile today. Or start a conversation. Or lend a shaky hand. Other people might be better qualified. More polished. More confident than you. Do it anyway. Smile at somebody. Make eye contact. Say hello. **Do it anyway.**
>
> But, but … what if you're not enough? **Just … do it anyway.**
>
> Life is hard. Harder for some than others. Weathering storms makes us more grateful for calmer waters when they eventually arrive. We learn to somehow stay afloat. Sometimes by clinging on for dear life to the nearest buoyant object, thrashing about and gasping for air. But what if each storm is pushing us forward? Teaching us to swim and not sink? To use our survival skills to build a raft? A raft to lift others out of the depths, to offer sanctuary and somewhere safe and dry for those who are frantically treading water behind us?
>
> It's connection that keeps us going. Support from others when we can barely stand, never mind swim.

On reflection, this is what I did when I taught a fellow patient in the psychiatric ward to knit and also when I blogged so regularly whilst grieving.

Some mothers have begun to regularly use social media, such as Facebook and Twitter, as a means of connection to help themselves and others through a challenging time. Rosey has created a weekly chat @PNDandMe for mothers and also writes in her blog at http://pndandme.wordpress.com/

Another popular form of creativity that can aid mood changing is music. I certainly use it as a medium to match or improve my mood as it is so closely linked to our emotions. At times if I want to allow myself to wallow in a sad place I shall purposefully play sad music. If I am feeling stressed or down and I want to change that mindset, I shall choose some music accordingly. Remember to keep listening out for the new perinatal music currently being composed and played by Jennie Muskett: www.withyouintheworld.com/index.html

Music can also be a personal or group choice. An all-women choir called Maternal Harmony, from Bridgend, South Wales, got together to support each other and raise awareness of PND/PTSD after childbirth.[14] They say that 'the choir boosts confidence and gives women some "me time", providing them with a sense of belonging.'

Also take a look at www.thegoodenoughmumsclub.com/ for a musical based on early motherhood.

In her thesis, 'The Effectiveness of Early-Intervention Music Therapy for a Mother with Postnatal Depression and her Family',[15] Rozana Whiteley cites:

> McMahon *et al.* (2005) observed that many women entirely stopped attending interventions that were directly related to depression, as they highlighted the condition that they were trying to be released from, which made them feel more restricted. This could indicate that it may beneficial for the focus of an intervention to be more creative, so as to give the mother a sense of enjoyment, and even an end product, which may provide an increased sense of achievement.

She continues to say that:

> Participants noted that music could be more accessible than words and therefore could be used as an alternative to increase communication between family members and to surface deeper and more hidden emotions which may resolve issues of the past. Music was also seen as a method for relaxation and to promote well-being, which was deemed to be important for women and their families when anxiety and stress levels were higher in the postnatal period.

For professionals, if you need further evidence or ideas of how creativity can help mental health, have a look at some of the preview pages[16] online taken from Le Navenec and Bridges book, *Creating Connections between Nursing*

Care and the Creative Arts Therapies: expanding the concept of holistic care.[17] A seven-year review of the effectiveness of Time 4U, a therapeutic group for women with postnatal depression, has been published too.[18]

Just because you have a diagnosis of poor mental health or you are striving to make it better, it is not a prescription to eliminate pleasure in your life. Quite the opposite in fact – you should actively seek and identify ways to bring and maintain joy. Those who support you should also encourage you to do these things.

> Each time a woman stands up for herself, without knowing it possibly, without claiming it, she stands up for all women.
>
> Maya Angelou

As this book is aimed at people who already have a child or children, I can hear some of the comments along the lines of 'You want me to sit and sew whilst I have a toddler at my feet and a baby on my breast?!' In the ideal world, of course, it would be wonderful to simply take yourself off for some 'me time' to be creative. If there is an organised group that you can attend, see where you can arrange child cover. Remember my suggestion that people do like to be asked and to be helpful? It may be possible for you to get that time. If you have a partner, suggest that you create specific 'daddy' time slots each week when he takes the children to do something fun, e.g. walk to the park, visit to his parents. That gives you the chance to focus on something for you whilst they enjoy time together. Also consider what activities you can do together as a family.

Another suggestion would be to include the children in the activity. My 5-year-old niece loves all of the creative activities and will spend hours with her grandma, sticking, painting, making bracelets, singing, etc. In recent years there has been a move towards acknowledging the therapeutic value of adult colouring books, with a growing number available to buy. Here are some other ideas:

- gardening
- dancing
- cooking, baking
- bead work and jewellery making
- making jam
- going to the library for story time then choosing new books to loan
- collage
- getting messy – have you tried mixing cornflour and water?
- make a den!
- scrapbooking
- card making
- film and photography.

One mum suggests that a good way to get your chores done is to tell your older child that you will 'craft' for so long then alternate with a task, e.g. 'whilst glue dries we'll hang out the washing'. It is good for children to learn how to sort washing and put things away, etc. as they will have to do it for themselves one day. Make it fun by putting music on! On the other hand, ask what is more important, some quality time for yourself and family or that dusting? Perhaps it is more about managing your expectation of yourself, rather than time management.

It may be that your pets are good for you. One mum told me that being with her collection of reptiles, including snakes, made her feel relaxed! A study published in November 2014 concluded that 'Pet therapy significantly reduced anxiety and depression in antepartum hospitalized women with high-risk pregnancies.'[19]

If you still need some inspiration, look at *101 Hobbies for Mom*.[20] Katie Norris describes some most unusual suggestions include being a secret shopper, doing puzzles and playing Bingo! She also says:

> I discovered that when I got back to my own identity, I became a much better and happier mom. Every mom needs a hobby. We need something we are passionate about, that can feed our individual souls so that we can embrace life. Our kids benefit from seeing Mom have a special talent or interest.

So what are you going to do? Stop looking for reasons why you cannot do something artistic and creative and look for reasons why and how you can.

TOP TIPS FOR PARENTS ON USING ARTS AND CREATIVITY IN THE PERINATAL PERIOD

1. Remember that perinatal mental illness can get better.
2. Even back in Victorian times, creative activities were recommended to help women to 'soothe their mind'.
3. The use of arts and creativity is as a means of expressing hidden thoughts and feelings – it is not about filling an art gallery.
4. They can be relaxing, a means of escapism, provide a sense of achievement through producing tangible items, and bring people together.
5. Arts and creative activities are vast – the choice is personal and can be done as a formal 'therapy' group, community lesson or at an individual level.
6. Some women have found that their activity started in the perinatal period has led to a new career or outcome, e.g. published book.
7. Use simple acts to make connections that benefit everyone involved.
8. Make arrangements to free you some time to enjoy your chosen activities.

TOP TIPS FOR HEALTHCARE PROFESSIONALS ON USING ARTS AND CREATIVITY IN THE PERINATAL PERIOD

1. Remind sufferers that just because they may have a diagnosis of poor mental health, it does not mean they are unable to have pleasure in their lives. It does give them a reason to actively find ways to smile again.

2. If you need to have further clinical evidence-based research, look at the suggested references.

3. Find out what is available in your locality for offering to families and individuals, e.g. by healthcare and third sector agencies along with community events.

4. Make a point of asking parents what hobbies and activities they usually enjoy, and discover ways they may be able to continue them.

5. What do you do for yourself in arts and creative activity? Read the final quote above by Katie again – what are you passionate about?

REFERENCES

1. www.hanzak.com/blog specifically February 2011 to February 2012.
2. Marland H. *Maternity and Madness: puerperal insanity in the nineteenth century.* Warwick: Centre for the History of Medicine, University of Warwick; 2003. Available at: www.nursing.manchester.ac.uk/ukchnm/publications/seminarpapers/maternityand madness.pdf
3. www.amazon.co.uk/Dangerous-Motherhood-Insanity-Childbirth-Victorian/dp/1403 920389
4. http://mindfulmysticmama.com/art-therapy-heals-postnatal-depression/
5. www.ncbi.nlm.nih.gov/pubmed/18243941
6. www.creativityworks.org.uk/what-we-do/for-mental-health/my-time-my-space/
7. www.bathnes.gov.uk/services/your-council-and-democracy/local-research-and-statistics/wiki/postnatal-depression
8. www.haltonlikeminds.co.uk/support-services-for-postnatal-depression/
9. www.smh.com.au/entertainment/art-and-design/hiromi-tango-finds-relief-from-postnatal-depression-in-her-craft-20140519-zrh1w.html
10. Doodlemum www.guardian.co.uk/lifeandstyle/2013/mar/06/drawing-family-helped-my-postnatal-depression
11. www.tworoadsbooks.com/books/doodlemum/
12. www.circleofmoms.com/top25/top-postpartum-depression-mom-blogs-2012
13. www.time-to-change.org.uk/blog/dealing-postnatal-depression-blogging-helped
14. https://twitter.com/MaternalHarmony
15. www.musability.co.uk/PNDresearch1.pdf
16. http://books.google.co.uk/books?id=N9O2rU9eYNsC&pg=PA141&lpg=PA141&dq=creative+arts+for+postnatal+depression&source=bl&ots=wSOG21O58R&sig=yHAarsIqfOhYR-yrLUvD4psbd6Q&hl=en&sa=X&ei=sZ7OU4qfIsi00QW14IDYCw&ved=0CFAQ6AEwCA#v=onepage&q=creative%20arts%20for%20postnatal%20depression&f=false

17. Le Navenec C-L, Bridges L. *Creating Connections Between Nursing Care and the Creative Arts Therapies: expanding the concept of holistic care.* Springfield, IL: Charles C Thomas; 2005.
18. www.ingentaconnect.com/content/cp/cp/2014/00000087/00000009/art00008
19. Lynch CE, Magann EF, Barringer SN, *et al.* Pet therapy program for antepartum high-risk pregnancies: a pilot study. *J Perinatol.* 2014; **34**: 816–18. Available at: www.chimat.org.uk/resource/view.aspx?RID=218823&src=pimh
20. www.mommywithselectivememory.com/2012/08/101-hobbies-for-mom.html

CHAPTER 31

And finally ...

The past is a source of knowledge and the future is a source of hope.

Stephen Ambrose

As we have arrived at the end of the book, I thought I would close by sharing some of the comments of lived experience by other people who have contemplated or succeeded in having another child after a previous perinatal mental health challenge. I hope that these may assist you in whichever decision you make or help others with. I asked the respondents of my survey for their top three tips to share with people. We have already covered them and I use them here as reminders. Here are some of the clear areas they recommend for action and their general comments.

PARTNER AND FAMILY

- Be in the right relationship.
- Are you and your partner strong enough to press for help if needed?
- Ensure that your relationship is a good supportive one.
- Make sure your partner and family are supportive and discuss warning signs/ red flags.
- Tell everyone around how bad it gets and they will look for you slipping.
- My husband says that regarding the decision to have another baby, he trusted my judgement on taking the risk, and was reassured by all the support that we'd be able to access if the worst happened again.
- Tell as many friends and family that you can about the mental health risks you'll face, let them know what support you'd find helpful from them, and tell them what to look out for as signs that you may be getting unwell or struggling to cope. Please don't let stigma stand in the way of being open with people.

TALK

- Speak to family and friends and tell them what you need and don't want.
- To talk to a professional about fears and feelings.
- Talk to your GP early; talk to your midwife; speak to your health visitor.
- Shout loudly! Make yourself heard.

PLAN

- There is help out there. Find it and put steps into place to access it quickly for when you need it. A bit like having a fire extinguisher close by a barbecue. You don't want to waste time having to look for one.
- Make plans for if it does happen but don't assume that it will.
- Plan, speak to a medical professional to help you plan throughout pregnancy, birth and after.
- Identify the right set of professionals (psychiatrist, etc.) and talk to them before and, if necessary, throughout pregnancy so they know you and can be ready to intervene if they need to.
- Prepare solutions to the problems you experienced first time, e.g. line up expert (e.g. breastfeeding support).
- Prepare your health professional team.
- Ensure you have a medical support team in place, e.g. your consultant or counsellor to discuss feelings.
- Co-operate with professionals and accept their help and input.
- Be confident to request anything (healthcare related) that you know will make you feel more comfortable and do not take no for an answer. If you do not look out for yourself, you cannot guarantee that anyone else will.

KNOWLEDGE

- Seek help before symptoms start.
- Make a diary of previous feelings.
- Find ways to prevent or limit similar damage next time.
- Identify any areas that trigger lows and plan to minimise them.

PRE-CONCEPTION

- The urge to have a child is huge, if you have that urge then talk to your GP and ask for a referral to someone in the perinatal mental health team. You don't want to get to the menopause and have regrets that you never even properly considered it. If it's right for you to stop and go no further then you will know you made an informed decision.

- Explore your previous issues thoroughly.
- Seek CBT/counselling before and after.
- Only do it if you feel ready.
- Talk to a psychologist to help you come to terms with your previous experience.
- Make sure you've completely got over it – it does bring back memories, and you need to be mentally strong to deal with them.
- See a psychiatrist before conception or while pregnant.

ASK

- As soon as you begin feeling poorly, seek immediate help.
- Seek help early if things start to deteriorate.
- Ask for help – be honest.
- Monitor your mood before and after the birth and be honest with professionals if you notice any signs of relapse in your mental health.
- Consider adoption.

MEDICATION

- To consider a safe medication.
- Consider medication during pregnancy if you need it.
- Weigh up the risks of meds and pregnancy carefully and make an informed decision.
- Stay on or change medication accordingly.
- Seriously consider how important breastfeeding the new baby is to you, thinking about the potential impact on your mental health and bonding with the baby. When you've made the decision whether to do it or not plan any medications accordingly with specialist medical advice.

SUPPORT

- Surround yourself with support and be realistic that it could happen again, but be confident that you can get through it like you did before.
- Do you know where to get help if needed?
- Have a list of specific help, i.e. emotional, practical, child care, housework, errands, etc.
- Find local support groups.
- Make a list of support sources with contact numbers.

- Have a network of family and friends as well as your health professional around you who you tell your story and tell them to ask and check on you regularly.

ATTITUDE

- Stay relaxed.
- Be 100% transparent about your feelings or anxieties. It makes a huge difference to have people on side.
- Keep positive.
- Take people's opinions with a pinch of salt – when they walk a day in your shoes then they can judge.
- Rest as much as you can before and after birth. Rest when baby rests, thinking of your own health too.
- Don't overbook visitors or activities for the first few weeks after the birth. Sleep really has to be your top priority.
- Look after yourself, and give yourself a break. The washing up can wait!
- Make more time for YOU; after all mommy holds the family together xx.
- Be very, very prepared and allow yourself to enjoy *this* pregnancy.
- Have faith in yourself.

What did you or would you do differently in your next pregnancy knowing that your mental health may be at risk?	
Mother	• Make more time for myself.
	• Sleep when baby does.
	• Attend CBT.
	• Was kinder to myself.
	• Be more open with some people about how I'm feeling.
	• Identified and used coping strategies.
Charity and community support	• Online and telephone support for someone to chat with – a kind of 'anchor person' to touch base with, every day, even with just a chat. Just someone to listen, to understand, be sympathetic and caring and giving me hope.
	• Practical support – ask for it and accept it graciously.
	• I joined a children's centre.
Family and friends	• My husband took more time off work.
	• I was able to talk to my husband about my feelings.
	• Put things in to place to care for first child if I was admitted again.
	• Arrange babysitting on a regular basis.
	• Talked with and prepared my family – asked for and accepted help.
	• Prepared a checklist of who could help in what way – practical helpers, emotional helpers. Discussed my warning signs for others to look out for.

(continued)

	What did you or would you do differently in your next pregnancy knowing that your mental health may be at risk?
Lifestyle	• Took more maternity leave, was more prepared, no one was allowed to touch my changing bag so I was prepared to leave the house with less delays. • No building work this time! • We moved to a more accessible property.
Healthcare professionals	• Put in support, made people listen. • Saw a psychologist pre-birth and a psychiatrist. • I asked for help antenatally but never got it. Afterwards I made sure they took me seriously straight away – I KNEW what it was and couldn't be fobbed off. • I was on medication. I think this helped. • I had to seek help and be admitted to the mother and baby unit despite not wanting to as I knew what I was suffering from. Previous to the birth I ensured everything was ready and organised for the birth. • Pushed for a referral to a psychiatrist while pregnant who told me he felt I was already getting depressed again and that getting PND was almost a dead cert. He recommended I go on antidepressants at about 30 weeks and stay on them forever! • Talked with and prepared my GP.
Birth	• The elective Caesarean was the main difference, and gave me the feeling of control that I needed. It also meant that my partner felt he could be present and I needed him there.
Knowledge	• I did nothing differently, I just knew what it was and actively sought help. • I did not read any books so that my instinct could be nurtured. • I planned my self-care before, during and after the pregnancy in great detail. I readied everything I would need in advance. I made sure my husband knew what to look for in me. I confided in friends and gave them my 'what to do' file, and I made sure everyone knew what had happened before and what I needed this time. I accessed in advance all the holistic care I knew I would need. Finally I did many things I knew would help to relax and prepare me and the household for the baby's arrival.
Attitude	• Nothing – I still insist my PND was hormone related and the lack of support made it worse. • More relaxed definitely.

There were a number of factors that parents felt helped particularly with the subsequent perinatal period:

- Knowing what to expect and knowing some triggers and signs.
- Being more organised – all of the prep was instrumental.
- Remaining on medication throughout /sooner – the medication made a huge difference before, during and after the birth. Drugs – drugs help a lot!!

- Being given CBT.
- Easier birth /planned C-section.
- Much more realistic expectations of newborns and their needs.
- Support from mental health team, midwives, GP, health visitor and family.
- Being taken seriously. I knew it would happen again, it was nice to find some-one who believed me. The difference between doing it all with and without the depressive symptoms is unbelievable!
- Transparency about my feelings with my husband, making him feel involved in my experiences and as much rest as possible.
- Being happy with husband.
- Relaxation – I had free reflexology from someone training to do it once a week and it helped me sleep afterwards – I have a big fear around not sleeping.
- Thanks to not reading, I am relaxed in going with my baby and not trying to conform to schedules, track milestones too closely etc.
- Nothing – it was going to happen regardless.
- Taking the baby out.
- Being admitted. Knowing that it DOES END. You DO get better. First time around that was the worst thing – you really do think that is you forever.

Here is a comment about the importance and influence healthcare professionals can have:

- HCPs can play a vital role in stopping things spiralling out of control when all does not go to plan. They really can make a difference. Many things contributed to me being unwell in the first place – lack of sleep, protracted labour, our baby getting stuck in labour etc. However, I am certain that 2 things could have been done to prevent me from being unwell, i.e.
  1. I was left in labour too long. (I had to flag up to the midwife that I had 'reached the end of the road' and could not continue to labour on my own)
  2. I needed a blood transfusion earlier than I got one.

  However, I am certain that the thing that tipped me over the edge from being unwell into paranoia, fear, terror and psychosis was the way I was looked after post-partum. These are controversial comments I know and this is only my perspective but I feel that with sensitivity, understanding, reassurance and some explanation of what had happened and how I was feeling, my decline into full-blown psychosis could have been prevented. The overriding feeling I have of the first few months of my daughter's life is absolute terror. I know many other mothers will feel robbed of this precious time too. This makes me feel incredibly sad. I hope that my comments and candid feedback will help the mums of the future avoid feeling like I did.

There are some wonderful healthcare professionals who are dedicated to the care of the families within their role. I applaud the work that they do and I trust that services will continue to develop and grow to assist people who wish to add to their families, or otherwise. Where I have highlighted examples of where and how care could have been improved, I do so in the light of learning and progress.

> We shall draw from the heart of suffering itself the means of inspiration and survival.
>
> Winston Churchill

I asked those who had another child if they had ever regretted it. All of them said no, with some additional thoughts and feelings.

- No – it's still the best decision.
- No! I am grateful every day for having my son, even or especially that he came along when he did.
- No. But I think my husband would still prefer not to have had a second, though he loves her for herself.
- No. I still would have done it. My son means the world to me and he was more than worth the months of illness, as my daughter is.
- Now he's here, I love my second son to bits and don't regret having him, but in hindsight I was so unwell this pregnancy (and am still struggling) that I don't think it was a wise decision. I guess I had to go through it this second time to know that I definitely won't put myself through it again.
- No. I never regretted having William. I do feel sad that I had to stop at 2 but that's what is best for me and my boys (not to mention I don't have anyone to father one anymore!!).
- While I was ill I regretted having another child but that was because my first child was my focus but this quickly stopped.
- If it didn't just happen as a surprise I probably wouldn't have had any more because I was so worried about getting the postnatal illness again.
- No, although my son has ASD and ADHD which presents massive challenges for all of us plus I had a second bout of PND, I could never regret the birth of my precious boy.
- I am so pleased it happened as I got to experience what having a baby can feel like.

GENERAL REFLECTIONS

- Remember all pregnancies are different.
- It won't nearly be the same story this time.

- Second time around can be very healing – but the flipside is that you realise even more how much you missed first time.
- Don't give up on your dream for another child. Don't let the risk destroy that.
- It might not happen again, I've met people who it didn't happen to next time around, but if it does you have the huge advantage that you have wrestled with this beast before and come out the other side. You know you are not actually going mad, that you will one day feel 'okay' again and that this is an illness and you will recover. This puts you at a huge advantage compared to people who suddenly find themselves in this strange land with no idea where they are or how to get back 'home'.
- Look at the bigger picture. The future following the illness you will have a beautiful new addition for the rest of your life.
- Not only is postpartum psychosis a risk, but you might find it hard to cope all the way until the child is five and more independent. Just wait to have children. Take your time. Everything changes after a baby and there's no going back.
- You have to be sure of your motivation to want another baby, and be honest with yourself. Is it just to assuage history and put the past right? I feel very strongly that as per my GP's advice, you have to consider the impact and views of the entire family – partner, other children.
- I think my first child was a huge lifestyle change and this added to my depression. Even in prenatal stages and I think this may have been one of the reasons my depression was worse. With the second child my lifestyle was already more family dominated and so my postnatal depression better although was still bad during pregnancy.
- Don't be put off from considering more children if you've always wanted a bigger family. You could feel more guilt and disappointment in the long run if you let the illness stop you, and there's a chance you could become unwell again even if you don't have another child. If you have unresolved issues about your illness seek counselling to talk these over and help you decide what's best for you regarding future children.
- I would recommend that any prospective 2nd time parents have full and frank discussions about coping and MH before conceiving another child. We did this and when we conceived our second my husband had a good idea of how things might go wrong, and I had a good idea of how I would recognise the signs and support myself, and enable him to support me. I also prepared trusted friends and family, gave out lists of numbers and names who to contact if they had concerns. I found it extremely helpful and reassuring and I know my husband was infinitely more aware – and much more confident. I strongly feel that the result of all this prep (which, in all, took a year to finalise) was that my second time was so much calmer and more reassured than the first.
- Although I have suffered this awful cruel illness twice and been to the darkest depths of despair, my children and partner are the light of my life and the year I

suffered following their births is nothing compared to the life of happiness these children give me every day. I adore them and feel a stronger person than ever.

No one but you and your partner have the right to say that you should or should not have another child. There is no guarantee that you will be able to. I set out to assist you, or in you helping others, to decide if the risks to their mental health with a subsequent pregnancy are high and if so, how they can be managed. There are so many factors, as we have looked at, regarding the decision to extend a family. No pregnancy is without risk to physical or mental health, yet the human race continues to expand. I feel that in the UK we are beginning to see steps forward in the parity of esteem for both mental and physical health around pregnancy. If we continue to work together to ensure that the correct treatments and provisions are in place, we can move forward with a greater confidence that families and healthcare professionals can minimise the effects of poor perinatal mental health.

If you have reached this final chapter and you are still unclear about your decision, there is the school of thought that says you should simply do nothing. Go to bed. Sleep on it. Try not to think about it. Apparently your body/subconscious mind has the ability to process without trying. You can wear yourself out chewing things over and get nowhere. If you can stand back from it and let it go, then just maybe it will become clear. Revisit the decision at a later date.

As you have read through all the chapters perhaps you have made notes and actions, to create your unique plan to determine your decision. You may now feel confident about what to do.

Whatever you decide, I wish you peace with your decision and a lifetime of happiness with your family, no matter what size it is!

There comes a time in your life when you have to choose to turn the page, write another book or simply close it.

Shannon L Alder

Resources and further information

Here are some additional sources of information. I shall keep an up-to-date and emerging list on my website at www.hanzak.com I also add useful new examples of good practice when I blog following an event I have been to. Please let me know if there is anything you feel I should include or find broken links via elaine@hanzak.com

Although I have found these references I have not fully evaluated them and I do not accept responsibility for the information or the quality of the information contained on these sites.

Abusive relationships
- http://thisisabuse.direct.gov.uk/
- www.nhs.uk/Livewell/abuse/Pages/violence-and-sexual-assault.aspx
- www.mind.org.uk/information-support/guides-to-support-and-services/abuse/

Antenatal depression
- www.netmums.com/pregnancy/pregnancy-problems/antenatal-depression
- www.nct.org.uk/pregnancy/antenatal-depression

Antenatal anxiety
- www.moodcafe.co.uk/media/14163/AntenatalAnxiety.pdf
- http://cope.org.au/pregnancy/mental-health-conditions-pregnancy/antenatal-anxiety/

Bereavement
- www.cruse.org.uk/
- www.preg.info/PostnatalBereavementNotes/
- www.bereavementadvice.org/
- www.compassionbooks.com mail order catalogue and internet resource

centre of professional books, videos and CDs related to loss and grief for children and adults across the lifespan

- Boyd-Webb N, editor. *Helping Bereaved Children: a handbook for practitioners.* New York: Guilford Press, 2010.
- www.winstonswish.org.uk/ for bereaved children

Bipolar disorder

- www.app-network.org/
- www.blackdoginstitute.org.au/public/bipolardisorder/inpregnancypost natal.cfm

Body dysmorphic disorder

- http://my.clevelandclinic.org/services/neurological_institute/center-for-behavorial-health/disease-conditions/hic-body-dysmorphic-disorder
- www.anxietyuk.org.uk/about-anxiety/anxiety-disorder-and-stress/body-dysmorphic-disorder-bdd

Eating disorders

- http://motherscircle.net/how-pregnancy-and-postpartum-are-affected-by-eating-disorders/
- www.nice.org.uk/guidance/cg192/ifp/chapter/eating-disorders

Hormonal conditions

- www.iblamethehormones.com/index.htm
- www.studd.co.uk/depression.php

Miscarriage and loss of a baby

- www.uk-sands.org/
- www.tommys.org/page.aspx?pid=693
- www.miscarriageassociation.org.uk/ *also see* www.miscarriageassociation.org.uk/support/trying-again/
- www.pregnancyafterlosssupport.com/

Panic attacks

- www.nhs.uk/conditions/stress-anxiety-depression/pages/understanding-panic-attacks.aspx
- www.panic-attacks.co.uk/
- www.mentalhealth.org.uk/help-information/mental-health-a-z/P/panic-attacks/

Pelvic pain (pelvic girdle pain (PPGP) or symphysis pubis dysfunction (SPD))
- www.nhs.uk/conditions/pregnancy-and-baby/pages/pelvic-pain-pregnant-spd.aspx
- www.babycentre.co.uk/a546492/pelvic-pain-spd

Postnatal (postpartum) anxiety
- www.anxietyuk.org.uk/
- www.parents.com/parenting/moms/healthy-mom/the-other-postpartum-problem-anxiety/

Postnatal (postpartum) depression
- www.nhs.uk/Conditions/Postnataldepression/Pages/Introduction.aspx
- www.mind.org.uk/information-support/types-of-mental-health-problems/postnatal-depression/
- www.rcpsych.ac.uk/healthadvice/problemsdisorders/postnataldepression.aspx
- www.netmums.com/parenting-support/postnatal-depression
- https://itunes.apple.com/gb/app/ppd-gone!/id529141505?mt=8

PTSD
- www.growingyourbaby.com/2012/09/30/can-childbirth-cause-post-traumatic-stress-disorder/
- www.midwiferytoday.com/articles/healing_trauma.asp
- www.postpartum.net/learn-more/postpartum-post-traumatic-stress-disorder/

Self-harming
- http://selfharm.co.uk/home
- www.rcpsych.ac.uk/healthadvice/problemsdisorders/self-harm.aspx
- www.inourhands.com/contact/ Dr Pooky Knightsmith has a wealth of knowledge, resources and expertise in this area

Substance misuse
- www.drugscope.org.uk/resources/pregnancyguide
- www.maternal-and-early-years.org.uk/topic/pregnancy/substance-use-and-misuse-in-pregnancy
- www.bestbeginnings.org.uk/drugs
- http://help4addiction.co.uk/resources/about-alcohol/alcohol-drinks-journal
- http://help4addiction.co.uk/wp-content/uploads/2014/12/Help4 Addictions-Online-Alcohol-Journal.pdf

Suicide

- www.samaritans.org/
- http://uk-sobs.org.uk/
- www.survivorsofsuicide.com/
- www.allianceofhope.org/
- www.soslsd.org/

Underactive thyroid

- www.postpartumprogress.com/is-your-thyroid-making-you-depressed

SUPPORT GROUP INFORMATION

- Bertram L. *Supporting Postnatal Women into Motherhood: a guide to therapeutic groupwork for health professionals.* Oxford: Radcliffe; 2008. I love the basis of this book that all mothers should be able to come together in the early days of new parenthood to have the opportunity to nip anxieties in the early stages. A great preventative approach, I feel.
- www.panda.org.au/learning-with-panda/panda-resources/support-group-guide PANDA's Guide to Postnatal Depression Support Groups is a unique resource that assists in structuring the set-up, monitoring and further development of a range of different support groups for women and their families. There can be a range of activities that take place in the group depending on the purpose of the group, the resources available and the skills of the facilitators.

Have a look at www.netmums.com/local-to-you/local/index/support-groups/antenatal-postnatal-support to find (or add) what is in your area. Examples:
- Beat the Blues – Stockport www.beattheblues-stockport.co.uk
- Burnham www.thewellatlentrise.org/pndsupport.htm
- Cedar House Support group, Surrey www.postnataldepression.com/cedar-house-support-group
- Mothers for Mothers – Bristol www.mothersformothers.co.uk/
- Macclesfield www.thesmilegroup.org/

GENERAL PERINATAL SUPPORT AND INFORMATION

- The Association for Postnatal Illness http://apni.org/ can put you in touch with a trained volunteer who is experienced in talking to women with PND.
- Visit the BabyCentre community http://community.babycentre.co.uk/ to talk to other mums who know how you are feeling.
- The British Association for Counselling and Psychotherapy (BACP) www.bacp.co.uk/ website has a search facility for finding a qualified counsellor or psychotherapist in your area.

- The charity Depression Alliance www.depressionalliance.org/ produces a leaflet and runs a helpline (0845 120 6162) for anyone affected by depression during and after pregnancy.
- www.joebingleymemorialfoundation.org.uk/, an organisation that aims to help women and their families by raising awareness and providing information about postnatal depression.
- Home-Start www.home-start.org.uk/, the family support organisation, will visit you at home and offer friendship, support and practical help. It can also put you in touch with other parents in your area.
- Your local National Childbirth Trust www.nct.org.uk/ may also be able to put you in touch with other women who have or have had PND.
- Parentline www.familylives.org.uk/ (0808 800 2222) is a telephone helpline which provides support and information for parents who are under stress.
- PNI.ORG.UK www.pni.org.uk/ is a useful forum with other families who are affected.
- Postpartum Support International is dedicated to helping women suffering from perinatal mood and anxiety disorders, including postpartum depression, the most common complication of childbirth. www.postpartum.net/.

OTHER ARTICLES OF INTEREST

- www.theguardian.com/society/2004/jan/18/mentalhealth.observer magazine
- www.netmums.com/parenting-support/depression-and-anxiety/having-another-baby-after-post-natal-depression

Handouts and short articles on depression in new mothers from www.uppity sciencechick.com/ppdhandouts.html:
- *Antidepressant Use in Pregnant and Breastfeeding Mothers* www.uppity sciencechick.com/kendall-tackett_antidep_bf_jhl.pdf
- *Non-Drug Treatments for Depression in Pregnant and Postpartum Women* www.uppitysciencechick.com/non_drug_treatments_of_trauma.pdf
- *Medication Use for Trauma Symptoms and PTSD in Pregnant and Postpartum Women* (www.uppitysciencechick.com/medication_use_for_ trauma_symptoms.pdf)
- *Non-Drug Treatments for Trauma Symptoms and PTSD* (www.uppity sciencechick.com/non_drug_treatments_of_trauma.pdf)
- *Exercise as a Treatment for Depression in New Mothers* (www.uppity sciencechick.com/exercise.pdf)
- *Can Fats Make You Happy? Omega-3s and Your Mental Health Pregnancy, Postpartum and Beyond* (www.uppitysciencechick.com/can_fats_make_ you_happy.pdf)

- *Bright Light Therapy for Depression* (www.uppitysciencechick.com/Bright_light_therapy.pdf)
- *Why Breastfeeding and Omega-3s Help Prevent Depression in Pregnant and Postpartum Women* (www.uppitysciencechick.com/why_bfand_omega_3s.pdf).

Depression, breastfeeding and related topics:
- *Should Mothers Avoid Night time Breastfeeding to Decrease Their Risk of Depression?* (www.uppitysciencechick.com/nighttime_breastfeeding.pdf)
- *Making Peace with Your Birth Experience* (www.uppitysciencechick.com/making_peace.pdf)
- *How Other Cultures Prevent Postpartum Depression: social structures that protect new mothers' mental health* (www.uppitysciencechick.com/how_other_cultures.pdf)
- *Breastfeeding after Sexual Trauma* (www.uppitysciencechick.com/Breastfeeding_after_Sexual_Trauma.pdf)
- *Why Breastfeeding Lowers Women's Risk of Cardiovascular and Metabolic Disease* (www.uppitysciencechick.com/bf_lowers_cardiovascular_and_meta.pdf).

Case studies of families with lived experience

I received almost 80 stories from people who have suffered from a perinatal mental health illness and have either considered or gone on to have another baby. Throughout the book I have included many anecdotes relevant to the different aspects of the decisions and actions they have made or are making. As time goes on I would love to be able to share more examples, so I invite people to continue to send any personal details that they wish to be used to help others (names can be changed if desired). On my website at www.hanzak.com I have created a section where these stories can be submitted and collated.

Here is one example from Claire:

After my first experience of postnatal psychosis with my son Bayley, second time round things have been completely different for me. I've learnt to relax more. I've learnt to make sure I eat regularly, exercise regularly and slow down to appreciate the present situation more. By living more 'in the now', I've become calmer with both children, looking for the positives rather than the negatives; not comparing my situation with others and appreciating my children and praising more rather than criticising. As a result my second child, Lily, is a confident, outgoing child that mixes with others well. Bayley has improved tonnes. It's been a long journey though and we did experience a lot of problems initially, including being sent down the avenue of ADHD Attention deficit hyperactivity disorder by the school. I made a decision to turn things around and he has calmed down considerably and is a creative, loving little boy. I know now that a lot of the issues were reflective of my own state of mind and actions after my illness.

Having my little girl Lily was a major decision for both myself and my husband. It was a big, scary decision to make and I had his full support. The birth second time round was the most beautiful birth experience I had always imagined and longed for. We had Lily at home; my midwife and the mental health team gave incredible support before, during and after the birth. I laboured in water, had soft music, lavender and candles. It was truly a magical experience and from the moment I set my eyes on her, I was overcome with love instead of fear. I would recommend anyone to go for it. If having another baby is your dream, your past does not need to dictate your future. I learnt a lot from my past experience and overcame adversity to make me a much stronger better person today. With love and support you can do anything.

There are an increasing number of families who are willing to share their stories online. For example, this is Natalie's story (www.thesmilegroup.org/our-story-natalie-nuttall/):

I look at my son and I cannot begin to articulate just how much I love him.

It is the kind of intense, infinite, unconditional love other mothers describe yet I knew very little of in the early days.

When I became a mum I mostly felt numb. Numb from the trauma of a brutal delivery and subsequent operation and blood transfusion. Numb with an exhaustion that didn't really abate until Oscar was about nine months old and had (finally) learnt the value of sleep.

Suspected baby blues turned into something far more sinister for me. I would wake with a familiar dread, wired with anxiety, panic, and worst of all, a sense of detachment from reality. Thankfully I took swift action. Help was at hand but it took a number of trips to find an empathetic GP and a tougher battle to secure CBT [cognitive behavioural therapy].

My recovery took months not weeks, but the biggest realisation for me was the lack of community support for people with PND. I met another mum in the same boat and together Ruth and I set up The SMILE Group.

The journey has been a tough one. Without doubt the hardest thing I've faced in my life. I don't regret it though. It gave me my beautiful son and hopefully it will help to bring others hope and support when they need it most.

The update to this is that Natalie has gone on to deliver a little girl (www.thesmilegroup.org/shes/):

It's 15.42. I am anxiously repeating the phrase 'I'm frightened' to my husband and trying to avoid the reflective lights in the operating theatre. My irrational fear is being the exception to the rule; the one to feel every slice of the knife despite the reassurance of a surgeon poised with the spinal block to administer.

15.47 and, consumed by rising nausea and sinking blood pressure, in the corner of my eye I see a baby being swiftly transferred from one blue uniform to another and then I realise. She is ours. Violet Martha is here. She is beautiful – full of wonderment and already mouthing to me in her quest for milk.

And there it is. The rush. A surge of love, not just for my baby girl but for her four year old brother. For our family and the togetherness that knits us, like a tightly woven fabric. For the pain of the past, the turmoil of doubt and fear and for the healing that followed which binds us irrevocably.

In those first fragile hours as darkness descends on the ward and Violet and I are alone in our curtained bay I am lost in exploration – marvelling at the intricate detail of her DNA … her tiny perfect features. In the small hours of Tuesday I am thankful for the decision to push through my fear of facing PND again and not letting it define my experience of early motherhood, regardless of what happens next. For in that moment I realise that what I am feeling is contentment.

Also have a look at:

- www.womenmakewaves.co.uk/postnatal-psychosis-story/ Keeley writes about her pregnancies and mental health challenges.
- www.liveitwell.org.uk/live-it-library/traceys-story/ Tracey talks about being unwell with puerperal psychosis and postnatal depression and how returning to work and getting good support from family and friends helped in her recovery.
- https://smalltimemum1.wordpress.com/2015/01/18/ Eve describes how she feels now her son is five years old.

Remember that if you would like to share your experiences please email me at elaine@hanzak.com or submit them via my website www.hanzak.com

Planning and screening tools

As every individual and their circumstances are unique to each decision in considering whether to have another baby, I feel that it is unlikely that one simple checklist would suit everyone. You may find it helpful to create your own lists or charts to identify the pros and cons for each area of this book that is relevant to you, to assist in your coming to your conclusion or making plans for actions. For example, using the guidance I outlined in Chapter 29 on ways to wellbeing, you could create something like this:

Identified area for improvement	My actions
Hope Identify your triggers for 'lows' What steps will you put in place to avoid them?	
Attitude Which words are you going to choose to reframe so that your self-talk is more positive?	
Needs • **Nurture:** What can you do to make others and yourself feel special? • **Education:** What do you need to learn about your potential condition? • **Exercise:** Which form of exercise are you going to commit to? • **Diet:** What three small changes can you make to become a new, healthier habit? • **Sleep:** Identify one way that you can gain at least an extra 30 minutes a day	
Zest Create a mental health 'first aid kit' of sensory sensations.	
Altogether Who will you connect with?	
Kindness What will you give?	

If you thrive on making lists and keeping records, have a look at www.psychologytools.org/download-therapy-worksheets.html for a wide range of downloadable worksheets relevant to mental health. They are not specific to the perinatal period but could be adapted.

If you require a more structured approach to the decision on whether or not to have another child, there is a personal decision guide at https://decisionaid.ohri.ca/docs/das/OPDG.pdf which you may find of use.

Another format would be to take yourselves through these steps:

- Listing all possible solutions/options.
- Setting a timescale and deciding who is responsible for the decision.
- Information gathering.
- Weighing up the risks involved.
- Deciding on values, or in other words what is important.
- Weighing up the pros and cons of each course of action.
- Making the decision.

Go to www.skillsyouneed.com/ips/decision-making2.html for more details.

SCREENING TOOLS

Screening for antenatal and postnatal depression and anxiety is a subject that appears to divide opinion with queries over its effectiveness, accuracy and delivery. If you are a healthcare professional and wish to investigate this further I would draw your attention to the following resources:

1. Austin MP; Marcé Society Position Statement Advisory Committee. Marcé International Society position statement on psychosocial assessment and depression screening in perinatal women. *Best Pract Res Clin Obstet Gynaecol.* 2014; **28**(1): 179–87. Available at: www.ncbi.nlm.nih.gov/pubmed/24138943
2. Milgrom J, Gemmill AW. *Identifying Perinatal Depression and Anxiety: evidence-based practice in screening, psychosocial assessment and management.* Foreword by John Cox and J Milgrom. Wiley Blackwell; in press 2015.
3. Sit DK, Wisner KL. The identification of postpartum depression. *Clin Obstet Gynecol.* 2009; **52**(3): 456–68. Available at: www.ncbi.nlm.nih.gov/pmc/articles/PMC2736559/
4. www.sign.ac.uk/guidelines/fulltext/60/section2.html
5. www.postpartumprogress.com/tools-for-professionalsclinicians
6. Beauchamp H. What factors influence the use of the Whooley questions by health visitors? *J Health Visiting.* 2014; **2**(7): 378–87. Available at: www.journalofhealthvisiting.com/cgi-bin/go.pl/library/abstract.html?uid=105784

Here are some of the tools that are used by different organisations:

1. The Centre for Epidemiologic Studies Depression Scale (CESD) is a general depression measurement and includes answering 20 questions about how you have been feeling in the last week. An example of a question is 'I felt that I could not shake off the blues even with help from my family or friends.' To answer the questions you have to choose from four options: 'rarely or none of the time', 'some or a little of the time', 'occasionally or a moderate amount of time' and 'most or all of the time'. These questions are designed to find out how often the feelings of depression occur and how long they last. This scale would only take 10 minutes for a patient to fill in. Statistics show that this scale is accurate at distinguishing between people with major depression and lesser symptoms of depression, but little research has been completed to show how accurate it is at identifying initial depressive symptoms which would be needed if a mother did not have a history of depression prior to the birth of her child.

2. The Beck Depression Inventory-II (BDI-II) is also a general depression questionnaire rather than one especially for people with postnatal depression. The BDI-II is a series of 21 questions which you have to answer by choosing the one of the four options that is most like how you have been feeling for the last day or two. An example question is 'Self-Dislike'; to complete this an answer must be chosen from 'I feel the same about myself as ever', 'I have lost confidence in myself', 'I am disappointed in myself' and 'I dislike myself'. This questionnaire is longer and would take about 20 minutes for someone to fill out. This scale has been used widely in research and with patients due to its reproducible results, but little published work has been completed using the BDI-II in a primary healthcare setting yet.

3. The Edinburgh Postnatal Depression Scale (EPDS), as its name suggests, is scale that has been made directly to assess postnatal depressive symptoms. This scale has a similar format to the previous two where you have to assess how you have been feeling in the last week, but this one only has 10 questions, so will be faster to use. An example of a question is 'I have been able to laugh and see the funny side of things' with answers to choose from being 'As much as I always could', 'Not quite so much now', 'Definitely not so much now' and 'Not at all'. Even though it is a specific postnatal depression scale, the only question which relates to the baby is asking how old the baby is – which is to find out how long the mother has been in the postnatal period; all the other questions relate to the mother. This scale has many good reviews due to its consistent, reliable nature. It is available in many languages.

4. The Two Question Screen Test or Whooley Questions (2-Q) is a measure specifically for identifying postnatal depression. It was originally made to be a pre-screening test, but it has, however, been shown to do its job well and be statistically very accurate at identifying postnatal depression. The

two questions the scale asks are 'During the past month, have you often been bothered by feeling down, depressed or hopeless?' and 'During the past month, have you often been bothered by having little interest in doing things?' A yes or no answer for each question is all that is required to complete this screening process. This scale is therefore very quick to administer and could very easily be used by any healthcare professional without specific training. Mothers are likely to be happier answering two questions which can be administered verbally rather than filling out a questionnaire, which involves more concentration and attention and is therefore usually considered more taxing, leading to fewer people completing the questionnaire. This ease of completion is more important in a maternal care setting as mothers are likely to be trying to manage their babies during the consultation. Due to the specific nature of postnatal depression and the importance of the illness for the mother, child, and family unit, if possible a scale should be used that is sensitive to these qualities. More specifically, when mothers suffer from postnatal depression they often become very self-critical and harbour a great deal of guilt because they feel they are causing trouble and not looking after their baby to the standard they think they should be. Being asked to respond to a questionnaire about their mental state may result in people opting not to take part or causing further distress to those who do. If a questionnaire appears to be a standard part of postnatal treatment it might be easier for a worried mother to accept. Furthermore, the Two Question Screen test can be administered in a more subtle conversational style, possibly eliciting a more honest or representative response, leading to more cases of postnatal depression being identified. It is for the aforementioned reasons that the Two Question Screen is widely used in the UK and endorsed by the National Institute for Health and Care Excellence.

5. The Hospital Anxiety and Depression Scale (HADS) was originally developed by Zigmond and Snaith (1983) and is commonly used by doctors to determine the levels of anxiety and depression that a patient is experiencing. The HADS is a 14-item scale that generates ordinal data. Seven of the items relate to anxiety and seven relate to depression. Available at: www.ncbi.nlm.nih.gov/pubmed/6880820

6. PHQ9 (Patient Health Questionnaire 9) is an easy to use patient questionnaire and is a self-administered version of the PRIME-MD diagnostic instrument for common mental disorders. www.patient.co.uk/doctor/patient-health-questionnaire-phq-9 Kroenke K, Spitzer RL, Williams JB. The PHQ-9: validity of a brief depression severity measure. *J Gen Intern Med.* 2001 Sep; **16**(9): 606–13.

7. GAD 7 (Generalised Anxiety Disorder) is an easy to use self-administered patient questionnaire used as a screening tool and severity measure for generalised anxiety disorder. www.patient.co.uk/doctor/

generalised-anxiety-disorder-assessment-gad-7 Swinson RP. The GAD-7 scale was accurate for diagnosing generalised anxiety disorder. *Evid Based Med.* 2006 Dec; **11**(6): 184. Spitzer RL, Kroenke K, Williams JB, *et al.* A brief measure for assessing generalized anxiety disorder: the GAD-7. *Arch Intern Med.* 2006 May 22; **166**(10): 1092–7.

UK policy drivers around antenatal and postnatal (perinatal) mental health

As perinatal mental health has become more prevalent, there is an increasing number of reports and resources emerging. To keep abreast with them, sign up to the email newsletter at www.chimat.org.uk/pimh for new information – The National Child and Maternal Health Observatory (ChiMat) provides information and intelligence to improve decision making for high-quality, cost-effective services. It supports policy makers, commissioners, managers, regulators and other health stakeholders working on children's, young people's and maternal health.

In addition, refer to the Maternal Mental Health Alliance resource page at http://everyonesbusiness.org.uk/?page_id=24 This is where all new, relevant information will be posted.

Here is a list of some of the most influential and significant reports. Healthcare providers and commissioners will find them to be useful. Parents may also find them useful to know what may be or could be available in their area.

- October 2014. Bauer A, Parsonage M, Knapp M, *et al. Costs of Perinatal Mental Health Problems.* Available at: www.centreformentalhealth.org.uk/publications/costs_perinatal_mh_problems.aspx?ID=711
- October 2013. *Perinatal Mental Health: experiences of women and health professionals: introduction from the Boots Family Trust.* London: Boots Family Trust; 2013. Available at: http://everyonesbusiness.org.uk/wp-content/uploads/2014/06/Boots-Family-Trust-Alliance-report.pdf
- 2013: NSPCC. *Prevention in Mind: all babies count: spotlight on perinatal mental health.* London: NSPCC; 2013. Available at: http://everyones business.org.uk/wp-content/uploads/2014/06/NSPCC-Spotlight-report-on-Perinatal-Mental-Health.pdf
- 2012. Joint Commissioning Panel for Mental Health: *Guidance for Commissioners of Perinatal Mental Health Services.* Practical Mental Health

Commissioning. London: Joint Commissioning Panel for Mental Health. Available at: www.jcpmh.info/resource/guidance-perinatal-mental-health-services/

- NHS Commissioning Board. *Specialised Commissioning Specifications: perinatal mental health services*. London: NHS Commissioning Board; 2012. Available at: www.england.nhs.uk/wp-content/uploads/2013/06/c06-spec-peri-mh.pdf
- Royal College of Psychiatrists. *Quality Network for Perinatal Mental Health Services*. London: Royal College of Psychiatrists; 2012.
- www.rcpsych.ac.uk/workinpsychiatry/qualityimprovement/qualityand accreditation/perinatal/perinatalqualitynetwork.aspx
- Scottish Intercollegiate Guidelines Network (SIGN). *Management of Perinatal Mood Disorders*. Edinburgh: SIGN; 2012. SIGN publication no. 127. [March 2012] www.sign.ac.uk/guidelines/fulltext/127/
- 2011: *Patients Association Report*. www.patients-association.org.uk/?s=postnatal
- 2011: 4Children. *Suffering in Silence*. London: 4Children; 2011. Available at: www.4children.org.uk/Resources/Detail/Suffering-in-Silence
- *RCOG Guidelines on Management of Women with Mental Health Issues during Pregnancy and the Postnatal Period*. Good Practice No. 14. London: RCOG; 2011. www.rcog.org.uk/globalassets/documents/guidelines/managementwomenmentalhealthgoodpractice14.pdf
- 2009: *New Horizons: a shared vision for mental health*. London, DoH; 2009. Available at: www.dh.gov.uk/en/Publicationsandstatistics/Publications/PublicationsPolicyAndGuidance/DH_109705
- 2008 Healthcare Commission. *Towards Better Births*. London, Healthcare Commission; 2008. Available at: http://webarchive.nationalarchives.gov.uk/20101014074803/http:/www.cqc.org.uk/_db/_documents/Towards_better_births_200807221338.pdf
- 2007 NSF Implementation. *Maternity Matters*. London, DoH; 2007. Available at: http://webarchive.nationalarchives.gov.uk/20130107105354/www.dh.gov.uk/prod_consum_dh/groups/dh_digitalassets/@dh/@en/documents/digitalasset/dh_074199.pdf
- 2007 NICE. *Clinical Guidelines: A & PMH*. London: NICE; 2007. Available at: http://guidance.nice.org.uk/CG45
- 2011, 2007, 2004, 2001 *CEMACH Saving Mothers' Lives Reports*. Available at: www.oaa-anaes.ac.uk/UI/Content/Content.aspx?ID=140
- DfES. *Every Child Matters*. London: DfES, Available at: www.dcsf.gov.uk/everychildmatters/
- 2004: Department of Health, Department for Education and Skills. *National Service Framework for Children, Young People and Maternity Services*. London: DoH; 2004.

- 2000 Royal College of Psychiatrists Reports (CR28, 1982, CR88). Available at: www.rcpsych.ac.uk/publications/collegereports/cr/cr88.aspx

Survey used as additional information for this book

'CONTEMPLATING PREGNANCY AFTER PERINATAL DEPRESSION' BY ELAINE A HANZAK

The publication of my book *Eyes without Sparkle: a journey through postnatal illness* (2005) resulted in me becoming a full-time speaker and 'expert by experience' on the subject. One question that has been often asked of me is what people should do if they are considering another pregnancy after suffering from a postnatal mental illness previously. I have been accepted by Radcliffe Publishing Ltd to write another book with this as the topic.

My second book will be designed to answer that dilemma and serve as a guide for both parents and professionals.

To that end initially I would be grateful for questions and examples of this dilemma faced by others to enable me to ensure that I cover all possible situations and provide guidance based up the experience of others. This questionnaire is aimed at mothers, with input from their partners where appropriate.

Currently there is no book written for parents and professionals in the UK that covers this topic. According to the NSPCC's 'All Babies Count report' there are approximately 122,000 babies under one in England living with a parent who has a mental health problem: www.nspcc.org.uk/inform/resourcesforprofessionals/underones/spotlight-mental-health_wdf96656.pdf

A large proportion of those parents are likely to consider the question of another child at some stage. My aim is to provide a guide to enable them to make a well-informed choice.

I would be most grateful if you would complete this questionnaire to assist me in identifying key areas which then will be used to help others. If you feel any questions are not relevant to you, simply leave them blank.

Please let me know (at the end) how much detail you are happy for me to use. I want to use direct quotes and stories as this will give a realistic balance.

These can be referenced to you or left as anonymous. **Many parents feel they are isolated in the decision to have another child after suffering from a previous postnatal illness. Knowing that others have been there before (and in the future) can be most helpful.** I will not share any information by name without seeking permission from you. I shall also be researching and using evidence-based clinical research and consulting relevant trained professionals, e.g. perinatal psychiatrists.

1. Your details:
   ‣ Your name
   ‣ Town
   ‣ County
   ‣ Email address
   ‣ Current age

Part 1

Previous pregnancy – (this refers to the first or previous pregnancy after which you were ill)

For you, which number pregnancy/children was this?

1. Planning
   ‣ Planned pregnancy – yes/no
   ‣ At this point did you plan on having more children?
   ‣ Stable relationship with father – yes/no
   ‣ Did your partner agree to the pregnancy?
   ‣ Previous mental health issues – yes/no
   ‣ If yes, please give outline details
   ‣ If yes, were you given any pre-conceptual counselling?
   ‣ If yes, were you recommended to change any medication?
   ‣ It might be interesting to ascertain whether they advised you to *begin to take* any medication as a precaution, e.g. alternative therapies, supplements. Was any provision made to pre-empt the likelihood of PND?
2. The pregnancy
   ‣ Did you conceive easily and quickly?
   ‣ Did you need to have assisted conception?
   ‣ Were you physically well? Yes/no – describe
   ‣ Were you mentally well? Yes/no – describe
   ‣ Did you have any sleep problems?
   ‣ Did you attend any antenatal classes?
   ‣ Did you find them helpful?
   ‣ How else did you prepare for the birth?
   ‣ What could have made your experience better?
   ‣ Did you know anything about postnatal illness during this first/previous pregnancy?
   ‣ If so, where from?

- ▸ Was it enough?
- ▸ What would you have found helpful in hindsight?
3. The birth
   - ▸ Home, hospital or other place of birth?
   - ▸ Your age at birth of child
   - ▸ Month and year of birth of child
   - ▸ Single or multiple birth?
   - ▸ Did you have a birth plan?
   - ▸ What kind of delivery did you have?
   - ▸ Describe what happened …
   - ▸ Were your expectations met?
   - ▸ What could have made your experience better?
4. The baby
   - ▸ Was the baby well?
   - ▸ Did he/she survive?
   - ▸ If not, please explain what happened, if you feel able to.
5. Early days post delivery
   - ▸ How soon did you go home (if in hospital) after delivery?
   - ▸ Were you happy with this timescale?
   - ▸ What were your initial feelings to motherhood?
   - ▸ Was the baby well?
   - ▸ How much support did you get from healthcare professionals?
   - ▸ How much support did you get from family and friends?
   - ▸ What did this involve?
   - ▸ What could have made your experience better?
6. Feeding your baby
   - ▸ Did you breastfeed or bottle-feed?
   - ▸ Did you want to breastfeed?
   - ▸ Did you get sufficient help with this?
   - ▸ How did you feel about bottle-feeding?
   - ▸ Do you feel that your choice of feeding helped or hindered your mental state? How?
7. The early weeks
   - ▸ Describe your living situation
   - ▸ Describe your feelings
8. Your previous experience of postnatal illness
   - ▸ When did you first realise that your feelings were not as you expected?
   - ▸ How did you realise this?
   - ▸ Did you get an immediate diagnosis? (Yes/No)
   - ▸ If no, how long afterwards did you get a diagnosis?
   - ▸ Did you remain undiagnosed and only realise much later?
   - ▸ Who identified that you were not feeling or behaving as expected?
   - ▸ How did they/you know?

- What, if any, treatments were offered to you?
- What, if anything, could have made your experience better?

9. Your partner
   - Are they male or female?
   - How did they feel about the pregnancy?
   - What role did they play during the labour and birth?
   - How did you feel about that?
   - How did they feel?
   - Was their mental health affected by your pregnancy and after the birth?
   - If so, please explain.

10. Other family and friends
    - Before the pregnancy when you were postnatally depressed, did you have any other children in your care?
    - How did they respond when you were ill?
    - What support for the children, if any, did you receive?
    - Were any other family members or friend of particular help? (no need to name)
    - If so, in what way?
    - Were any other family members or friends of hindrance or did you feel pressured or criticised? (no need to name)
    - If so, in what way?
    - How could critical members of family and friends have been more helpful?
    - How do you feel any relationships changed or developed due to post-natal illness?

11. Recovery
    - Do you feel you have recovered?
    - How long after you first noticed symptoms do you feel it took you to recover?
    - Have you been left with any long-term effects? Please describe …
    - Were you able to go back to work (if relevant)?
    - If yes, how did you feel about and manage this?

Part 2

If you have already had another baby after suffering from postnatal illness after a previous baby

1. Contemplating another pregnancy (in the past)
   a) My partner and I both wanted another baby
   b) Neither my partner nor I wanted another baby
   c) I wanted another baby, my partner did not
   d) My partner wanted another baby, I did not
   e) Our feelings and/or situation changed over time (describe)
   f) I got unexpectedly pregnant again

g) I previously had a miscarriage/stillbirth

h) Other (describe)

Did you have any pre-conceptual counselling or discussions with health professionals about your previous PNI?

During the pregnancy how did you feel?

Did health professionals have any input in your birth plan based on your past experience?

2. What was the outcome of the next pregnancy?
   ‣ Did you have (please tick all that apply):
     – no issues
     – physical issues
     – mental health issues
     – physical and mental health issues
     – relationship issues
     – other issues (please state)?

How did your prior experiences of PNI help or hinder your understanding of your emotions following this birth?
   ‣ Did your baby have:
     – no issues
     – physical issues
     – mental health issues
     – physical and mental health issues?

How did you cope emotionally and physically with caring for and loving another child with relation to their existing siblings?

3. What did you differently this time, knowing that you might suffer from postnatal illness?

4. What do you think helped?

5. What do you think did not?

6. Was there anything you would have found helpful? How did your partner's behaviour/feelings differ following this pregnancy in the light of your previous experience?

7. In hindsight, would you have made a different decision about having another child or not?

8. Has this changed over time? If so, please explain.

9. What three main tips would you give to others who face the dilemma of risking PNI in order to have another child?

Part 3

1. Contemplating another pregnancy (currently). Where would you consider yourself to be? Please tick all that apply

a) My partner and I both want another baby
b) Neither my partner nor I want another baby
c) I want another baby, my partner does not
d) My partner wants another baby, I do not
e) Our feelings and/or situation changed over time (describe)
f) I am unexpectedly pregnant again
g) I previously had a miscarriage/stillbirth
h) Other (describe)
2. What are your biggest concerns about another possible pregnancy?
3. What do you think might help to ease these concerns?
4. What plans, if any, have you put into place to make it easier this time?
5. Have you found any help or support that you lacked last time?
6. What help or support are you looking for which appears to be unavailable?

Index

CPD with Radcliffe

You can now use a selection of our books to achieve CPD (Continuing Professional Development) points through directed reading.

We provide a free online form and downloadable certificate for your appraisal portfolio. Look for the CPD logo and register with us at: www.radcliffehealth.com/cpd

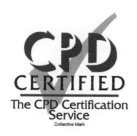

Printed and bound by CPI Group (UK) Ltd, Croydon, CR0 4YY

25/10/2024

01779633-0001